Preterm Birth

Editors

RONALD J. WONG
GARY M. SHAW
DAVID K. STEVENSON

CLINICS IN PERINATOLOGY

www.perinatology.theclinics.com

Consulting Editor
LUCKY JAIN

June 2024 • Volume 51 • Number 2

ELSEVIER

1600 John F. Kennedy Boulevard • Suite 1800 • Philadelphia, Pennsylvania, 19103-2899

http://www.theclinics.com

CLINICS IN PERINATOLOGY Volume 51, Number 2
June 2024 ISSN 0095-5108, ISBN-13: 978-0-443-13081-6

Editor: Kerry Holland
Developmental Editor: Nitesh Barthwal

Clinics in Perinatology (ISSN 0095-5108) is published quarterly by Elsevier Inc., 360 Park Avenue South, New York, NY 10010-1710. Months of issue are March, June, September, and December. Business and Editorial Offices: 1600 John F. Kennedy Blvd., Ste. 1800, Philadelphia, PA 19103-2899. Customer Service Office: 3251 Riverport Lane, Maryland Heights, MO 63043. Periodicals postage paid at New York, NY and additional mailing offices. Subscription prices are $351.00 per year (US individuals), $398.00 per year (Canadian individuals), $475.00 per year (international individuals), $100.00 per year (US and Canadian students), and $195.00 per year (International students). For institutional access pricing please contact Customer Service via the contact information below. International air speed delivery is included in all Clinics subscription prices. All prices are subject to change without notice. **POSTMASTER:** Send address changes to Clinics in Perinatology, Elsevier Health Sciences Division, Subscription Customer Service, 3251 Riverport Lane, Maryland Heights, MO 63043. **Customer Service: Telephone: 1-800-654-2452** (U.S. and Canada); **1-314-447-8871** (outside U.S. and Canada). **Fax: 1-314-447-8029. E-mail: journalscustomerservice-usa@elsevier.com** (for print support); **journalsonlinesupport-usa@elsevier.com** (for online support).

Reprints. For copies of 100 or more, of articles in this publication, please contact the Commercial Reprints Department, Elsevier Inc., 360 Park Avenue South, New York, NY 10010-1710. Tel. 212-633-3874; Fax: 212-633-3820; E-mail: reprints@elsevier.com.

Clinics in Perinatology is also published in Spanish by McGraw-Hill Interamericana Editores S.A., P.O. Box 5-237, 06500 Mexico D.F., Mexico.

Clinics in Perinatology is covered in MEDLINE/PubMed (Index Medicus) Current Contents, Excepta Medica, BIOSIS and ISI/BIOMED.

Contributors

CONSULTING EDITOR

LUCKY JAIN, MD, MBA
Pediatrician-in-Chief, Children's Healthcare of Atlanta, George W. Brumley Jr. Professor and Chair, Emory University School of Medicine, Department of Pediatrics, Executive Director, Emory+Children's Pediatric Institute, Atlanta, Georgia, USA

EDITORS

RONALD J. WONG, PhD
Senior Research Scientist, Department of Pediatrics, Division of Neonatal and Developmental Medicine, Stanford University School of Medicine, Stanford, California, USA

GARY M. SHAW, DrPH
Associate Chair for Clinical Research, Professor (by courtesy), Epidemiology and Population Health, Obstetrics and Gynecology – Maternal Fetal Medicine, NICU Nurses Endowed Professor, Department of Pediatrics, Department of Pediatrics, Division of Neonatal and Developmental Medicine, Stanford University School of Medicine, Stanford, California, USA

DAVID K. STEVENSON, MD
Senior Associate Dean for Maternal and Child Health, Co-Director, Stanford Child Health Research Institute, Principal Investigator, March of Dimes Prematurity Research Center, Harold K. Faber Professor, Department of Pediatrics, Division of Neonatal and Developmental Medicine, Stanford University School of Medicine, Stanford, California, USA

AUTHORS

NIMA AGHAEEPOUR, PhD
Associate Professor, Department of Anesthesiology, Perioperative and Pain Medicine, Stanford University School of Medicine, Department of Pediatrics, Division of Neonatal and Developmental Medicine, Stanford University School of Medicine, Department of Biomedical Data Science, Stanford University, Stanford, California, USA

FOUZIA ZAHID ALI KHAN, MBBS, MSPH
Gynecologist, Department of Gynecology and Obstetrics, Johns Hopkins University School of Medicine, Baltimore, Maryland, USA

MARTIN S. ANGST, MD
Professor, *Department of Anesthesiology, Perioperative and Pain Medicine*, Stanford University School of Medicine, Stanford, California, USA

PETRA C. ARCK, MD
Professor, Department of Obstetrics and Fetal Medicine, Hamburg Center for
Translational Immunology, University Medical Center Hamburg-Eppendorf,
Martinistrasse, Hamburg, Germany

THALYSSA-LYN AUGUSTIN
Université de Montréal, Pavillion Roger-Gaudry, Research Center, Centre de recherche
du CHU Sainte-Justine, Montreal, Quebec, Canada

FERNANDO C. BARROS, PhD
Professor, Catholic University of Pelotas, Rua Félix da Cunha, Pelotas, Rio Grande do Sul,
Brazil

MARTIN BECKER, PhD
Professor, Department of Computer Science and Electrical Engineering, Institute for
Visual and Analytic Computing, Universität Rostock, Rostock, Germany

ERIKA BLACKSHER, PhD
John B. Francis Endowed Chair in Bioethics, Center for Practical Bioethics, Kansas City;
and Research Professor, Department of History and Philosophy of Medicine, University of
Kansas Medical Center, Kansas City, Kansas, USA

TONIA BRANCHE, MD, MPH
Assistant Professor, Department of Pediatrics, Northwestern University, Division of
Neonatology, Ann & Robert H. Lurie Children's Hospital of Chicago, Chicago, Illinois,
USA

WYLIE BURKE, MD, PhD
Professor Emeritus, Department of Bioethics and Humanities, University of Washington,
Seattle, Washington, USA

PAOLO IVO CAVORETTO, MD, PhD
Head of Maternal Fetal Medicine, Department of Obstetrics and Gynaecology, School of
Medicine, IRCCS San Raffaele Scientific Institute, Vita-Salute San Raffaele University,
Milan, Italy

PRANESH CHAKRABORTY, MD
Medical Director, Newborn Screening Ontario, Children's Hospital of Eastern Ontario,
Professor, Department of Pediatrics, University of Ottawa, Ottawa, Ontario, Canada

SYLVAIN CHEMTOB, MD, PhD
Professor, Université de Montréal, Pavillion Roger-Gaudry, Research Center, Centre de
recherche du CHU Sainte-Justine, Montreal, Quebec, Canada

GWENDOLINE CHIMHINI, MMed, MPH
Paediatrician, Department of Child Adolescent and Women's Health, Faculty of Medicine
and Health Sciences, University of Zimbabwe, Harare, Zimbabwe

JAMES W. COLLINS Jr, MD, MPH
Professor, Department of Pediatrics, Northwestern University, Division of Neonatology,
Ann & Robert H. Lurie Children's Hospital of Chicago, Chicago, Illinois, USA

FRANCE CÔTÉ, BS
Université de Montréal, Pavillion Roger-Gaudry, Research Center, Centre de recherche
du CHU Sainte-Justine, Montreal, Quebec, Canada

ALISON D. COWAN, MD, MSCR
Head of Medical Affairs, Mirvie, Inc., South San Francisco, California, USA

GARY L. DARMSTADT, MD, MS
Associate Dean for Maternal and Child Health, Professor, Department of Pediatrics, Division of Neonatal and Developmental Medicine, Stanford University School of Medicine, Stanford, California, USA

MICHAL A. ELOVITZ, MD
Professor, Department of Obstetrics and Gynecology, Women's Health Research, Icahn School of Medicine at Mount Sinai; Director, Women's Biomedical Research Institute, New York, New York, USA

SARAH K. ENGLAND, PhD
Vice Chair, Research, Alan A. and Edith L. Wolff Professor of Medicine, Obstetrics and Gynecology, Director, Center for Reproductive Health Sciences, Washington University School of Medicine, St Louis, Missouri, USA

CAMILO ESPINOSA, MPhil
PhD Student, Immunology Program, Departments of Anesthesiology, Perioperative and Pain Medicine, and Pediatrics, Stanford University School of Medicine; Department of Biomedical Data Science, Stanford University, Stanford, California, USA

BÉATRICE FERRI, BS
Université de Montréal, Pavillion Roger-Gaudry, Research Center, Centre de recherche du CHU Sainte-Justine, Montreal, Quebec, Canada

DORIEN FEYAERTS, PhD, MSc
Postdoctoral Scholar, Department of Anesthesiology, Perioperative and Pain Medicine, Stanford University, Stanford, California, USA

BRICE GAUDILLIÈRE, MD, PhD
Associate Professor, Department of Anesthesiology, Perioperative and Pain Medicine, Stanford Department of Pediatrics (courtesy), Stanford University School of Medicine, Stanford University, Stanford, California, USA

SYLVIE GIRARD, PhD
Chair, Division of Research, Department of Obstetrics & Gynecology, Associate Professor of Obstetrics and Gynecology, Mayo Clinic, Rochester, Minnesota, USA

DANA E. GOIN, PhD
Assistant Professor, Department of Epidemiology, Mailman School of Public Health, Columbia University, New York, New York, USA

NARDHY GOMEZ-LOPEZ, PhD
Professor, Department of Obstetrics and Gynecology and Department of Pathology and Immunology, Center for Reproductive Health Sciences, Washington University School of Medicine, St Louis, Missouri, USA

DAVID.J.X. GONZALEZ, PhD
Assistant Professor, Division of Environmental Health Sciences, School of Public Health, University of California, Berkeley, Berkeley, California, USA

TIFFANY HABELRIH, BS
Vanier Scholar, Université de Montréal, Pavillion Roger-Gaudry, Research Center, Centre de recherche du CHU Sainte-Justine, Montreal, Quebec, Canada

STEVEN HAWKEN, PhD
Senior Scientist, Clinical Epidemiology Program, Ottawa Hospital Research Institute, Centre for Practice Changing Research, Associate Professor, School of Epidemiology and Public Health, University of Ottawa, Ottawa, Ontario, Canada

BJARNE C. HILLER, MS
PhD Student, Department of Computer Science and Electrical Engineering, Institute for Visual and Analytic Computing, Universität Rostock, Rostock, Germany

BO JACOBSSON, MD, PhD
Professor, Chief Physician, Department of Obstetrics and Gynaecology, Sahlgrenska Academy, Institute of Clinical Sciences, University of Gothenburg, Gothenburg, Sweden; Senior Researcher, Department of Genetics and Bioinformatics, Health Data and Digitalization, Norwegian Institute of Public Health, Oslo, Norway

MANEESH JAIN, PhD
CEO and Co-Founder, Mirvie, Inc., South San Francisco, California, USA

STEPHEN H. KENNEDY, MD
Professor, Nuffield Department of Women's and Reproductive Health, Oxford Maternal & Perinatal Health Institute, Green Templeton College, University of Oxford, Oxford, United Kingdom

CHRISTINA KIM, MD
Fellow, Department of Pediatrics, Northwestern University, Physician, Division of Neonatology, Ann & Robert H. Lurie Children's Hospital of Chicago, Chicago, Illinois, USA

ANNE CC LEE, MD, MPH
Attending Pediatrician, Department of Pediatric Newborn Medicine, Brigham and Women's Hospital, Boston, Massachusetts, USA

WILLIAM D. LUBELL, PhD
Professor, Département de Chimie, Université de Montréal, Complexe des Sciences, Montreal, Quebec, Canada

IVANA MARIĆ, PhD
Assistant Professor, Department of Pediatrics, Division of Neonatal and Developmental Medicine, Stanford University School of Medicine, Stanford, California, USA

NANA MATOBA, MD, MPH
Associate Clinical Professor, Department of Pediatrics, University of California San Diego, Division of Neonatology, Rad Children's Hospital San Diego, San Diego, California

AMIN MIRZAEI, MS
Research Assistant, Department of Computer Science and Electrical Engineering, Institute for Visual and Analytic Computing, Universität Rostock, Rostock, Germany

NAGENDRA MONANGI, MD
Associate Professor, Department of Pediatrics, University of Cincinnati College of Medicine, Center for Prevention of Preterm Birth, Perinatal Institute, Cincinnati Children's Hospital Medical Center, March of Dimes Prematurity Research Center Ohio Collaborative; Attending Neonatologist, Division of Neonatology, Cincinnati Children's Hospital Medical Center, Cincinnati, Ohio, USA

LOUIS J. MUGLIA, MD, PhD
Adjunct Professor, Division of Human Genetics, Cincinnati Children's Hospital Medical Center, Center for Prevention of Preterm Birth, Perinatal Institute, March of Dimes Prematurity Research Center Ohio Collaborative, Department of Pediatrics, University of Cincinnati College of Medicine, Cincinnati, Ohio, USA; The Burroughs Wellcome Fund, Research Triangle Park, North Carolina, USA

HILDA A. MUJURU, MMed, MSc
Professor, Department of Child Adolescent and Women's Health, Faculty of Medicine and Health Sciences, University of Zimbabwe, Harare, Zimbabwe

DAVID M. OLSON, PhD, DSc
Professor, Departments of Obstetrics and Gynecology, Pediatrics, and Physiology, University of Alberta, Edmonton, Alberta, Canada

NANCY A. OTIENO, PhD
Research Officer and Deputy Chief, Kenya Medical Research Institute (KEMRI), Center for Global Health Research, Nairobi, Kenya

AMY M. PADULA, PhD
Associate Professor, Department of Obstetrics, Gynecology and Reproductive Sciences, University of California San Francisco, San Francisco, California, USA

ARIS T. PAPAGEORGHIOU, MD
Professor, Nuffield Department of Women's and Reproductive Health, Oxford Maternal & Perinatal Health Institute, Green Templeton College, University of Oxford, Oxford, United Kingdom

ANNA MAYA POWELL, MD, MSCR
Assistant Professor, Department of Gynecology and Obstetrics, Johns Hopkins University School of Medicine, Baltimore, Maryland, USA

JELMER R. PRINS, MD, PhD
Assistant Professor, Department of Obstetrics and Gynecology, University of Groningen, University Medical Center Groningen, Groningen, The Netherlands

MORTEN RASMUSSEN, PhD
VP of Research and Development, Mirvie, Inc., South San Francisco, California, USA

JACQUES RAVEL, PhD
Professor, Department of Microbiology and Immunology, Institute for Genome Sciences, Baltimore, Maryland, USA

VIDHYA RAVICHANDRAN, MBBS
Research Scholar, Divisions of Human Genetics and Neonatology, Cincinnati Children's Hospital Medical Center, Cincinnati, Ohio, USA

ROBERTO ROMERO, D(Med)Sc, MD
Chief, Pregnancy Research Branch, Head of the Program for Perinatal Research and Obstetrics, Division of Intramural Research, Eunice Kennedy Shriver National Institute of Child Health and Human Development, National Institutes of Health, United States Department of Health and Human Services, Bethesda, Maryland, USA; Department of Obstetrics and Gynecology, University of Michigan, Ann Arbor, Michigan, USA; Department of Epidemiology and Biostatistics, Michigan State University, East Lansing, Michigan, USA

JULIANE SÉVIGNY
Département de Biologie, Université de Sherbrooke, Sherbrooke, Quebec, Canada

KEVIN SAWAYA
Research Center, Centre de recherche du CHU Sainte-Justine, Department of Microbiology and Immunology, McGill University, Montreal, Quebec, Canada

DAVID SEONG, BA
MD-PhD Student, Immunology Program, Medical Scientist Training Program, Departments of Microbiology and Immunology, and Anesthesiology, Perioperative and Pain Medicine, Stanford University School of Medicine, Stanford, California, USA

GARY M. SHAW, DrPH
Associate Chair for Clinical Research, Professor (by courtesy), Epidemiology and Population Health, Obstetrics and Gynecology – Maternal Fetal Medicine, NICU Nurses Endowed Professor, Department of Pediatrics, Division of Neonatal and Developmental Medicine, Stanford University School of Medicine, Stanford, California, USA

POL SOLÉ-NAVAIS, MSc, PhD
Research Associate, Department of Obstetrics and Gynaecology, Sahlgrenska Academy, Institute of Clinical Sciences, University of Gothenburg, Gothenburg, Sweden

AMIT K. SRIVASTAVA, PhD
Research Associate, Division of Human Genetics, Cincinnati Children's Hospital Medical Center, Cincinnati, Ohio, USA

INA A. STELZER, PhD, MSc
Assistant Professor, Department of Pathology, University of California San Diego, La Jolla, California, USA; Department of Microbiology and Immunology, Stanford University School of Medicine, Stanford, California, USA

DAVID K. STEVENSON, MD
Senior Associate Dean for Maternal and Child Health, Co-Director, Stanford Child Health Research Institute, Principal Investigator, March of Dimes Prematurity Research Center, Harold K. Faber Professor, Department of Pediatrics, Division of Neonatal and Developmental Medicine, Stanford University School of Medicine, Stanford, California, USA

YUQI TAN, PhD
Postdoctoral Fellow, Department of Microbiology and Immunology, Stanford University School of Medicine, Stanford, California, USA

KRISTIN THIELE, PhD
Postdoctoral Fellow, Division of Experimental Feto-Maternal Medicine, Department of Obstetrics and Fetal Medicine, University Medical Center Hamburg-Eppendorf, Hamburg, Germany

RACHEL M. TRIBE, PhD
Professor, Department of Women and Children's Health, School of Life Course and Population Sciences, King's College London, Thomas's Hospital Campus, London, United Kingdom

SUSAN BROWN TRINIDAD, MA, PhD
Assistant Professor, Department of Bioethics and Humanities, University of Washington, Seattle, Washington, USA

JOSE VILLAR, MD
Professor, Nuffield Department of Women's and Reproductive Health, Oxford Maternal & Perinatal Health Institute, Green Templeton College, University of Oxford, Oxford, United Kingdom

VICTORIA C. WARD, MD
Clinical Associate Professor, Department of Pediatrics, Stanford University School of Medicine, Stanford, California, USA

KARI A. WEBER, PhD, MHS
Assistant Professor, Department of Epidemiology, Fay W. Boozman College of Public Health, University of Arkansas for Medical Sciences, Little Rock, Arkansas, USA

KUMANAN WILSON, MD, MSc
Professor, Department of Medicine, University of Ottawa, Clinical Epidemiology Program, Ottawa Hospital Research Institute, Centre for Practice Changing Research; CEO, Bruyère Research Institute, Ottawa, Ontario, Canada

VIRGINIA D. WINN, MD, PhD
Associate Professor, *Department of Obstetrics and Gynecology*, Divisions of Reproductive, Stem Cell and Perinatal Biology and Maternal Fetal Medicine and Obstetrics, Stanford University School of Medicine, Stanford, California, USA

RONALD J. WONG, PhD
Senior Research Scientist, Department of Pediatrics, Division of Neonatal and Developmental Medicine, Stanford University School of Medicine, Stanford, California, USA

GE ZHANG, MD, PhD
Professor, Division of Human Genetics, Center for the Prevention of Preterm Birth, Perinatal Institute, Cincinnati Children's Hospital Medical Center, Cincinnati, Ohio, USA

Contents

> Solving the puzzle of preterm birth has been challenging and will require novel integrative solutions as preterm birth likely arises from many etiologies. It has been demonstrated that many sociodemographic and psychological determinants of preterm birth relate to its complex biology. It is this understanding that has enabled the development of a novel preventative strategy, which integrates the omics profile (genome, epigenome, transcriptome, proteome, metabolome, microbiome) with sociodemographic, environmental, and psychological determinants of individual pregnant people to solve the puzzle of preterm birth.

> Preterm birth (PTB) is the leading cause of morbidity and mortality in children globally, yet its prevalence has been difficult to accurately estimate due to unreliable methods of gestational age dating, heterogeneity in counting, and insufficient data. The estimated global PTB rate in 2020 was 9.9% (95% confidence interval: 9.1, 11.2), which reflects no significant change from 2010, and 81% of prematurity-related deaths occurred in Africa and Asia. PTB prevalence in the United States in 2021 was 10.5%, yet with concerning racial disparities. Few effective solutions for prematurity prevention have been identified, highlighting the importance of further research.

> Preterm birth (PTB) is the leading cause of infant mortality and morbidity. For several decades, extensive epidemiologic and genetic studies have highlighted the significant contribution of maternal and offspring genetic factors to PTB. This review discusses the challenges inherent in conventional genomic analyses of PTB and underscores the importance of adopting nonconventional approaches, such as analyzing the mother–child pair as a single analytical unit, to disentangle the intertwined maternal and fetal genetic influences. We elaborate on studies investigating PTB phenotypes through 3 levels of genetic analyses: single-variant, multi-variant, and genome-wide variants.

Social determinants of health have received increasing attention in public health, leading to increased understanding of how social factors—individual and contextual—shape the health of the mother and infant. However, racial differences in birth outcomes persist, with incomplete explanation for the widening disparity. Here, we highlight the social determinants of preterm birth, with special attention to the social experiences among African American women, which are likely attributed to structural racism and discrimination throughout life.

Multiple studies have hinted at a complex connection between maternal stress and preterm birth (PTB). This article describes the potential of computational methods to provide new insights into this relationship. For this, we outline existing approaches for stress assessments and various data modalities available for profiling stress responses, and review studies that sought either to establish a connection between stress and PTB or to predict PTB based on stress-related factors. Finally, we summarize the challenges of computational methods, highlighting potential future research directions within this field.

Preterm birth (PTB) is associated with substantial mortality and morbidity. We describe environmental factors that may influence PTB risks. We focus on exposures associated with an individual's ambient environment, such as air pollutants, water contaminants, extreme heat, and proximities to point sources (oil/gas development or waste sites) and greenspace. These exposures may further vary by other PTB risk factors such as social constructs and stress. Future examinations of risks associated with ambient environment exposures would benefit from consideration toward multiple exposures – the exposome – and factors that modify risk including variations associated with the structural genome, epigenome, social stressors, and diet.

Spontaneous preterm birth (sPTB) is a complex and clinically heterogeneous condition that remains incompletely understood, leading to insufficient interventions to effectively prevent it from occurring. Cell-free ribonucleic acid signatures in the maternal circulation have the potential to identify biologically relevant subtypes of sPTB. These could one day be used to predict and prevent sPTB in asymptomatic individuals, and to aid in prognosis and management for individuals presenting with threatened preterm labor and preterm prelabor rupture of membranes.

The complexity of preterm birth (PTB), both spontaneous and medically indicated, and its various etiologies and associated risk factors pose a significant challenge for developing tools to accurately predict risk. This
review focuses on the discovery of proteomics signatures that might be
useful for predicting spontaneous PTB or preeclampsia, which often results in PTB. We describe methods for proteomics analyses, proteomics
biomarker candidates that have so far been identified, obstacles for discovering biomarkers that are sufficiently accurate for clinical use, and
the derivation of composite signatures including clinical parameters to increase predictive power.

Preterm birth (PTB) is a leading cause of morbidity and mortality in children
aged under 5 years globally, especially in low-resource settings. It remains
a challenge in many low-income and middle-income countries to accurately measure the true burden of PTB due to limited availability of accurate measures of gestational age (GA), first trimester ultrasound dating
being the gold standard. Metabolomics biomarkers are a promising area
of research that could provide tools for both early identification of high-
risk pregnancies and for the estimation of GA and preterm status of newborns postnatally.

This review illuminates the complex interplay between various maternal
microbiomes and their influence on preterm birth (PTB), a driving and persistent contributor to neonatal morbidity and mortality. Here, we examine
the dynamics of oral, gastrointestinal (gut), placental, and vaginal microbiomes, dissecting their roles in the pathogenesis of PTB. Importantly, focusing on the vaginal microbiome and PTB, the review highlights (1) a
protective role of *Lactobacillus* species; (2) an increased risk with select
anaerobes; and (3) the influence of social health determinants on the composition of vaginal microbial communities.

Throughout pregnancy, the maternal peripheral circulation contains valuable information reflecting pregnancy progression, detectable as tightly
regulated immune dynamics. Local immune processes at the maternal–fetal interface and other reproductive and non-reproductive tissues are likely
to be the pacemakers for this peripheral immune "clock." This cellular immune status of pregnancy can be leveraged for the early risk assessment

and prediction of spontaneous preterm birth (sPTB). Systems immunology approaches to sPTB subtypes and cross-tissue (local *and* peripheral) interactions, as well as integration of multiple biological data modalities promise to improve our understanding of preterm birth pathobiology and identify potential clinically actionable biomarkers.

Preterm birth (PTB) and its associated morbidities are a leading cause of infant mortality and morbidity. Accurate predictive models and a better biological understanding of PTB-associated morbidities are critical in reducing their adverse effects. Increasing availability of multimodal high-dimensional data sets with concurrent advances in artificial intelligence (AI) have created a rich opportunity to gain novel insights into PTB, a clinically complex and multifactorial disease. Here, the authors review the use of AI to analyze 3 modes of data: electronic health records, biological omics, and social determinants of health metrics.

Preterm birth (PTB) is a complex syndrome traditionally defined by a single parameter, namely, gestational age at birth (ie, ˂37 weeks). This approach has limitations for clinical usefulness and may explain the lack of progress in identifying cause-specific effective interventions. The authors offer a framework for a functional taxonomy of PTB based on (1) conceptual principles established a priori; (2) known etiologic factors; (3) specific, prospectively identified obstetric and neonatal clinical phenotypes; and (4) postnatal follow-up of growth and development up to 2 years of age. This taxonomy includes maternal, placental, and fetal conditions routinely recorded in data collection systems.

This review examines the complexities of preterm birth (PTB), emphasizes the pivotal role of inflammation in the pathogenesis of preterm labor, and assesses current available interventions. Antibiotics, progesterone analogs, mechanical approaches, nonsteroidal anti-inflammatory drugs, and nutritional supplementation demonstrate a limited efficacy. Tocolytic agents, targeting uterine activity and contractility, inadequately prevent PTB by neglecting to act on uteroplacental inflammation. Emerging therapies targeting toll-like receptors, chemokines, and interleukin receptors exhibit promise in mitigating inflammation and preventing PTB.

Preterm birth (PTB) occurs disproportionately among women who are minoritized and who live and work in poverty. This disadvantage occurs as a result of societal norms and policies that affect how people are treated and determine their access to a broad range of resources. Research that takes social context into account offers the best opportunity for identifying approaches to prevent PTB. The experience and knowledge of women from groups experiencing high rates of PTB can provide important insights for research design and for determining the feasibility and acceptability of potential interventions.

PROGRAM OBJECTIVE

The goal of *Clinics in Perinatology* is to keep practicing perinatologists, neonatologists, obstetricians, practicing physicians and residents up to date with current clinical practice in perinatology by providing timely articles reviewing the state of the art in patient care.

TARGET AUDIENCE

Perinatologists, neonatologists, obstetricians, practicing physicians, residents and healthcare professionals who provide patient care utilizing findings from *Clinics in Perinatology*.

LEARNING OBJECTIVES

Upon completion of this activity, participants will be able to:

1. Recognize that multiple factors contribute to preterm birth (PTB) increasing the need for integrative solutions.
2. Discuss innovative solutions for preventing preterm births.
3. Review preterm birth (PTB) and gain an understanding of its associated morbidities, which are critical in reducing their adverse effects.

ACCREDITATION

The Elsevier Office of Continuing Medical Education (EOCME) is accredited by the Accreditation Council for Continuing Medical Education (ACCME) to provide continuing medical education for physicians.

The EOCME designates this journal-based CME activity for a maximum of 15 *AMA PRA Category 1 Credit*(s)™. Physicians should claim only the credit commensurate with the extent of their participation in the activity.

All other health care professionals requesting continuing education credit for this enduring material will be issued a certificate of participation.

DISCLOSURE OF CONFLICTS OF INTEREST

The EOCME assesses conflict of interest with its instructors, faculty, planners, and other individuals who are in a position to control the content of CME activities. All relevant conflicts of interest that are identified are thoroughly vetted by EOCME for fair balance, scientific objectivity, and patient care recommendations. EOCME is committed to providing its learners with CME activities that promote improvements or quality in healthcare and not a specific proprietary business or a commercial interest.

The planning committee, staff, authors, and editors listed below have identified no financial relationships or relationships to products or devices they or their spouse/life partner have with commercial interest related to the content of this CME activity:

Sylvain Chemtob, MD, PhD; Nima Aghaeepour, PhD; Martin S. Angst, MD; Petra C. Arck, MD; Thalyssa Augustin; Fernando C. Barros, PhD; Nitesh Barthwal; Martin Becker, PhD; Erika Blacksher, PhD; Tonia Branche, MD, MPH; Wylie Burke, MD, PhD; Paolo Ivo Cavoretto, MD, PhD; Pranesh Chakraborty, MD; Gwendoline Chimhini, Mmed, MPH; James W. Collins Jr, MD, MPH; France Côté; Gary L. Darmstadt, MD, MS; Michal A. Elovitz, MD; Sarah K. England, PhD; Camilo Espinosa, MPhil; Béatrice Ferri; Dorien Feyaerts, PhD, MSc; Brice Gaudillière, MD, PhD; Sylvie Girard, PhD; Dana E. Goin, PhD; Nardhy Gomez-Lopez, PhD; David J.X. Gonzalez, PhD; Tiffany Habelrih; Steven Hawken, PhD; Bjarne Hiller, MS; Kerry Holland; Lucky Jain, MD, MBA; Bo Jacobsson, MD, PhD; Stephen H. Kennedy, MD; Fouzia Zahid Ali Khan, MBBS, MSPH; Christina Kim, MD; Anne CC Lee, MD, MPH; Michelle Littlejohn; William D. Lubell, PhD; Ivana Marić, PhD; Nana Matoba, MD, MPH; Mohammad Amin Mirzaei, MS; Nagendra Monangi, MD; Louis J. Muglia, MD, PhD; Hilda A. Mujuru, MMed, MSc; David M. Olson, PhD, DSc; Nancy Otieno, MA; Amy M. Padula, PhD; Aris T. Papageorghiou, MD; Anna Maya Powell, MD, MSc; Jelmer R. Prins, MD, PhD; Jacques Ravel, PhD; Vidhya Ravichandran, MBBS; Kevin Sawaya; David Seong; Juliane Sévigny; Gary M. Shaw, DrPH; Pol Solé-Navais, MSc, PhD; Amit K. Srivastava, PhD; Ina A. Stelzer, PhD; David K. Stevenson, MD; Jeyanthi Surendrakumar; Yuqi Tan, PhD; Kristin Thiele, PhD; Rachel M. Tribe, PhD; Susan Brown Trinidad, MA, PhD; Jose Villar, MD; Victoria C. Ward, MD; Kari A. Weber, PhD, MHS; Kumanan Wilson, MD, MSc; Virginia D. Winn, MD, PhD; Ronald J. Wong, PhD; Ge Zhang, MD, PhD

The planning committee, staff, authors, and editors listed below have identified financial relationships or relationships to products or devices they or their spouse/life partner have with commercial interest related to the content of this CME activity:

Alison D. Cowan, MD, MSCR: Employee: Mirvie, Inc.

Maneesh Jain, PhD: Employee: Mirvie, Inc.

Morten Rasmussen, PhD: Employee: Mirvie, Inc.

UNAPPROVED/OFF-LABEL USE DISCLOSURE

The EOCME requires CME faculty to disclose to the participants:

1. When products or procedures being discussed are off-label, unlabelled, experimental, and/or investigational (not US Food and Drug Administration [FDA] approved); and

2. Any limitations on the information presented, such as data that are preliminary or that represent ongoing research, interim analyses, and/or unsupported opinions. Faculty may discuss information about pharmaceutical agents that is outside of FDA-approved labelling. This information is intended solely for CME and is not intended to promote off-label use of these medications. If you have any questions, contact the medical affairs department of the manufacturer for the most recent prescribing information.

TO ENROLL

To enroll in the *Clinics in Perinatology* Continuing Medical Education program, call customer service at 1-800-654-2452 or sign up online at http://www.theclinics.com/home/cme. The CME program is available to subscribers for an additional annual fee of USD 254.00.

METHOD OF PARTICIPATION

In order to claim credit, participants must complete the following:

1. Complete enrolment as indicated above.
2. Read the activity.
3. Complete the CME Test and Evaluation. Participants must achieve a score of 70% on the test. All CME Tests and Evaluations must be completed online.

CME INQUIRIES/SPECIAL NEEDS

For all CME inquiries or special needs, please contact elsevierCME@elsevier.com.

CLINICS IN PERINATOLOGY

SERIES OF RELATED INTEREST

Obstetrics and Gynecology Clinics of North America
https://www.obgyn.theclinics.com

THE CLINICS ARE AVAILABLE ONLINE!
Access your subscription at:
www.theclinics.com

Foreword

The Complex Puzzle of Preterm Births

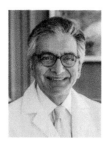

Lucky Jain, MD, MBA
Consulting Editor

Preterm birth is a complex medical issue with immense health and economic consequences worldwide.[1,2] Even in economically well-resourced nations with advanced obstetric and neonatal services, preterm births account for nearly three-fourths of all neonatal deaths and over half of cases with long-term disability. Efforts to improve perinatal outcomes in the past have (paradoxically) resulted in higher preterm births.[3] Some of this increase is attributed to an increase in medically indicated early births with an intention to reduce the impact of perinatal complications, such as hypertensive disorders, intrauterine growth retardation, fetal distress, and so forth, which can result in fetal injury or demise. Similar trends in early term and medically indicated Cesarean births have been reported from many parts of the world, although recent efforts to find an optimal balance have stemmed the increase.

Overall, the epidemiology of preterm births is daunting. Nearly one in 10 births occur before 37 weeks; that is a whopping 15 million preterm births worldwide.[1,2] In the United States, the rate is not only higher but also disproportionately impacts women of color, perpetuating health disparities that sometimes persist a lifetime. The economic toll is equally daunting: precious health care dollars (>$25 billion) that could be devoted to preventive care are consumed in managing preterm births and neonatal morbidity. Cost of managing long-term physical and neurologic disabilities in preterm babies would make these numbers even more staggering.

Meanwhile, science has advanced our understanding of what triggers various types of preterm births (**Fig. 1**).[4] Approaches such as genomics and metabolomics coupled with computational science have begun to yield targets for intervention that could eventually change the face of this malady.[4] However, thorny and vexing issues remain. Social determinants of mental and physical health are unsolved issues whose

Clin Perinatol 51 (2024) xxi–xxiii
https://doi.org/10.1016/j.clp.2024.03.003
0095-5108/24/© 2024 Published by Elsevier Inc.

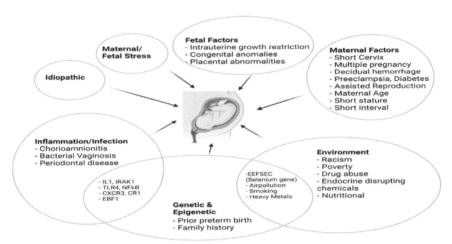

Fig. 1. Causes and interaction among various factors leading to preterm birth. (*From* Jain V, Monangi N, Zhang G, Muglia LJ. Genetics, epigenetics, and transcriptomics of preterm birth. Am J Reprod Immunol 2022; 88(4): e13600. https://doi.org/10.1111/aji.13600.)

contribution to prematurity may have intensified in the post-COVID era. There is also a paucity of diagnostic and therapeutic options to identify and prevent preterm births.

As Drs Wong, Shaw, and Stevenson point out in the preface, new etiologically based functional taxonomy of preterm birth and a brand-new precision medicine approach to prevention may hold the key to future advances. Neonatologists and perinatologists will welcome this news given how much health care resources are consumed in this (supposedly, albeit in part) preventable malady. Indeed, this bodes well for the field of neonatal-perinatal medicine given the opportunity to create a comprehensive set of strategies with long-term impact on reproductive health and outcomes.

Drs Wong, Shaw, and Stevenson are to be congratulated for assembling a true state-of-the-art offering on this subject. As always, I am grateful to the authors for their valuable contributions and to my publishing partners at Elsevier (Kerry Holland and Nitesh Barthwal) for their help in bringing this valuable resource to you. We may still be far from solving the "puzzle" of premature birth; however, a clearer understanding of the issues is critical if we are to move in the right direction!

Lucky Jain, MD, MBA
Emory University School of Medicine, and
Children's Healthcare of Atlanta
1760 Haygood Drive, W409
Atlanta, GA 30322, USA

E-mail address:
ljain@emory.edu

REFERENCES

1. Barfield WD. Public health implications of very preterm birth. Clin Perinatol 2018; 45(3):567–77.

2. Goldenberg RL, Culhane JF, Iams JD, et al. Epidemiology and causes of preterm birth. Lancet 2008;371:75–84.
3. Ananth CV, Joseph KS, Oyelesa Y, et al. Trends in preterm birth and perinatal mortality among singletons: United States, 1989 through 2000. Obstet Gynecol 2005; 105:1084–91.
4. Jain V, Monangi N, Zhang G, et al. Genetics, epigenetics, and transcriptomics of preterm birth. Am J Reprod Immunol 2022;88(4):e13600. https://doi.org/10.1111/aji.13600.

Preface

Preterm Birth

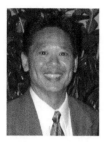
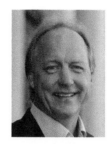
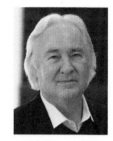

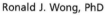

Ronald J. Wong, PhD	Gary M. Shaw, DrPH	David K. Stevenson, MD
	Editors	

This special issue of *Clinics in Perinatology* covers the topic of "Premature Birth" and includes a range of articles by experts with various perspectives. The articles discuss the complexities of solving the puzzle of preterm birth (PTB); the overall burden of PTB globally and in the United States; recent advances in genomics studies of gestational duration; the role of social determinants; computational approaches used to connect maternal stress and PTB; the impact of the ambient environment and epidemiology of PTB; prediction of PTB using cell-free RNA, proteomics, metabolomics, microbiomics, and immunomics; computational approaches to predicting PTB and newborn outcomes; introduction of a new etiologically based functional taxonomy of PTB; exploration of innovative prevention strategies for PTB; and ethical considerations of prediction and prevention of PTB. Indeed, this special issue is a collection of perspectives from experts on the topic of PTB, a plaguing human condition that results in substantial newborn death and developmental consequences well into early life for those who survive.

DISCLOSURES

The authors have no conflicts of interest to disclose.

FUNDING

This work was supported, in part, by the Prematurity Research Fund, the March of Dimes Prematurity Research Center at Stanford University, the Charles B. and Ann L. Johnson Research Fund, the Christopher Hess Research Fund, the Providence

Clin Perinatol 51 (2024) xxv–xxvi
https://doi.org/10.1016/j.clp.2024.03.002
0095-5108/24/© 2024 Elsevier Inc. All rights reserved.

perinatology.theclinics.com

Foundation Research Fund, the Roberts Foundation Research Fund, Bill and Melinda Gates Foundation, and the Stanford Maternal and Child Health Research Institute.

Ronald J. Wong, PhD
Department of Pediatrics
Division of Neonatal and
Developmental Medicine
Stanford University School of Medicine
Biomedical Innovations Building
240 Pasteur Drive, Room 2652
Stanford, CA 94305-5139, USA

Gary M. Shaw, DrPH
Department of Pediatrics
Division of Neonatal and
Developmental Medicine
Stanford University School of Medicine
Center for Academic Medicine
453 Quarry Road
Stanford, CA 94304-5660, USA

David K. Stevenson, MD
Department of Pediatrics
Division of Neonatal and
Developmental Medicine
Stanford University School of Medicine
Biomedical Innovations Building
240 Pasteur Drive, Room 2456
Stanford, CA 94305-5139, USA

E-mail addresses:
rjwong@stanford.edu (R.J. Wong)
gmshaw@stanford.edu (G.M. Shaw)
dstevenson@stanford.edu (D.K. Stevenson)

Solving the Puzzle of Preterm Birth

David K. Stevenson, MD[a,1,*], Virginia D. Winn, MD, PhD[b,1],
Gary M. Shaw, DrPH[a], Sarah K. England, PhD[c],
Ronald J. Wong, PhD[a]

KEYWORDS

- Preterm birth • Omics • Bioengineering • Sleep/circadian • AI/machine learning

KEY POINTS

- Preterm birth (PTB) represents a worldwide health concern.
- Understanding the biology of immunotolerance and rejection during a normal pregnancy may provide insight into the mechanisms of adverse pregnancy outcomes, such as PTB.
- Computational approaches for integrating systems-wide analyses of omics profiles of term and preterm pregnancies throughout gestation in combination with demographic, environmental, and psychosocial data may guide the development of preventive strategies.

Preterm birth (historically defined as delivery before 37 weeks completed gestation) represents a substantial global health problem and is responsible for more deaths under the age of 5 years than any other single cause.[1]

While many factors have been associated with preterm birth (PTB), the causal mechanisms, especially those that instigate spontaneous PTB at very early gestational ages, are not known in roughly 50% of cases.[2] Through evolutionary adaptation, nature has "worked out" the biology of tolerance in human pregnancy — to allow a woman and her fetus to be immunologically tolerant of each other for an amount of time to ensure the appropriate maturational disposition of her fetus — and also the biology of regulated rejection—so as to avoid "inflammatory" injury to either the

[a] Department of Pediatrics, Division of Neonatal and Developmental Medicine, Stanford University School of Medicine, Biomedical Innovations Building (BMI), 240 Pasteur Drive, Room 2652, Stanford, CA 94305, USA; [b] Department of Obstetrics and Gynecology, Division of Reproductive, Stem Cell and Perinatal Biology, Stanford University of School of Medicine, Biomedical Innovations Building (BMI), 240 Pasteur Drive, Module 2700, Stanford, CA 94305, USA; [c] Department of Obstetrics and Gynecology, Center for Reproductive Health Sciences, Washington University School of Medicine, 425 S. Euclid Avenue, CB 8064, St. Louis, MO 63110, USA
[1] Shared first authorship.
* Corresponding author.
E-mail address: dstevenson@stanford.edu

Clin Perinatol 51 (2024) 291–300
https://doi.org/10.1016/j.clp.2024.02.001
0095-5108/24/© 2024 Elsevier Inc. All rights reserved.
perinatology.theclinics.com

woman or fetus, which is effectively what normal labor and delivery represent.[3,4] Thus, an understanding of the biology of immunologic tolerance and rejection in pregnancy might provide insight into the causes of normal as well as abnormal parturition, such as PTB. A side benefit of this scientific inquiry of immune tolerance and growth might be an improved comprehension of other undesirable biologic phenomena, such as very early fetal loss, cancer, autoimmunity, cardiovascular diseases, and even aging.

Although PTB is a syndrome with multiple etiologies, a **common pathway of parturition** has been proposed for both term and preterm labor (**Fig. 1**).[3,5] Obstetricians have known for some time about pro-labor signals. The "inflammatory" nature of these signals, working in combination with progesterone receptor (PR)-A leads to the release of various proteins and lipids (eg, hormones), which eventually cause myometrial contractions, cervical ripening, and ultimately membrane rupture and expulsion of a fetus.[6,7] Normally, progesterone, acting through PR-B, results in a "progesterone block" of the inflammatory signaling pathways, leading to the upregulation of pro-gestation genes, myometrial relaxation, and uterine quiescence.[8] In humans, when the "progesterone block" threshold is exceeded by the proinflammatory signaling and a change in progesterone sensitivity, term labor occurs.[9] Sometimes, this "progesterone block" is overcome too early and preterm labor occurs with the delivery of an immature fetus.

Some of the proposed mechanisms implicated in preterm labor include uterine overdistension, infection, premature placental aging, drop in progesterone effect, cervical dysfunction, diminution of maternal-fetal tolerance, and many other contributors including stress, environmental exposures, and genomic background are likely to be in the causal pathway[3] (as reviewed by Stevenson and colleagues[10,11]). To solve the causal puzzle of PTB, most investigations focus on risk factors, but their identification alone is insufficient for disentangling the complex etiologic puzzle of PTB and a full understanding the biology of pregnancy. As researchers continue to explore the etiologies of PTB, further investigations into the intersection between biology and social disadvantage will be necessary to move this field forward. This is highlighted by the fact that PTB disproportionally affects certain populations. As reported by the March of Dimes, in 2021, 10.5% of livebirths were preterm in the United States, but more Black infants were born preterm (14.4%) than infants of any other racial or ethnic background, with Whites having the lowest rate (9.3%). Thus, we need to identify how factors relate to the underlying biology and social determinants correlate with various biomarkers (proteins and other molecules), the genes and their transcripts, and ultimately cell signaling at the tissue level.

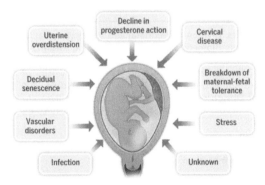

Fig. 1. Preterm labor: a syndrome with multiple etiologies. (Used with permission Romero R, Dey SK, Fisher SJ. Preterm labor: one syndrome, many causes. Science 2014;345(6198):760–5.)

For this purpose, our group at Stanford in collaboration with investigators at other institutions have undertaken an integrated approach for a systems-wide analysis of term and preterm pregnancies (and other pregnancy-related disorders), profiling individual pregnant people throughout gestation for various biologic measures, as well as demographic and psychosocial data using a variety of computational approaches.[12-22] Our goal has been to create integrative personal omics profiles (**Fig. 2**) of normal and abnormal pregnancies,[23] including data on the genome,[24,25] epigenome,[26] transcriptome,[27-29] proteome,[30,31] metabolome,[32,33] immunome,[34,35] microbiome,[36-38] and exposome.[39-41] We began with a question, **"Is it possible to noninvasively monitor the developmental gene expression program of a human fetus and pregnant person simultaneously?"** We now know that the answer to this question is "yes"—simply by longitudinally drawing samples of blood from the pregnant person throughout gestation.

The public is now aware of the utility of cfDNA for diagnosing aneuploidy and some single gene defects,[42,43] but few are aware of the utility of cfRNA, which circulates in the blood of pregnant people.[28] This cfRNA comes from the pregnant person, fetus, and placenta, from various cell types, and reflects gene expression from these sources.[44-46] The measurement of cfRNA in a blood sample from a pregnant person provides us with the equivalent of a biologic dialogue between the pregnant person, the fetus, and the placenta at a point in time during gestation[28]—but it can also be used to track what is changing during gestation through multiple blood samplings over the pregnancy.[27,45] Indeed, we were the first to describe a "transcriptomics clock," identifying over 400 genes displaying temporal changes across gestation.[47] Many of the genes are involved in immunologic pathways, suggesting the existence of an "immune clock."[35,48] Moreover, we also identified some genes that are expressed uniquely in pregnancies that would end prematurely, and early in gestation (12–16 weeks of gestation), long before any signs that labor might happen early.[27] The prediction of

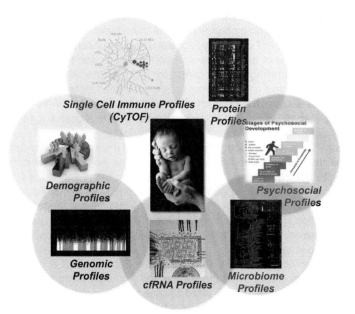

Fig. 2. Integrative personal omics profiling.

spontaneous PTB could be made based on only 7 genes, and gestational age could be estimated based on only 9.

Indeed, there is an "immune clock" of pregnancy, and the immune balance during pregnancy is nature's way of regulating of gestational time.[35,48,49] The technology that we have used for describing this "immune clock" of pregnancy is mass cytometry by time-of-flight mass spectrometry (CyTOF), which uses mass labeling of antibodies for precise phenotyping of individual immune cells and simultaneous interrogation of intracellular responses.[50–52] We validated "surface" markers and changes in the peripheral immune cell distribution and validated "functional" markers of pregnancy-induced changes in cell function.[48] This approach has facilitated the understanding of the timing of immunologic events in normal and pathologic pregnancies. Most recently, we have used this technology not only to date a pregnancy (estimate gestational age), but predict the timing of "onset of labor," based on changes in cell signaling.[53] A breakpoint of omics trajectories was found to demarcate the transition from a pregnancy maintenance state to a pre-labor biology, suggesting a regulatory "braking" of the normal progression of systemic immune inflammatory escalation at the tissue level. This regulatory shift in systemic cellular signaling seems to be true for not only term, but also preterm labor, although the findings for preterm birth are preliminary. The potential utility of CyTOF for identifying those who may be at risk for spontaneous PTB is apparent from the observation that people with a history of PTB, who otherwise appear normal from an immunologic perspective, demonstrate exacerbated myeloid differentiation factor 88 (MyD88) responses in myeloid dendritic cells (mDCs) and classical monocytes (cMCs) when their cells are stimulated, thus revealing a possible target for intervention.[52] Such an immunologic 'stress test" may be a way to uncover biologic vulnerabilities. Once identified, an allosteric interleukin (IL)-1 receptor (IL-1R) antagonist might provide a way to prevent PTB, while preserving defense immunity against infection[54,55] — or less novel, low-dose aspirin could be used for this purpose.[56]

We have explored whether a similar approach could be taken for preventing preeclampsia, a major cause of maternal morbidity and medically-induced PTB.[18,34] Our studies have suggested a change in signal transducer and activator of transcription 5 (STAT5) signaling in T cells early in gestation, suggesting a loss in tolerance, long before the appearance of any clinical signs of preeclampsia, may harbinger its later onset, while also identifying another target for a preventive intervention.[34] This sets the stage for developing a more targeted and simplified assay to identify those at risk for preeclampsia, and then treating them with low-dose IL-2, which can modulate this important step in T-regulatory cell development, as has been suggested in some autoimmune conditions.[57,58]

The risk for PTB would be incompletely understood if we did not consider the role of the microbiome. Humans are "super-organisms." The human microbiome is represented by all the microbes, including bacteria, archea, fungi, and viruses, that inhabit the human body. The combined genomes of these microbial symbionts contain more than 5 million unique genes — our "second," and much larger, genome. The microbiome fulfills critical roles for health, for example, nutrient and energy acquisition, immune programming, and protection against pathogen invasion. Although our individual microbiomes are alike in many respects as humans, we each have a unique microbiome, a microbial signature, that can distinguish us, and it is a dynamic signature, reflecting our interaction with the environment. Taking advantage of a longitudinal cohort of pregnant people, we identified changes in the vaginal microbiome early in pregnancy that could predict the later onset of preterm labor.[37,59] Community state type (CST) IV was found more frequently in those who delivered preterm.[37] In fact,

CST IV exhibited a dose-response relationship with PTB, that is, an increase in the proportion of time points that were in the diverse state correlated with a lower gestational age at delivery. However, we also learned that populations could differ in how CST IV would reflect the risk for PTB, suggesting that genetic or environmental factors are also important to consider for the purpose of knowing the relationship between the microbiome and PTB.[59] A very intriguing observation is the relationship between the persistence of a diverse vaginal microbiome after either vaginal or cesarean birth and cytokine profiles suggesting local inflammation. The timeframe for returning to a *Lactobacillus*-dominated microbiome fits with the epidemiologic observation of the risk for PTB associated with a short interpregnancy interval.[37] In addition, we have recently shown the vaginal ecosystem can be influenced by reproductive history and childbirth and that the timing and degree of recovery from delivery may impact the long-term health as well as subsequent pregnancies.[36] Collectively, the vaginal microbiome data suggest that an intervention to alter the microbial communities in the vagina might be possible, using prebiotic and probiotic approaches.[60]

The previous paragraphs highlight our work toward exploring new pathways and processes leading to PTB. The collection of articles in this edition of *Clinics in Perinatology* highlights the progress of others that have been made in understanding PTB. However, it is clear is that PTB is multifactorial and complex. Most studies remain siloed in their approaches. New omics approaches are leading the way using unbiased approaches to better understand the integration of pathways leading to PTB. Another consideration is the possibility of overarching systems, like circadian rhythms, that impact multiple pathways and processes. The understanding of the molecular foundation of biological clocks has progressed with the awarding of the Nobel Prize in 2017;[61] however, understanding the link between circadian mechanisms and clinical outcomes of pregnancy is only in the early phases. Circadian mechanisms have been shown in various species to influence the timing of birth, including humans as labor onset most commonly occurs during the late night or early morning in both term and PTBs.[62–65] Additionally, uterine contractile activity develops a diurnal pattern in the later stages of the second trimester with a majority of contractions occurring during the night.[66] Because circadian rhythms can regulate physiologic processes in response to environmental triggers, chronodisruption (or disruption of circadian rhythms) has been proposed to be 1 contributor to PTB, likely due to dysregulation of systems discussed in this issue that are circadian regulated (ie, immune and endocrine systems, metabolic pathways, and maternal activity).[67] Our collaborative findings indicated that disruptions of the normal "clock" of physical activity and sleep during pregnancy strongly correlated with pregnancy outcomes and provide hope that monitoring using wearable devices may provide clinical utility. Furthermore, light has been speculated to be beneficial in overcoming preterm deliveries by resetting or establishing stronger circadian rhythms.[68] Further studies in this area will hopefully identify if such easy interventions, like light therapy, could be easily implemented not only in the United States, but also in low-income and middle-income countries.

In summary, the puzzle of PTB has not been solved, as it likely has many causes and will require many solutions. However, having a better understanding of how the many sociodemographic, environmental, and psychological determinants of PTB relate to the underlying biology has brought us closer to introducing rational approaches for the prevention of this complex condition.[10] An integrative personalized omics profiling of a pregnant person, considering the genome, epigenome, transcriptome, proteome, metabolome, microbiome, exposome in combination with the lived experience has at least begun to put us in a better position of evolving from a simply reactive approach to PTB to having a more actionable preventive approach to this complex process of PTB.[69]

DISCLOSURE

The authors have nothing to disclose.

Best Practices

What is the current practice for preterm birth?

Currently, there is no best practice for the prevention for preterm birth (PTB).

What changes in current practice are likely to improve outcomes?

Computational approaches for integrating systems-wide analyses of omics (genome, epigenome, transcriptome, proteome, metabolome, microbiome) profiles of term and preterm pregnancies throughout gestation in combination with demographic, environmental, and psychosocial data may guide the development of preventive therapeutic strategies for PTB.

Bibliographic sources

1. Becker M, Dai J, Chang AL, et al. Revealing the impact of lifestyle stressors on the risk of adverse pregnancy outcomes with multitask machine learning. Front Pediatr 2022;10:933,266.

2. Espinosa C, Becker M, Maric I, et al. Data-driven modeling of pregnancy-related complications. Trends Mol Med 2021;27(8):762-76.

3. Ghaemi MS, DiGiulio DB, Contrepois K, et al. Multiomics modeling of the immunome, transcriptome, microbiome, proteome and metabolome adaptations during human pregnancy. Bioinformatics 2019;35(1):95 to 103.

4. Le BL, Iwatani S, Wong RJ, et al. Computational discovery of therapeutic candidates for preventing preterm birth. JCI Insight 2020;5(3):e133761.

5. Stanley N, Stelzer IA, Tsai AS, et al. VoPo leverages cellular heterogeneity for predictive modeling of single-cell data. Nat Commun 2020;11(1):3738.

6. Culos A, Tsai AS, Stanley N, et al. Integration of mechanistic immunologic knowledge into a machine learning pipeline improves predictions. Nat Mach Intell 2020;2(10):619-28.

7. Maric I, Contrepois K, Moufarrej MN, et al. Early prediction and longitudinal modeling of preeclampsia from multiomics. Patterns (NY) 2022;3(12):100,655.

8. Maric I, Tsur A, Aghaeepour N, Montanari A, Stevenson DK, Shaw GM, et al. Early prediction of preeclampsia via machine learning. Am J Obstet Gynecol MFM 2020;2(2):100,100.

9. Espinosa CA, Khan W, Khanam R, et al. Multiomic signals associated with maternal epidemiologic factors contributing to preterm birth in low- and middle-income countries. Sci Adv 2023;9(21):eade7692.

10. Ozen M, Aghaeepour N, Maric I, et al. Omics approaches: interactions at the maternal-fetal interface and origins of child health and disease. Pediatr Res 2023;93(2):366-75.

REFERENCES

1. Goldenberg RL, Culhane JF, Iams JD, et al. Epidemiology and causes of preterm birth. Lancet 2008;371(9606):75–84.

2. Wallenstein MB, Shaw GM, Stevenson DK. Preterm birth as a calendar event or immunologic anomaly. JAMA Pediatr 2016;170(6):525–6.

3. Romero R, Dey SK, Fisher SJ. Preterm labor: one syndrome, many causes. Science 2014;345(6198):760–5.
4. Muglia LJ, Katz M. The enigma of spontaneous preterm birth. N Engl J Med 2010; 362(6):529–35.
5. Romero R, Espinoza J, Kusanovic JP, et al. The preterm parturition syndrome. BJOG 2006;113(Suppl 3):17–42.
6. Ozen M, Zhao H, Lewis DB, et al. Heme oxygenase and the immune system in normal and pathological pregnancies. Front Pharmacol 2015;6:84.
7. Peters GA, Yi L, Skomorovska-Prokvolit Y, et al. Inflammatory stimuli increase progesterone receptor-A stability and transrepressive activity in myometrial cells. Endocrinology 2017;158(1):158–69.
8. Patel B, Peters GA, Skomorovska-Prokvolit Y, et al. Control of progesterone receptor-A transrepressive activity in myometrial cells: implications for the control of human parturition. Reprod Sci 2018;25(2):214–21.
9. Druckmann R, Druckmann MA. Progesterone and the immunology of pregnancy. J Steroid Biochem Mol Biol 2005;97(5):389–96.
10. Stevenson DK, Aghaeepour N, Maric I, et al. Understanding how biologic and social determinants affect disparities in preterm birth and outcomes of preterm infants in the NICU. Semin Perinatol 2021;45(4):151408.
11. Stevenson DK, Gotlib IH, Buthmann JL, et al. Stress and its consequences-biological strain. Am J Perinatol 2022. https://doi.org/10.1055/a-1798-1602.
12. Becker M, Dai J, Chang AL, et al. Revealing the impact of lifestyle stressors on the risk of adverse pregnancy outcomes with multitask machine learning. Front Pediatr 2022;10:933266.
13. Espinosa C, Becker M, Maric I, et al. Data-driven modeling of pregnancy-related complications. Trends Mol Med 2021;27(8):762–76.
14. Ghaemi MS, DiGiulio DB, Contrepois K, et al. Multiomics modeling of the immunome, transcriptome, microbiome, proteome and metabolome adaptations during human pregnancy. Bioinformatics 2019;35(1):95–103.
15. Le BL, Iwatani S, Wong RJ, et al. Computational discovery of therapeutic candidates for preventing preterm birth. JCI Insight 2020;5(3):e133761.
16. Stanley N, Stelzer IA, Tsai AS, et al. VoPo leverages cellular heterogeneity for predictive modeling of single-cell data. Nat Commun 2020;11(1):3738.
17. Culos A, Tsai AS, Stanley N, et al. Integration of mechanistic immunological knowledge into a machine learning pipeline improves predictions. Nat Mach Intell 2020;2(10):619–28.
18. Maric I, Contrepois K, Moufarrej MN, et al. Early prediction and longitudinal modeling of preeclampsia from multiomics. Patterns (NY) 2022;3(12):100655.
19. Maric I, Tsur A, Aghaeepour N, et al. Early prediction of preeclampsia via machine learning. Am J Obstet Gynecol MFM 2020;2(2):100100.
20. Espinosa CA, Khan W, Khanam R, et al. Multiomic signals associated with maternal epidemiological factors contributing to preterm birth in low- and middle-income countries. Sci Adv 2023;9(21):eade7692.
21. Ozen M, Aghaeepour N, Maric I, et al. Omics approaches: interactions at the maternal-fetal interface and origins of child health and disease. Pediatr Res 2023;93(2):366–75.
22. Ravindra NG, Espinosa C, Berson E, et al. Deep representation learning identifies associations between physical activity and sleep patterns during pregnancy and prematurity. NPG Digit Med 2023;6(1):171.
23. Jehan F, Sazawal S, Baqui AH, et al. Multiomics characterization of preterm birth in low- and middle-income countries. JAMA Netw Open 2020;3(12):e2029655.

24. Stevenson DK, Wong RJ, Shaw GM, et al. The contributions of genetics to premature birth. Pediatr Res 2019;85(4):416–7.

25. Sun T, Cruz GI, Mousavi N, et al. HMOX1 genetic polymorphisms display ancestral diversity and may be linked to hypertensive disorders in pregnancy. Reprod Sci 2022;29(12):3465–76.

26. Li J, Oehlert J, Snyder M, et al. Fetal *de novo* mutations and preterm birth. PLoS Genet 2017;13(4):e1006689.

27. Ngo TTM, Moufarrej MN, Rasmussen MH, et al. Noninvasive blood tests for fetal development predict gestational age and preterm delivery. Science 2018; 360(6393):1133–6.

28. Moufarrej MN, Wong RJ, Shaw GM, et al. Investigating pregnancy and its complications using circulating cell-free RNA in women's blood during gestation. Front Pediatr 2020;8:605219.

29. Moufarrej MN, Vorperian SK, Wong RJ, et al. Early prediction of preeclampsia in pregnancy with cell-free RNA. Nature 2022;602(7898):689–94.

30. Ghaemi MS, Tarca AL, Romero R, et al. Proteomic signatures predict preeclampsia in individual cohorts but not across cohorts – implications for clinical biomarker studies. J Matern Fetal Neonatal Med 2022;35(25):5621–8.

31. Hao S, You J, Chen L, et al. Changes in pregnancy-related serum biomarkers early in gestation are associated with later development of preeclampsia. PLoS One 2020;15(3):e0230000.

32. Contrepois K, Chen S, Ghaemi MS, et al. Prediction of gestational age using urinary metabolites in term and preterm pregnancies. Sci Rep 2022;12(1):8033.

33. Zhang Y, Sylvester KG, Jin B, et al. Development of a urine metabolomics biomarker-based prediction model for preeclampsia during early pregnancy. Metabolites 2023;13(6):715.

34. Han X, Ghaemi MS, Ando K, et al. Differential dynamics of the maternal immune system in healthy pregnancy and preeclampsia. Front Immunol 2019;10:1305.

35. Peterson LS, Stelzer IA, Tsai AS, et al. Multiomic immune clockworks of pregnancy. Semin Immunopathol 2020;42(4):397–412.

36. Costello EK, DiGiulio DB, Robaczewska A, et al. Abrupt perturbation and delayed recovery of the vaginal ecosystem following childbirth. Nat Commun 2023;14(1): 4141.

37. DiGiulio DB, Callahan BJ, McMurdie PJ, et al. Temporal and spatial variation of the human microbiota during pregnancy. Proc Natl Acad Sci USA 2015; 112(35):11060–5.

38. Kowarsky M, Camunas-Soler J, Kertesz M, et al. Numerous uncharacterized and highly divergent microbes which colonize humans are revealed by circulating cell-free DNA. Proc Natl Acad Sci USA 2017;114(36):9623–8.

39. Weber KA, Yang W, Lyons E, et al. Greenspace, Air Pollution, Neighborhood factors, and preeclampsia in a Population-based Case-control study in California. Int J Environ Res Public Health 2021;18(10):5127.

40. Sindher SB, Chin AR, Aghaeepour N, et al. Advances and potential of omics studies for understanding the development of food allergy. Front Allergy 2023; 4:1149008.

41. Becker M, Mayo JA, Phogat NK, et al. Deleterious and protective psychosocial and stress-related factors predict risk of spontaneous preterm birth. Am J Perinatol 2023;40(1):74–88.

42. Fan HC, Blumenfeld YJ, Chitkara U, et al. Noninvasive diagnosis of fetal aneuploidy by shotgun sequencing DNA from maternal blood. Proc Natl Acad Sci USA 2008;105(42):16266–71.

43. Fan HC, Quake SR. Sensitivity of noninvasive prenatal detection of fetal aneuploidy from maternal plasma using shotgun sequencing is limited only by counting statistics. PLoS One 2010;5(5):e10439.
44. Koh W, Pan W, Gawad C, et al. Noninvasive *in vivo* monitoring of tissue-specific global gene expression in humans. Proc Natl Acad Sci USA 2014;111(20): 7361–6.
45. Pan W, Ngo TTM, Camunas-Soler J, et al. Simultaneously monitoring immune response and microbial infections during pregnancy through plasma cfRNA sequencing. Clin Chem 2017;63(11):1695–704.
46. Koh W, Wu A, Penland L, et al. Single cell gene transcriptomes derived from human cervical and uterine tissue during pregnancy. Adv Biosyst 2019;3:1800336.
47. Aghaeepour N, Lehallier B, Baca Q, et al. A proteomic clock of human pregnancy. Am J Obstet Gynecol 2018;218(3):347 e1–e14.
48. Aghaeepour N, Ganio EA, McIlwain D, et al. An immune clock of human pregnancy. Sci Immunol 2017;2(15):eaan2946.
49. Ando K, Hedou JJ, Feyaerts D, et al. A peripheral immune signature of labor induction. Front Immunol 2021;12:725989.
50. Bandura DR, Baranov VI, Ornatsky OI, et al. Mass cytometry: technique for real time single cell multitarget immunoassay based on inductively coupled plasma time-of-flight mass spectrometry. Anal Chem 2009;81(16):6813–22.
51. Bendall SC, Simonds EF, Qiu P, et al. Single-cell mass cytometry of differential immune and drug responses across a human hematopoietic continuum. Science 2011;332(6030):687–96.
52. Gaudilliere B, Ganio EA, Tingle M, et al. Implementing mass cytometry at the bedside to study the immunological basis of human diseases: Distinctive Immune features in patients with a history of term or preterm birth. Cytometry 2015;87(9): 817–29.
53. Stelzer IA, Ghaemi MS, Han X, et al. Integrated trajectories of the maternal metabolome, proteome, and immunome predict labor onset. Sci Transl Med 2021; 13(592):eabd9898.
54. Nadeau-Vallee M, Quiniou C, Palacios J, et al. Novel noncompetitive IL-1 receptor-biased ligand prevents infection- and inflammation-induced preterm birth. J Immunol 2015;195(7):3402–15.
55. Quiniou C, Sapieha P, Lahaie I, et al. Development of a novel noncompetitive antagonist of IL-1 receptor. J Immunol 2008;180(10):6977–87.
56. Hoffman MK, Goudar SS, Kodkany BS, et al. Low-dose aspirin for the prevention of preterm delivery in nulliparous women with a singleton pregnancy (ASPIRIN): a randomised, double-blind, placebo-controlled trial. Lancet 2020;395(10220): 285–93.
57. Klatzmann D, Abbas AK. The promise of low-dose interleukin-2 therapy for autoimmune and inflammatory diseases. Nat Rev Immunol 2015;15(5):283–94.
58. Rosenzwajg M, Lorenzon R, Cacoub P, et al. Immunological and clinical effects of low-dose interleukin-2 across 11 autoimmune diseases in a single, open clinical trial. Ann Rheum Dis 2019;78(2):209–17.
59. Callahan BJ, DiGiulio DB, Goltsman DSA, et al. Replication and refinement of a vaginal microbial signature of preterm birth in two racially distinct cohorts of US women. Proc Natl Acad Sci USA 2017;114(37):9966–71.
60. Elovitz MA, Gajer P, Riis V, et al. Cervicovaginal microbiota and local immune response modulate the risk of spontaneous preterm delivery. Nat Commun 2019;10(1):1305.

61. Callaway E, Ledford H. Medicine Nobel awarded for work on circadian clocks. Nature 2017;550(7674):18.
62. Cagnacci A, Soldani R, Melis GB, et al. Diurnal rhythms of labor and delivery in women: modulation by parity and seasons. Am J Obstet Gynecol 1998;178(1 Pt 1):140–5.
63. Cooperstock M, England JE, Wolfe RA. Circadian incidence of labor onset hour in preterm birth and chorioamnionitis. Obstet Gynecol 1987;70(6):852–5.
64. Lindow SW, Jha RR, Thompson JW. 24 hour rhythm to the onset of preterm labour. BJOG 2000;107(9):1145–8.
65. Vatish M, Steer PJ, Blanks AM, et al. Diurnal variation is lost in preterm deliveries before 28 weeks of gestation. BJOG 2010;117(6):765–7.
66. Moore TR, Iams JD, Creasy RK, et al. Diurnal and gestational patterns of uterine activity in normal human pregnancy. The Uterine Activity in Pregnancy Working Group. Obstet Gynecol 1994;83(4):517–23.
67. Mark PJ, Crew RC, Wharfe MD, et al. Rhythmic three-part harmony: the complex interaction of maternal, placental and fetal circadian systems. J Biol Rhythms 2017;32(6):534–49.
68. McCarthy R, Jungheim ES, Fay JC, et al. Riding the rhythm of melatonin through pregnancy to deliver on time. Front Endocrinol 2019;10:616.
69. Stevenson DK, Wong RJ, Aghaeepour N, et al. Towards personalized medicine in maternal and child health: integrating biologic and social determinants. Pediatr Res 2021;89(2):252–8.

Overview of the Global and US Burden of Preterm Birth

Victoria C. Ward, MD[a],*, Anne CC Lee, MD, MPH[b,c],
Steven Hawken, PhD[d], Nancy A. Otieno, PhD[e],
Hilda A. Mujuru, MMed, MSc[f], Gwendoline Chimhini, MMed, MPH[f],
Kumanan Wilson, MD, MSc[d,g,h], Gary L. Darmstadt, MD, MS[i]

KEYWORDS

- Preterm birth • Gestational age dating • Maternal health • Newborn health
- Neonatal mortality • Health disparities • Global burden of disease • Global health

KEY POINTS

- Preterm birth (PTB) is the leading cause of morbidity and mortality for under-5 children globally, including respiratory, infectious, metabolic and neurodevelopmental sequelae.
- The true global prevalence of PTB has been difficult to determine due to inadequate access to reliable gestational age dating methods; the global PTB rate was estimated to be 9.9% in 2020, unchanged over the last decade, and the PTB rate in the US was 10.5% in 2021, with important racial disparities for black women compared with white and Hispanic women.
- Global guidelines for high-quality care of preterm infants have recently been released, and access to these preventive, promotive, treatment, and family support measures should be ensured.
- Further research is required to better understand the causes of PTB in order to develop effective preventive interventions.
- Improved methods are needed for identification of preterm infants for purposes of population-level estimation and health resource allocation and for individual patient care.

[a] Department of Pediatrics, Stanford University School of Medicine, 291 Campus Drive, Li Ka Shing Building, Stanford, CA 94305, USA; [b] Department of Pediatrics, Global Advancement of Infants and Mothers, Brigham and Women's Hospital, 75 Francis St, Boston, MA 02115, USA; [c] Department of Pediatrics, Harvard Medical School, 77 Avenue Louis Pasteur, Boston, MA 02115, USA; [d] Clinical Epidemiology Program, Ottawa Hospital Research Institute, Center for Practice Changing Research, 501 Smyth Road, Box 201-B, Ottawa, Ontario K1H 8L6, Canada; [e] Kenya Medical Research Institute (KEMRI), Centre for Global Health Research, Division of Global Health Protection, Box 1578 Kisumu 40100, Kenya; [f] Department of Child Adolescent and Women's Health, Faculty of Medicine and Health Sciences, University of Zimbabwe, MP 167, Mount Pleasant, Harare, Zimbabwe; [g] Department of Medicine, University of Ottawa, 501 Smyth Road, Ottawa, ON K1H 8L6, Canada; [h] Bruyère Research Institute, 43 Bruyère Street, Ottawa, ON K1N 5C8, Canada; [i] Department of Pediatrics, Stanford University School of Medicine, 453 Quarry Road, Palo Alto, CA 94304, USA
* Corresponding author.
E-mail address: vward@stanford.edu

Clin Perinatol 51 (2024) 301–311
https://doi.org/10.1016/j.clp.2024.02.015
0095-5108/24/© 2024 Elsevier Inc. All rights reserved.

INTRODUCTION

In this review, we aim to provide a comprehensive overview of the prevalence of preterm birth (PTB), examining its trends and variations across different geographic regions and populations. We also address the multifaceted impacts of PTB, encompassing the immediate health challenges for infants born preterm as well as the long-term physical, developmental, and socioeconomic consequences. Through analyses of current research, we highlight the need for enhanced preventative interventions, improved access to antenatal and intrapartum care, better sexual and reproductive health services, and supportive policies for resource allocation and research to decrease PTB rates. Furthermore, improved access to postnatal care and key interventions for the care of preterm infants can mitigate the profound effects of PTB on individuals, families, communities, and nations.

DEFINITIONS AND TYPES OF PRETERM BIRTH

The PTB rate is defined as all live births prior to 37 weeks gestational age (GA) divided by all livebirths. Prematurity can be classified as late preterm between 34 and less than 37 weeks, moderate preterm between 32 and less than 34 weeks, very preterm between 28 and less than 32 weeks, and extremely preterm less than 28 weeks GA.[1] An important limitation of these population-based estimates is that stillbirths are not captured in the numerator or denominator of the PTB rate and contribute to a substantial burden of pregnancy loss, particularly in low and middle-income countries (LMICs) where misclassification of stillbirths as PTBs, and vice versa, is common.[2] In these settings, it is challenging to distinguish between intrapartum stillbirths from the births of infants born alive but too small or too early for life-sustaining measures.[3] Furthermore, the variability in application of the threshold of viability (22 vs 28 weeks GA) also affects the denominators used and classification of which babies are considered live births.[4] On average, idiopathic preterm labor and preterm premature rupture of membranes account for about two-thirds of preterm deliveries while provider-induced deliveries for indications such as preeclampsia or placental abruption account for the other third.[5] Preterm infants who survive into the post-neonatal period or even fall under 5 mortality categories may not be counted as preterm-associated mortality, despite it being the root cause of their deaths.

ACCURACY OF METHODS OF GESTATIONAL AGE ESTIMATION

Multiple challenges hinder accurate estimation of GA and thereby estimation of rates of PTB. Currently, the gold standard for GA assessment includes first trimester ultrasound with its accuracy estimated to be within ±1 week.[6] Ultrasound may not be reliably accurate, however, for women who present to antenatal care beyond the first trimester, which is common practice in many LMIC settings. Furthermore, in low-resource settings, ultrasound is often not available prenatally. Thus, less-expensive but less-accurate methods are more commonly used, such as a maternal report of the first day of her last menstrual period (LMP). LMP typically dates pregnancies to within ±35 to 40 days of ultrasound[7,8] and is influenced by maternal education, literacy, and recall period.[4,9,10] Symphysis fundal height is also commonly used in clinical settings to date pregnancies in LMICs when other methods are not available. In a systematic review, however, symphysis fundal height was determined to be biased, systematically underestimating GA, and only accurate to ±42 days of early ultrasound dating.[10] Increasing access to early ultrasonography less than 24 weeks is a priority not only for GA dating of pregnancy but also clinical care. While ultrasound in later pregnancy has traditionally been less accurate (±4 weeks), new algorithms and use of artificial intelligence are promising.[11–13] Postnatally, scoring systems based on clinical examination, such as Ballard, New Ballard, and Dubowitz, are also commonly used, yet these are time intensive, require good clinical acumen, and frequently date pregnancies to ±2 to 4 weeks of ultrasound dating.[14] New simplified models with newborn characteristics using machine learning are accurate (±15 days), though need further validation. Methods of GA dating that are reliant on examination can be particularly challenging when infants are born small, as it can be difficult to differentiate whether an infant is preterm or small-for-GA (SGA)—defined as a birthweight of less than the 10th percentile for GA[15]—or both. A recent Lancet series emphasized the importance of appropriate differentiation of PTB from fetal growth restriction.[16,17] Given the importance of individual identification of preterm infants as well as the importance of estimating population representative PTB rates, metabolomics analyses have been increasingly explored for both GA dating and estimation of risk of PTB as well as identification of infants who are SGA.[18–21]

At the individual level, accurate identification of PTB is critical given the significant health and developmental sequelae occurring as a result, and the need for early and immediate interventions. Complications of PTB are extensive and depend on the severity of prematurity and the quality of care provided. Most commonly, infants may suffer long-term neurodevelopmental delays,[22,23] hearing and visual defects, chronic lung disease, and vulnerability to infections. Early identification of infants in need of clinical interventions as well as long-term services to optimize neurodevelopmental outcomes is crucial for survival and future health and productivity. For instance, treatment with antenatal corticosteroids for women with a high likelihood of PTB can prevent acute respiratory failure as well as long-term sequelae of respiratory disease.[24] Similarly, access to continuous positive pressure ventilation postnatally can be life saving for a preterm infant at risk of or displaying respiratory distress.[25] From a long-term perspective, early developmental interventions for high-risk infants can be profoundly helpful for a child's lifelong development, and yet are rarely available in many low-resource settings.[26]

At the population level, understanding the burden of PTB from a public health perspective is needed for resource allocation and policymaking. Among major causes of the childhood burden of disease, PTB and its associated complications account for the largest percentage of neonatal and under-5 morbidity and mortality.[27] And yet, it is a critical public health problem that too often is left unattended and underfunded. Furthermore, there are profound equity gaps related to exposure to risk factors and unequal access to the perinatal care that is required to prevent PTB and manage its long-term impacts on survival, health, and neurodevelopment.

GLOBAL PREVALENCE

Previously published global PTB rates by the World Health Organization (WHO) in 2015 leveraged data from 1990 to 2014 and estimated that on average over this time period: 14.84 million infants were born preterm annually (95% confidence interval [CI]: 12.65 million, 16.73 million livebirths). This reflects an average global PTB rate of approximately 10.6% (95% CI: 9.0, 12.0%).[28]

More recently, Ohuma and colleagues[29] reviewed global administrative and study data for 2010 to 2020 from across 103 countries, and used Bayesian modeling to estimate PTB rates and time trends. They estimated that 13.4 million infants were born preterm in 2020, accounting for 9.9% of all births (95% CI: 9.1, 11.2). This demonstrated almost no change when compared with 2010, when there were an estimated

13.4 million PTBs, or approximately 9.8% of all births (95% CI: 9.0, 11.0).[29] In 2020, while 55.6% of total livebirths were in South Asia and Sub-Saharan Africa, 65% of PTBs were identified in these 2 regions.

When examining geographic trends, 91% of PTBs occurred in LMICs. Further geographic disaggregation of the data demonstrates that 52.9% of PTBs occurred in South Asia and 28.2% in Sub-Saharan Africa.[29] Remarkably, over 50% of all PTBs in 2020 occurred in just 8 countries: India (30,016,700 or 13.0% livebirths), Pakistan (914,000, 14.4%), Nigeria (774,100, 9.9%), China (752,100, 6.1%), Ethiopia (495,900, 12.9%), Bangladesh (488,600, 16.2%), Democratic Republic of the Congo (487,500, 12.4%), and the United States (366,200, 10.0%).[29]

U S DOMESTIC PREVALENCE

In the United States, trends of overall PTB have demonstrated disappointing patterns. Between 1990 and 2005, the domestic PTB rate rose from 10.6% to 12.7%.[30] This was thought to be secondary to increased use of in vitro fertilization and higher proportions of multiple pregnancies which are at higher risk of being preterm, as well as improved intrapartum fetal care preventing stillbirth.[31] Rates subsequently declined back to 10.1% in 2020, but rose again during the coronavirus disease 2019 pandemic to 10.5% in 2021 likely due to increased maternal stress as well as compromises in access to prenatal and intrapartum care and decreased management of risk factors for PTB such as infection management, addressing undernutrition and micronutrient supplementation, use of progesterone, and provision of cervical cerclage among other effective interventions.[32]

It is important to note that there are also significant racial disparities in PTB rates in the United States population. In 2022, the PTB rate among black women was 14.6% compared with 9.4% among whites and 10.1% among Hispanics.[32] This is similar to differences observed in 2015, when 13.3% of black infants were born preterm, compared with 9.4% of white infants.[33] While the causes for this disparity are still unknown and likely multifactorial, many surmise that factors such as maternal stress associated with structural racism, environmental exposures, and limitations in access to health care play important roles.[33–35]

When compared to the PTB rates in other high-income countries, the United States is an outlier with substantially higher rates. In Europe, for instance, the PTB rate is approximately 6.5%.[28] While America's relatively high PTB rate may be both more accurately counted as a result of widespread access to early ultrasound dating and life-saving interventions for those born extremely premature that might otherwise be classified as stillbirth, the overall prevalence remains notably high and requires careful attention, especially for those mothers who are disproportionately affected due to racial and/or socioeconomic disparities.

CONSEQUENCES OF PRETERM BIRTH

PTB and its complications are the largest contributors to morbidity and mortality for children under the age of 5 years. In the 2014 Every Newborn Lancet series, Lawn and colleagues[36] found that PTB or SGA, or both, is the biggest risk factor for an estimated 80% or more of neonatal deaths, and in the postnatal period increases the risk of mortality, growth failure, and adult-onset non-communicable diseases. Of the 5.3 million deaths in children under 5 around the world in 2019, 17.7% (95% CI: 16.1, 19.5%), or 0.94 million total (95% CI: 0.86, 1.06), were due to PTB complications, the leading cause of mortality for all children globally.[27] A pooled analysis by Katz and colleagues[37] estimates that preterm infants have a relative risk (RR) of more than 6-fold for neonatal mortality (RR: 6.82; 95% CI: 3.56, 13.07) and nearly 3-fold (RR: 2.50; 95% CI:

1.48, 4.22) for post-neonatal mortality when compared to term infants. This can be further examined for mortality RR based on the severity of prematurity. In 2013, the RR of neonatal mortality for being born late preterm (34–37 weeks, 50%–96% of all PTBs) was 3.05 (95% CI: 2.02, 4.60), while for those born early preterm (<32 weeks), the RR was 28.82 (95% CI: 15.51, 53.56), compared with the full-term group. The adverse consequences of being born both preterm and SGA was the subject of a recent Lancet series on the small vulnerable newborn (SVN), finding that in 2020, 55.3% of the 2.4 million neonatal deaths were attributable to SVNs (almost 1.4 million), with 32·8% (50% CI: 23.1, 33.7%) attributed to preterm non-SGA, 14.7% (50% CI: 12.5, 15.8%) attributed to term SGA, and 7.7% (50% CI: 6.2, 16.9%) attributed to preterm SGA.[16] This echoes similar research by Suárez-Idueta and colleagues[17] who note that "though the prevalence of infants born both preterm and SGA is low (median: 0.6%, interquartile range: 0.6, 0.8%), these infants are at higher risk of mortality and chronic diseases later in life compared with those born either preterm only or SGA only."[17]

With regard to geographic differences in the mortality associated with being born preterm, the highest neonatal and infant mortality rates occur in Asia and Africa, with 81.1% of PTB-related deaths on these 2 continents.[28] Furthermore, more than 90% of under-5 mortality and 95% of maternal mortality in 2015 occurred in LMICs.[38] When assessing the US infant mortality rate, the infant death rate in 2021 was 543.6 infant deaths per 100,000 livebirths and PTB and low birthweight (LBW) accounted for approximately 15% of infant deaths.[39]

When examining the morbidity and mortality, in 2010 PTB was estimated to result in 77 million disability-adjusted life years globally due to newborn death and impairment associated with prematurity, 3.1% of the global total.[22] Studies by Saigal and colleagues[40] demonstrated that due to improved survival rates for early preterm infants following technological advances and increased health care capacity, infants have become more likely to survive prematurity, thus leading to increased health and developmental sequelae of prematurity occurring in a relatively larger percentage of infants. Similarly, using global data, Lawn and colleagues[36] reported in 2014 that in middle-income countries where progress was being achieved in reducing neonatal deaths and the neonatal mortality rate had reached 5 to 15 deaths per 1000 livebirths, and where neonatal intensive care was scaling up, rates of disability among infants born at 26 to 32 weeks GA was twice that of high-income countries, highlighting the need for improvements in the quality of care. A systematic review of global data demonstrated that in 2010 of the 13 million surviving PTBs, approximately 2.7% were estimated to have moderate or severe neurodevelopmental impairment and 4.4% had mild impairment.[22] Yet, neurodevelopmental delays is only 1 category in an extensive list of long-term adverse outcomes attributed to PTB, which broadly include impacts such as increased respiratory diseases, infections, retinopathy of prematurity, metabolic disorders, and growth faltering.[41–43]

PREVENTION OF PRETERM BIRTH

Despite being the leading cause of child mortality, the prevalence of PTB remains profoundly unattended to. In order to make progress, the prevention of PTB and the management of its complications are critical. Interventions during preconception, pregnancy, and the first 1000 days have strong evidence and yet implementation remains weak. Darmstadt and colleagues[44] demonstrated in 2014 that of 16 interventions proven to be effective in saving newborn lives globally in 2005, population-based data were available for only five interventions, and trend data showing change over time was available for just one.[45] Risk factors for PTB are known, and include both modifiable and non-modifiable risk factors. Bryce and colleagues[42] analyzed risk factors for spontaneous PTB in 81 countries and identified 24 risk factors which accounted for 77% of the population attributable fraction (PAF), or the proportional reduction in spontaneous PTB in the population if those with the risk factor did not have that risk factor. Their research suggests that the highest RRs (>2.0) are associated with short cervical length, twin pregnancies, and maternal syphilis infection, and the most common risk factors included in the model were maternal anemia (13.1%), indoor air pollution (9.7%), bacterial vaginosis (9.5%), chronic hypertension (4.9%), and maternal age greater than 35 years, and parity greater than 3 (3.3%). While these risk factors contribute to the greatest PAF of PTB, interventions targeting some of these risk factors have often failed to impact PTB rates. Certain interventions have demonstrated efficacy in PTB prevention such as smoking cessation, progesterone supplementation, medically indicated cervical cerclage,[46,47] and aspirin.[48] Hofmeyr and colleagues[49] estimated that implementation of 8 evidence-based preventive interventions ("inclusive of multiple micronutrient supplementation, balanced protein and energy supplementation, low-dose aspirin, progesterone provided vaginally, education for smoking cessation, malaria prevention, treatment of asymptomatic bacteriuria, and treatment of syphilis") across 81 LMICs could prevent 5.2 million births of small vulnerable newborns and 0.56 million stillbirths per year. Furthermore, they estimate that adding antenatal corticosteroids and delayed cord clamping to reduce the complications of PTB could avert 0.476 million neonatal deaths annually.

New technologies are also emerging for the prediction of those at highest risk for PTB, which may lead to even more targeted and cost-effective prevention efforts. For instance, utilization of prediction mechanisms such as antenatal metabolomic analysis[50] or temporal deep-learning models[51] can identify those at high risk for PTB and enable early intervention. These promising interventions are described in other articles in this series.

Given the significant impacts on morbidity and mortality, reduction of PTB rates would not only have extensive health benefits, but significant gains in human capital as well. Estimates provided by the National Academy of Sciences suggested that the annual societal economic burden associated with PTB in the United States was at least $26.2 billion USD.[52] Recently, Blakstad and colleagues[53] undertook a modeling study to estimate the long-term impacts on human capital of decreasing the prevalence of PTB across 121 countries and found that a reduction in PTB from 15% to a theoretic minimum of 5.5% would lead to a gain of 9.8 million school years (95% CI: 1.5, 18.4) and $41.9 billion USD (95% CI: 6.1, 80.9) in lifetime income.

TREATMENT FOR COMPLICATIONS OF PREMATURITY

Evidence supporting the importance of high-quality care for infants born preterm in averting neonatal death and preventing long-term sequelae is strong. Darmstadt and colleagues[44] modeled the potential impact of evidence-based interventions on neonatal mortality in 2005, and found that if all interventions were implemented at full coverage (99%), an estimated 41% to 72% of neonatal deaths could be averted. Bhutta and colleagues[54] showed in 2014 in an expanded analysis that available interventions had the potential to avert 71% of neonatal deaths, including 58% of deaths among preterm infants, with an annual cost reduction of $5.65 billion USD. Recent WHO guidelines were released with recommendations for effective care for preterm or LBW infants including 25 recommendations, 14 of which were strong (applicable to all preterm or LBW infants) and 11 were conditional (applicable to specific populations or settings), and most (n = 16) were for preventive and promotive care. Recommendations include kangaroo mother care and exclusive breastfeeding for at least 6 months, several feeding and micronutrient recommendations, and treatment with caffeine for preterm infants experiencing apneic events as well as the use of continuous positive airway pressure for management of respiratory distress. Additional recommendations that should be considered include micronutrient supplementation, probiotic administration, emollient therapy, and caffeine for prevention of apnea in infants less than 34 weeks GA.[25] Notably, WHO recommended family involvement during the hospital stay and home-visit support of families in caring for preterm or LBW infants. Ensuring access to key life-saving and health-promoting interventions along the continuum of care is estimated by the WHO to be able to save 1.7 million newborn lives each year.[55]

LIMITATIONS

The true prevalence of PTB remains difficult to reliably capture. The low availability and poor quality of GA data are significant problems, particularly in LMICs where antenatal care access is lacking, as are inaccurate methods of GA dating as described earlier. Furthermore, there is poor differentiation for SVNs between growth restricted and PTBs.[17] There also exists heterogeneity in the inclusion of infants born too early or too small for survival and those who are stillborn. Therefore, there are inherent challenges in accurately estimating the true potential impacts of preventive and therapeutic interventions.

DISCUSSION

While the extent of their impacts might be underrepresented, the morbidity and mortality associated with PTB remains the most significant threat to infant survival and long-term thriving, and thus a primary contributor to the well-being of humanity. Multiple studies have aimed to accurately describe the scope of the problem, including the recent Lancet series on small, vulnerable newborns, suggesting that over 13 million infants were born prematurely in 2020, 15% of which were born at less than 32 weeks of gestation thus requiring a significant amount of extra care.[16] Research has also demonstrated significant disparities in rates of PTB, demonstrating that over 90% of PTBs occur in LMICs.[29] In the United States specifically, there remain significant disparities in PTB rates between black mothers (14.6%) and white and Hispanic mothers (9.4% and 10.1%, respectively.)[32] Many of these differences are ascribed to a combination of maternal risk factors as well as disparities in access to health care services.

While it is critically important to ensure better and more accurate data to more reliably elucidate the scope of the PTB problem, it clearly remains the most detrimental cause of morbidity and mortality amongst infants. Infants must first be accurately identified as preterm, rather than simply small or weak. Better yet, mothers should be accurately assessed for their risk of going into preterm labor. But for those who are identified as preterm, strong evidence exists for high-quality interventions to avert most deaths of preterm infants, and both preventive and therapeutic interventions are relatively cost-efficient and effective. Yet, resources must be mobilized to ensure that access to them is equitable. In this way, the prevalence of PTB sets up one of the great opportunities to improve human life, but must be pursued universally and equitably across all socioeconomic and geographic sections of the world.

DISCLOSURE

The authors have no disclosures to report.

Best Practices

What is the current practice for PTB?

- First-trimester ultrasound for GA dating.

What changes in current practice are likely to improve outcomes?

- Use of multiomics and machine learning are likely to lead to improvements in identification of infants at risk of PTB and complications of prematurity.
- Disparities in PTB rates mandate addressing social determinants, systemic racism and discrimination, environmental exposures, and limitations in access to health care.
- Implementation of WHO recommendations for care of preterm or LBW infants.

Bibliographic source:

WHO recommendations for care of the preterm or low birth weight infant [Internet]. Geneva: World Health Organization; 2022. Licence: CC BY-NC-SA 3.0 IGO.

REFERENCES

1. World Health Organization. Preterm birth. 2023. Available at: https://www.who.int/news-room/fact-sheets/detail/preterm-birth. [Accessed 6 February 2024].
2. Sanders MR, Donohue PK, Oberdorf MA, et al. Impact of the perception of viability on resource allocation in the neonatal intensive care unit. J Perinatol 1998;18(5):347–51.
3. Lawn JE, Gravett MG, Nunes TM, et al. Global report on preterm birth and stillbirth (1 of 7): definitions, description of the burden and opportunities to improve data. BMC Pregnancy Childbirth 2010;10(Suppl 1):S1.
4. Blencowe H, Cousens S, Chou D, et al. Born too soon: the global epidemiology of 15 million preterm births. Reprod Health 2013;10(Suppl 1):S2.
5. Gotsch F, Gotsch F, Romero R, et al. The preterm parturition syndrome and its implications for understanding the biology, risk assessment, diagnosis, treatment and prevention of preterm birth. J Matern Fetal Neonatal Med 2009;22(Suppl 2):5–23.
6. Committee Opinion No 700: Methods for estimating the due date. Obstet Gynecol 2017;129(5):e150–4.
7. Karl S, Li Wai Suen CSN, Unger HW, et al. Preterm or not – an evaluation of estimates of gestational age in a cohort of women from Rural Papua New Guinea. PLoS One 2015;10(5):e0124286.
8. Alliance for Maternal and Newborn Health Improvement AMANHI Gestational Age Study Group, Alliance for Maternal and Newborn Health Improvement AMANHI GA Study Group. Alliance for maternal and newborn health improvement (AMANHI) gestational age study group; alliance for maternal and newborn health improvement (AMANHI) GA study group. Simplified models to assess newborn gestational age in low-middle income countries: findings from a multi-country, prospective cohort study. BMJ Glob Health 2021;6(9):e005688.
9. Rosenberg RE, Ahmed ASMNU, Ahmed S, et al. Determining gestational age in a low-resource setting: validity of last menstrual period. J Health Popul Nutr 2009;27(3):332–8.

10. Whelan R, Schaeffer L, Olson I, et al. Measurement of symphysis fundal height for gestational age estimation in low-to-middle-income countries: a systematic review and meta-analysis. PLoS One 2022;17(8):e0272718.
11. WHO Alliance for Maternal and Newborn Health Improvement Late Pregnancy Dating Study Group. Performance of late pregnancy biometry for gestational age dating in low-income and middle-income countries: a prospective, multi-country, population-based cohort study from the WHO Alliance for Maternal and Newborn Health Improvement (AMANHI) Study Group. Lancet Global Health 2020;8(4):e545–54.
12. Papageorghiou AT, Kemp B, Stones W, et al. Ultrasound-based gestational-age estimation in late pregnancy. Ultrasound Obstet Gynecol 2016;48(6):719–26.
13. Pokaprakarn T, Prieto JC, Price JT, et al. AI estimation of gestational age from blind ultrasound sweeps in low-resource settings. NEJM Evid 2022;1(5). https://doi.org/10.1056/evidoa2100058.
14. Lee AC, Panchal P, Folger L, et al. Diagnostic accuracy of neonatal assessment for gestational age determination: a systematic review. Pediatrics 2017;140(6):e20171423.
15. Battaglia FC, Lubchenco LO. A practical classification of newborn infants by weight and gestational age. J Pediatr 1967;71(2):159–63.
16. Lawn JE, Ohuma EO, Bradley E, et al. Small babies, big risks: global estimates of prevalence and mortality for vulnerable newborns to accelerate change and improve counting. Lancet 2023;401(10389):1707–19.
17. Suárez-Idueta L, Yargawa J, Blencowe H, et al. Vulnerable newborn types: analysis of population-based registries for 165 million births in 23 countries. BJOG 2000-2021;2023.
18. Hawken S, Ward V, Bota AB, et al. Real world external validation of metabolic gestational age assessment in Kenya. PLOS Glob Public Health 2022;2(11):e0000652.
19. Wilson K, Hawken S, Potter BK, et al. Accurate prediction of gestational age using newborn screening analyte data. Am J Obstet Gynecol 2016;214(4):513.e1–9.
20. Ryckman KK, Berberich SL, Dagle JM. Predicting gestational age using neonatal metabolic markers. Am J Obstet Gynecol 2016;214(4):515.e1–13.
21. Jelliffe-Pawlowski LL, Norton ME, Baer RJ, et al. Gestational dating by metabolic profile at birth: a California cohort study. Am J Obstet Gynecol 2016;214(4):511.e1–13.
22. Blencowe H, Lee ACC, Cousens S, et al. Preterm birth-associated neurodevelopmental impairment estimates at regional and global levels for 2010. Pediatr Res 2013;74(Suppl 1):17–34.
23. Martin-Herz SP, Otieno P, Laanoi GM, et al. Growth and neurodevelopmental outcomes of preterm and low birth weight infants in rural Kenya: a cross-sectional study. BMJ Open 2023;13(8):e064678.
24. McGoldrick E, Stewart F, Parker R, et al. Antenatal corticosteroids for accelerating fetal lung maturation for women at risk of preterm birth. Cochrane Database Syst Rev 2020;12(12):CD004454.
25. Care of Preterm or Low Birthweight Infants Group. New World Health Organization recommendations for care of preterm or low birth weight infants: health policy. EClinicalMedicine 2023;63:102155.
26. Sutton PS, Darmstadt GL. Preterm birth and neurodevelopment: a review of outcomes and recommendations for early identification and cost-effective interventions. J Trop Pediatr 2013;59(4):258–65.

27. Perin J, Mulick A, Yeung D, et al. Global, regional, and national causes of under-5 mortality in 2000–19: an updated systematic analysis with implications for the Sustainable Development Goals. Lancet Child Adolesc Health 2022;6(2):106–15.

28. Chawanpaiboon S, Vogel JP, Moller AB, et al. Global, regional, and national estimates of levels of preterm birth in 2014: a systematic review and modelling analysis. Lancet Global Health 2019;7(1):e37–46.

29. Ohuma EO, Moller AB, Bradley E, et al. National, regional, and global estimates of preterm birth in 2020, with trends from 2010: a systematic analysis. Lancet 2023;402(10409):1261–71.

30. Hamilton BE, Martin JA, Ventura SJ. Births: preliminary data for 2005. Natl Vital Stat Rep 2006;55(11):1–18.

31. Goldenberg RL, Culhane JF, Iams JD, et al. Epidemiology and causes of preterm birth. Lancet 2008;371(9606):75–84.

32. Martin JA, Hamilton BE, Osterman MJK. Births in the United States, 2022. NCHS Data Brief 2023;(477):1–8.

33. Purisch SE, Gyamfi-Bannerman C. Epidemiology of preterm birth. Semin Perinatol 2017;41(7):387–91.

34. Braveman P, Heck K, Egerter S, et al. Worry about racial discrimination: a missing piece of the puzzle of Black-White disparities in preterm birth? PLoS One 2017; 12(10):e0186151.

35. Blebu BE, Waters O, Lucas CT, et al. Variations in maternal factors and preterm birth risk among Non-Hispanic Black, White, and mixed-race Black/White women in the United States, 2017. Wom Health Issues 2022;32(2):140–6.

36. Lawn JE, Blencowe H, Oza S, et al. Every newborn: progress, priorities, and potential beyond survival. Lancet 2014;384(9938):189–205.

37. Katz J, Lee AC, Kozuki N, et al. Mortality risk in preterm and small-for-gestational-age infants in low-income and middle-income countries: a pooled country analysis. Lancet 2013;382(9890):417–25.

38. Countdown to 2030 Collaboration. Countdown to 2030: tracking progress towards universal coverage for reproductive, maternal, newborn, and child health. Lancet 2018;391(10129):1538–48.

39. Xu J, Murphy SL, Kochanek KD, et al. Mortality in the United States, 2021. NCHS Data Brief 2022;(456):1–8.

40. Saigal S, Doyle LW. An overview of mortality and sequelae of preterm birth from infancy to adulthood. Lancet 2008;371(9608):261–9.

41. Ashorn P, Ashorn U, Muthiani Y, et al. Small vulnerable newborns-big potential for impact. Lancet 2023;401(10389):1692–706.

42. Bryce E, Gurung S, Tong H, et al. Population attributable fractions for risk factors for spontaneous preterm births in 81 low- and middle-income countries: a systematic analysis. J Glob Health 2022;12:04013.

43. Howson CP, Kinney MV, Lawn JE. March of dimes, the partnership for maternal, newborn, & child health, save the children, world health organization. Born too soon: the global action Report on preterm birth. Geneva (Switzerland): World Health Organization; 2012.

44. Darmstadt GL, Bhutta ZA, Cousens S, et al. Evidence-based, cost-effective interventions: how many newborn babies can we save? Lancet 2005;365(9463):977–88.

45. Darmstadt GL, Kinney MV, Chopra M, et al. Who has been caring for the baby? Lancet 2014;384(9938):174–88.

46. Chang HH, Larson J, Blencowe H, et al. Preventing preterm births: analysis of trends and potential reductions with interventions in 39 countries with very high human development index. Lancet 2013;381(9862):223–34.
47. Barros FC, Papageorghiou AT, Victora CG, et al. The distribution of clinical phenotypes of preterm birth syndrome: implications for prevention. JAMA Pediatr 2015;169(3):220–9.
48. Hoffman MK, Goudar SS, Kodkany BS, et al. Low-dose aspirin for the prevention of preterm delivery in nulliparous women with a singleton pregnancy (ASPIRIN): a randomised, double-blind, placebo-controlled trial. Lancet 2020;395(10220): 285–93.
49. Hofmeyr GJ, Black RE, Rogozińska E, et al. Evidence-based antenatal interventions to reduce the incidence of small vulnerable newborns and their associated poor outcomes. Lancet 2023;401(10389):1733–44.
50. Jehan F, Sazawal S, Baqui AH, et al. Multiomics characterization of preterm birth in low- and middle-income countries. JAMA Netw Open 2020;3(12):e2029655.
51. Gao C, Osmundson S, Velez Edwards DR, et al. Deep learning predicts extreme preterm birth from electronic health records. J Biomed Inf 2019;100:103334.
52. Institute of Medicine (US), Committee on understanding premature birth and assuring healthy outcomes. In: Behrman RE, Butler AS, editors. Preterm birth: causes, consequences, and prevention. Washington (DC): National Academies Press (US); 2007.
53. Blakstad MM, Perumal N, Bliznashka L, et al. Large gains in schooling and income are possible from minimizing adverse birth outcomes in 121 low- and middle-income countries: a modelling study. PLOS Glob Public Health 2022; 2(6):e0000218.
54. Bhutta ZA, Das JK, Bahl R, et al. Can available interventions end preventable deaths in mothers, newborn babies, and stillbirths, and at what cost? Lancet 2014;384(9940):347–70.
55. World Health Organization UNCF (UNICEF). Every newborn progress report 2019; 2020.

Recent Advances in Genomic Studies of Gestational Duration and Preterm Birth

Amit K. Srivastava, PhD[a,1], Nagendra Monangi, MD[b,c,1],
Vidhya Ravichandran, MBBS[a,c,1], Pol Solé-Navais, MSc, PhD[d],
Bo Jacobsson, MD, PhD[d,e], Louis J. Muglia, MD, PhD[a,b,f],
Ge Zhang, MD, PhD[a,b],*

KEYWORDS

- Genomics • Genetic association • Genome-wide association • Polygenic score
- Mendelian randomization • Genetic architecture • SNP-heritability
- Genetic correlation

Continued

INTRODUCTION

Preterm birth (PTB), defined as live birth before 37 weeks of completed gestation, is the leading cause of mortality in children aged under 5 years, and it remains one of the greatest adverse public health outcomes globally.[1] Worldwide, an estimated 13.4 million neonates are born prematurely every year, and nearly 1 million of these children die each year due to complications of prematurity.[2]

Despite the significant global health implications and the recognition that preventing PTB is the best way to improve health outcomes for children affected by prematurity-related complications, progress in preventing prematurity has been limited. Based on the clinical definition, PTB can be broadly grouped into medically indicated PTB, idiopathic PTB, and preterm premature rupture of membranes.[3] Likewise, the World Health Organization subcategorizes PTB based on the gestational age (GA) at birth:

[a] Division of Human Genetics, Cincinnati Children's Hospital Medical Center, 3333 Burnet Avenue, Cincinnati, OH 45229, USA; [b] Department of Pediatrics, University of Cincinnati College of Medicine, Center for Prevention of Preterm Birth, Perinatal Institute, Cincinnati Children's Hospital Medical Center and March of Dimes Prematurity Research Center Ohio Collaborative; [c] Division of Neonatology, Cincinnati Children's Hospital Medical Center, 3333 Burnet Avenue, Cincinnati, OH 45229, USA; [d] Department of Obstetrics and Gynaecology, Sahlgrenska Academy, Institute of Clinical Sciences, University of Gothenburg, Box 100, Gothenburg 405 30, Sweden; [e] Department of Genetics and Bioinformatics, Health Data and Digitalization, Norwegian Institute of Public Health, Lovisenberggata 8, Oslo 0456, Norway; [f] The Burroughs Wellcome Fund, 21 Tw Alexander Drive, Research Triangle Park, NC 27709, USA
[1] Authors contributed equally.
* Corresponding author.
E-mail address: ge.zhang@cchmc.org

Continued

KEY POINTS

- There is a significant genetic influence on the risk of preterm birth (PTB), with maternal genetics playing a dominant role.
- Analyzing mother–child pairs as a single analytical unit enables distinguishing between maternal and fetal genetic effects.
- Conducting genomic analyses at single-variant, multi-variant, and genome-wide levels can address different genetic questions, including identifying risk variants, understanding causal relationships, and deciphering the genetic architecture of human birth timing.
- There is a critical necessity to increase ancestral diversity in genomic studies to address observed demographic disparities in PTB.
- An integrative approach that combines genomic research with refined phenotyping and other omics technologies is essential to fully capture the complex etiology of PTB.

extreme PTB (<28 weeks), very preterm (28 to <32 weeks), and moderate or late PTB (32 to <37 weeks).[4]

A substantial body of research indicates a genetic influence on the risk of PTB and, more broadly, the duration of gestation. The most direct evidence is that a history of preterm delivery in a mother is the strongest predictor of PTB in her subsequent pregnancies.[5] Numerous epidemiologic studies have demonstrated the involvement of both maternal and fetal genetics, with maternal genetics often playing a more substantive role.[6–9]

Human genome-wide genetic studies provide an unbiased way to detect associated genes and biological pathways of birth timing. This is of particular importance because each species has its own reproductive strategy and animal studies cannot provide complete information about a human pregnancy.[10] The findings from genomic research could have multiple translational values including genomic prediction of PTB, mechanistic insights, and identification of potential interventional targets that may lead to novel approaches to reduce adverse pregnancy outcomes and their long-term sequelae. In the past, various reviews have comprehensively covered different aspects of the genetics of PTB, such as genetic epidemiology,[11] candidate gene association,[12] genome-wide association (GWA), rare variants, and copy number associations along with transcriptional and epigenetic regulation of PTB.[13–18]

In this review, we focused on recent genomic research on human birth timing in mothers and their children, aiming to distinguish between maternal and fetal genetic effects. Our discussion includes studies at 3 distinct levels: single-variant, multi-variant, and genome-wide variation analyses, each targeting different genetic questions. Additionally, we highlight some challenges in this field, particularly the lack of population diversity in genomic studies of pregnancy outcomes. We also explore the prospects and opportunities that lie ahead for new research directions.

GESTATIONAL DURATION AND SPONTANEOUS PRETERM BIRTH: THE FOCUS OF GENETIC STUDIES
The Phenotype (Outcome)

The success of genomic research heavily depends on the precise definition and measurements of outcomes. In the context of genetic analyses of PTB, gestational duration is a widely studied outcome. However, collecting accurate data on gestational duration is challenging, especially in underresourced and ethnically diverse communities. An early ultrasound along with fetal measurements, preferably in the first trimester is the most accurate way to assess GA with an error window of 5 to 7 days. However, many low-income and middle-income countries and communities with limited healthcare facilities and practitioners still depend on the date of the last menstrual period (LMP) in calculating the expected date of delivery. LMP method has low accuracy due to irregular and large variations in the length of the menstrual cycle, conception occurring up to several days after ovulation, and inability to recall the date of LMP.[4] Many developed countries and research studies combine ultrasound and LMP methods to estimate GA. This combined relatively new method of assessment referred to as "best obstetric estimate" can have better accuracy than either of the 2 methods.[4,19]

The diagnosis of PTB, defined by dichotomization of gestational duration, is a common practice in clinical research to simplify statistical analyses and interpretation of results. However, such simplicity is achieved at the cost of loss in statistical power to detect true genetic associations.[20] Genetic epidemiology studies suggest a model of similar genetic and environmental contributions across the range of GAs. This supports the notion that considering gestational duration as a continuous variable could provide greater statistical power than dichotomizing preterm and term pregnancies in genetic studies.[9] Indeed, most PTB-associated genetic loci identified to date are also associated with gestational duration with higher statistical significance. Recent research further indicated the overall genetic control of birth timing appears to be shared in the term and preterm.[21]

Genomic Studies in Mother–Child Pairs

Being genetically controlled by both maternal and fetal genomes is a distinctive characteristic of human birth timing and other pregnancy-related phenotypes. Consequently, genomic studies of these phenotypes must encompass both mothers and infants. With the growing volume of genomic data from mothers and infants across many birth cohort studies, new opportunities arise to dissect the relative contributions of maternal and fetal genomes.

Conventional genetic studies often consider each individual as the analytical unit, examining the association between an individual's genotype (usually comprising 2 alleles) and their phenotypes. This approach has several limitations when applied to pregnancy phenotypes. Firstly, distinguishing between maternal and fetal genetic effects becomes problematic due to the sharing of alleles transmitted from mother to fetus, especially when only maternal or fetal samples are analyzed. Secondly, analyzing mothers and infants separately fails to reveal the complex phenotypic and genetic interplay between the mother and her fetus. To address these challenges, Zhang and colleagues[13,22] developed a novel approach that treats the mother–child pair (or a pregnancy) as a single analytical unit with 3 alleles: the maternally transmitted allele (h1), the maternally non-transmitted allele (h2), and the paternally transmitted allele (h3) (**Fig. 1**). Each of these alleles influences pregnancy outcomes differently: h1 can affect outcomes either through the mother or through the fetus or both; h2 exclusively influences through the mother; and h3 acts solely through the fetus. The method is also referred to as a haplotype-based approach due to the joint estimation of haplotypic (allelic) effects of h1, h2, and h3. By considering the mother–child pair as one unit, this method enables a clear distinction between maternal and fetal genetic effects on pregnancy phenotypes.[13] This approach can also be extended to parent–offspring trios with 4 alleles (h1, h2, h3, and h4—paternally non-transmitted allele). Zhang and colleagues[13] also proposed 3 different levels of genetic analyses (**Fig. 2**)—single variant analysis, multi-variant analysis, and analysis of genome-wide variants under this analytical framework.

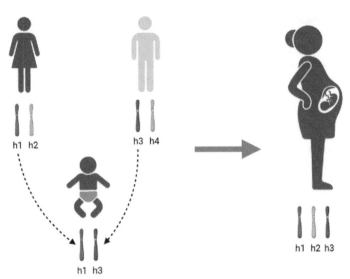

Fig. 1. Genomic analyses of pregnancy phenotypes. (Left) The conventional approach analyzes mothers and infants separately, which complicates the distinction between maternal and fetal genetic effects due to the sharing of transmitted alleles (h1). (Right) An integrated approach treats the mother–child pair as a single analytical unit with 3 alleles: the maternally transmitted allele (h1), the maternally non-transmitted allele (h2), and the paternally transmitted allele (h3). The paternally non-transmitted allele (h4) can be included in the model if consider parent–offspring trio as a single unit. (Created with BioRender.com.).

An alternative approach to estimate both maternal and fetal effects is the structural equation modeling method proposed by Warrington and colleagues.[23] To facilitate the genome-wide application of adjusted maternal and fetal effect estimates, they introduced a weighted linear model (WLM), which calculates unbiased estimates of maternal and fetal effects from GWA summary results obtained separately from mothers and infants.[24]

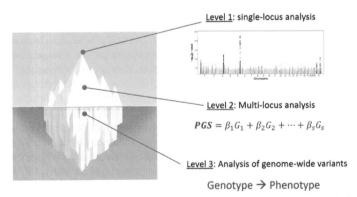

Level 1: single-locus analysis

Level 2: Multi-locus analysis

$$PGS = \beta_1 G_1 + \beta_2 G_2 + \cdots + \beta_s G_s$$

Level 3: Analysis of genome-wide variants

Genotype → Phenotype

Fig. 2. Genetic make-up of a complex phenotype depicted as an iceberg: Single-locus GWA analysis (Level 1) uncovers only the tip of the iceberg. Multilocus analysis (Level 2) captures the cumulative effects of multiple variants that are above the detection threshold. Analysis of genome-wide variants (Level 3) includes both the visible and submerged variants, offering a broader overview of the genetic architecture.

GENOMIC STUDIES OF BIRTH TIMING AT 3 LEVELS
Single-variant Analysis: Genome-wide Scan for Single-variant Associations

GWA studies (GWAS) have been instrumental in identifying specific genetic variants and genes associated with gestational duration and PTB.[13–18] Similar to other complex traits or diseases, these phenotypes are affected by numerous genetic variants, each with a modest effect.[13,25,26] While genetic association studies typically examine thousands to millions of genetic variations, analyses are conducted individually for each tested variant.[25] The significantly associated genetic variants or genes, particularly the causal ones, can provide valuable information about the biology of the studied phenotype.[27]

The first successful GWAS of gestational duration and PTB was published in 2017.[28] This study identified and replicated 6 genomic loci associated with gestational duration in over 50,000 mothers of European ancestry. Three of these loci were also associated with PTB with genome-wide significance. Parallel observations of the same associations in infant samples, albeit with smaller effect sizes, indicated the maternal origin of the identified genetic associations. The associated loci are linked to relevant biological pathways including uterine development, maternal nutrition, and vascular control. Promising results from this initial GWAS encouraged even larger GWAS aiming to identify more genetic associations and to reveal additional biological and mechanistic insights.

Recently, Sole-Navais and colleagues[29] conducted a comprehensive genome-wide meta-analysis on gestational duration (n = 195,555) and spontaneous PTB (sPTB; n = 276,218) across 18 cohorts of European ancestry. This study identified 24 independent genetic variants at 22 loci associated with gestational duration (**Table 1**) and 7 loci associated with sPTB. This research corroborated the 6 loci previously reported by Zhang and colleagues.[28] Using a haplotype-based analytical method, the study differentiated between maternal and fetal genetic effects, revealing that the majority of the identified loci (15 out of 22) exerted their effects through the maternal genome. Furthermore, the study unveiled an intriguing pattern: alleles that increase gestational duration through maternal effects tend to decrease birth weight via fetal effects. This observation suggests that the maternal and fetal genomes might coadapt[30] to achieve an optimal balance between gestational duration and birth weight, enhancing overall fitness between the mother and her baby.

GWA meta-analysis[31] of gestational duration (n = 68,732) and sPTB (n = 98,370) with participants from Finland and summary results from 23andMe identified and replicated 15 loci associated with gestational duration and 4 loci associated with sPTB, many overlapping with those reported by Sole-Navais and colleagues[29] (see **Table 1**). The functional roles of these genes highlight the intricate nature of spontaneous birth as a trait and emphasize the importance of reproductive and immune tissues.

To explore the fetal genetics on the timing of birth, Liu and colleagues[32] conducted a large fetal genome-wide meta-analysis of gestational duration, early preterm (<34 weeks), preterm (<37 weeks), and postterm births in 84,689 infants. This study identified a single nucleotide polymorphism (SNP; rs7594852), located at 2q13 locus within the *CKAP2L* gene, which is implicated in the proinflammatory pathway. A joint maternal–fetal genetic association analysis using the WLM method in mother–child pairs revealed that the association at the leading SNP was driven by fetal genotype.

Another fetal GWAS[33] in a Finnish population included 247 infants with sPTB (<36 weeks) and 419 term controls (38–41 weeks). The SNP, rs116461311, within

Table 1
Gestational duration associated loci reported in 2 recent large-scale genomic studies

Study[a]	Locus[b]	SNP[c]	CHR	POS	Overlap[d]
Solé-Navais et al,[29] 2023 (n = 195,555)	WNT4[e]	rs12037376	1	22462111	X
	HIVEP3	rs625036	1	42270779	—
	FAF1	rs72898946	1	50959262	—
	TET3	rs34555419	2	74235926	X
	LSM3	rs9823520	3	14293832	—
	ADCY5[e]	rs28654158	3	123112292	X
	EEFSEC[e]	rs2659685	3	128122396	X
	MRPS22	rs62270785	3	139004333	—
	ZBTB38	rs7650602	3	141147414	X
	KCNAB1	rs4359773	3	155862524	X
	KDR	rs113828443	4	55895282	—
	HAND2	rs6831441	4	174733296	X
	EBF1[e]	rs2963463	5	157895049	X
	HLA-DQA1	rs3129768	6	32595083	—
	GDAP1	rs6472846	8	75315146	—
	FBXO32	rs143530128	8	124603784	—
	COL27A1	rs7023208	9	116935764	X
	TFAP4	rs2387280	16	4339684	—
	MYOCD	rs17713682	17	12416363	—
	TCEA2	rs6090040	20	62692060	—
	AGTR2[e]	rs5991030	X	115129904	X
	RAP2C[e]	rs5930554	X	131312089	—
Pasanen et al,[31] 2023 (n = 68,732)	WNT3A	rs708119	1	228015567	—
	RHAG	rs10948514	6	49592080	—
	KCNN2	rs13175113	5	114208039	—
	COBL	rs151143987	7	51940143	—
	GNAQ	rs11145617	9	77936015	—

Abbreviations: CHR, chromosome; POS, position.
[a] For the first study, all 22 significant loci are listed. For the second study, only the 5 loci out of the total 15 that do not overlap with those identified in the first study are listed.
[b] Locus is annotated by the gene b symbol of closest protein coding gene.
[c] Index SNP: most significant SNP at a locus.
[d] If the locus was also identified in the second study (Pasanen et al.)[31].
[e] Replicated loci from previous GWAS (Zhang et. al., 2017)[28].

the gene encoding slit guidance ligand 2 (*SLIT2*) showed the strongest association with sPTB. The *SLIT2* gene and its receptor *ROBO1* were upregulated in the placenta of PTB infants which played a vital role in inflammation, decidualization, and fetal growth.[33]

Post-GWAS functional studies using in vitro and in vivo models have elucidated novel molecular mechanisms through which significantly associated genetic loci influence gestational duration and risk of PTB. For example, functional studies demonstrated that a leading variant within the *WNT4* gene disrupts the interaction with the estrogen receptor (ESR1), suggesting a mechanism that can impact various reproductive problems.[28,34] Gene expression analyses revealed that the maternal blood mRNA levels of *EBF1* were reduced in mothers who delivered preterm as early as the second trimester.[35] Bioinformatic and functional investigations indicated that a risk variant proximal to *AGTR2* could potentially modulate the risk of PTB by altering the expression of *AGTR2*, particularly in uterine tissues.[36] Integrative analyses combining transcriptional and gene regulation datasets revealed that the *HAND2* gene may regulate transcriptional programs involved in endometrium decidualization.[37] Additionally, assessments of tissue-specific expression enrichment and refined linkage disequilibrium-score regression of the top GWA genes highlighted the endometrium and other female reproductive and muscular tissues.[29]

Multi-variant Analysis: Examining the Cumulative Effects of Multiple Variants

A complex trait is influenced by many genetic variants with small effects.[38,39] Multi-variant analysis aims to capture the cumulative effects of hundreds to thousands of genetic variations significantly associated with a disease. A multi-variant analysis approach uses polygenic scores (PGS).[40] Such scores are commonly obtained by computing the sum of risk alleles weighted by their estimated effect sizes of many genetic variants associated with a phenotype. These scores can be used to predict the genetic risks of complex diseases.[40,41] The recently developed PGS for gestational duration accounts for 2.2% of the variance in gestational duration.[29] While this percentage remains relatively small for clinical prediction purposes, it surpasses the variance explained by any single known environmental risk factor. Notably, the average gestational duration differs by 5 days between mothers in the lowest and highest deciles according to their PGS. This demonstrates the potential of PGS to predict gestational duration with greater precision than traditional environmental risk factors alone.

Another application of PGS is to use it as a genetic instrument to investigate the causal effect of one phenotype (exposure) on another phenotype (outcome)—an approach called Mendelian randomization (MR).[42] By aggregating the cumulative genetic association of multiple variants with the exposure of interest, PGS can enhance the power of MR analysis.[43] In the framework of integrated maternal–fetal analysis, haplotype PGS can be developed based on h1, h2, and h3. These haplotype PGS can be used to dissect maternal and fetal genetic effects and to investigate the causal associations between maternal traits and pregnancy outcomes.[13] Over the past decade, many studies adopted this methodology to study the causal links between maternal phenotypes and pregnancy outcomes.

An initial study leveraging this method explored the potential causal links between maternal anthropometric traits and key pregnancy outcomes, including gestational duration, birth weight, and birth length.[22] The research utilized haplotype PGS related to maternal height to distinguish between maternal and fetal genetic influences. The findings demonstrated significant associations of birth length and weight with both h1 and h3, indicating a pronounced fetal genetic impact on these growth parameters. In contrast, the duration of gestation was significantly linked to the h2 PGS, suggesting a causal effect of maternal height on gestational duration.

The same group further investigated the causal associations of maternal phenotypes such as height, body mass index (BMI), blood pressure, and blood glucose level with pregnancy outcomes in 10,734 mother–child pairs.[44] The study showed that both maternal height and fetal growth are important factors in shaping the duration of gestation. The authors confirmed that taller maternal height was associated with longer gestational duration. They also demonstrated that fetal growth was influenced by both maternal and fetal genetic effects. For example, elevated maternal BMI and glucose levels were positively associated with birth weight due to maternal effects. Conversely, fetal alleles linked to heightened metabolic risk were found to negatively affect fetal growth.

Another significant finding from this research was the association of rapid fetal growth with shorter gestational duration and increased maternal blood pressure, a phenomenon known as "fetal drive." This pattern was confirmed in multiple subsequent studies.[29,45–47] Overall, these studies underscore the profound impact of both maternal and fetal genetic effects in shaping the relationship between maternal characteristics and birth outcomes, as well as the life-course associations between these birth outcomes and adult phenotypes. The findings support the fetal insulin hypothesis,[48] which emphasizes genetic determinants in linking early growth with the risk of metabolic diseases later in life.[44,49]

Analysis of Genome-wide Variants: Studying the Genetic Architecture

The third level of analysis focuses on exploring the genetic architecture using genome-wide variants. Genetic architecture broadly refers to mapping one's genotype to phenotype, including aspects like the proportion of phenotypic variance attributable to genetics, the distribution of allelic effects, and the genetic correlations with other phenotypes. A key method in this context is estimating heritability from genome-wide SNP data, known as SNP-based heritability.[50] This approach has been instrumental in understanding the genetic basis of complex traits and addressing the issue of "missing heritability."[51] Various methods have been developed to estimate the additive genetic variance of a complex trait using genome-wide SNP data.[52–54] However, these methods cannot be directly applied to the analysis of pregnancy phenotypes. This is because, unlike other complex traits, pregnancy outcomes are influenced by both maternal and fetal genomes. To avoid the confounding by shared alleles between mother and child, Srivastava and colleagues[55] developed a haplotype-based approach (haplotype-based genome-wide complex trait analysis [H-GCTA]) to estimate the genetic variance attributable to h1, h2, and h3. Their findings indicate that gestational duration is primarily genetically determined by the maternal genome, whereas fetal growth measurements such as birth weight, birth length, and head circumference are mainly influenced by the fetal genome.

Eaves and colleagues[56] introduced a contemporary method, maternal genome-wide complex trait analysis (M-GCTA), through the joint analysis of mother–child genotypes. Using this approach, they studied the genetic contribution of the maternal and fetal genomes on birth length. Later, Warrington and colleagues[24] estimated the SNP-heritability of birth weight. The results demonstrated the genetic variance in birth weight is mainly attributable to fetal genetics. Similar results were obtained by Qiao and colleagues.[57] These studies, facilitated by methods such as H-GCTA and M-GCTA, revealed that both maternal and fetal genomes significantly influence pregnancy outcomes, with maternal genetics predominantly determining gestational duration and fetal genetics mainly affecting fetal growth measurements.

Analysis of genome-wide variants can also shed light on the shared genetic architecture between 2 phenotypes. Genetic correlation estimates the proportion of genetic variance shared by 2 phenotypes due to common genetic factors.[58] Recently, Solé-Navais and colleagues[29] showed a strong genetic correlation between sex hormones with gestational duration and PTB. Specifically, testosterone and calculated bioavailable testosterone are negatively correlated with gestational duration, while sex hormone-binding globulin shows a positive correlation. These findings suggest the importance of sex hormone regulations in shaping gestational duration. In addition, the study also detected negative genetic correlations between gestational duration with pre-eclampsia and endometriosis suggesting shared gene pathways in these reproductive disorders. Genetic correlations might stem from either genetic pleiotropy or direct causal relationships. Indeed, Solé-Navais and colleagues[29] provided evidence for the genetic causality of sex hormones on birth timing.

CHALLENGES AND FUTURE DIRECTIONS
Reducing Disparities in Preterm Birth: Increasing Diversity is the Key

Significant disparities exist in PTB across various racial/ethnic, socioeconomic, and geographic populations. In the United States, African-American/Black women experience PTB at a rate that is approximately 1.5 to 1.6 times higher than that of Whites.[59,60] Extensive research indicates that these disparities are primarily driven by social health determinants and systemic racism.[60–62] In addressing these disparities, genomic research in diverse populations becomes critically important.[63] The objective is not about finding genetic differences that account for varying susceptibilities to PTB. Instead, the goal is to discover population-specific risk variants and gene-environmental interactions (G × E), thereby enriching our understanding of the biological mechanisms underlying PTB. Such research can also shed light on the intricate interactions between social and environmental risk factors and genetic predispositions across different populations.[64]

One of the first multi-ancestry GWAS on early sPTB examined nearly 1000 cases of mother–infant pairs and a similar number of control pairs, including over 20% of African Americans.[65] Although several maternal and fetal candidate loci were identified in the discovery phase, none were replicated in a smaller validation cohort. Another multiethnic GWAS[66] investigated 1349 extreme preterm infants (25 and 30 weeks of gestation) against 12,595 ancestry-matched controls, focusing on fetal genomic signals, and identifying 2 inter-genic loci. The authors also attempted replication using several datasets. However, they found no evidence supporting these findings.

A recent maternal GWAS in the Indian population,[67] including 521 PTB mothers and 1042 matched controls, identified 15 SNPs that reached a relaxed significance threshold ($P < 2E-6$). However, none of the genes implicated showed overlap with the top associated genes from much larger European studies. In a separate study, Juvinao-Quintero and colleagues[68] conducted a GWAS on PTB and gestational duration among 2212 Peruvian women, uncovering several suggestive signals ($P < 1E-5$); again, none of them overlapped with any signals previously identified in European populations. Interestingly, this study replicated 2 genetic variants within the *WNT4* gene, significantly associated with gestational duration in European datasets. These findings reinforce the need for larger sample sizes to ensure robust and replicable results across diverse populations.

Given the importance of social and other environmental contributors to PTB risk, Hong and colleagues[69] investigated G × E. The authors conducted genome-wide G × E analyses of PTB in 1733 African-American women from the Boston Birth Cohort and they found a significant interaction between a variant in the *COL24A1* gene with maternal pre-pregnancy overweight/obesity on PTB risk. This interaction was replicated in African-American mothers but not replicated in mothers of European ancestry. This finding highlights the importance of taking non-genetic factors into account when conducting genetic association studies of PTB.

Despite these research efforts across diverse populations, it is important to note that most of the replicated genomic findings related to gestational duration and PTB predominantly come from studies in European cohorts,[28,29,31,32] which often have significantly larger sample sizes. This implies that the benefits of genomic research, including understanding pathogenesis, early screening for adverse outcomes, better diagnosis, improving clinical care, and managing comorbidities during pregnancy may be eluded in those underrepresented and usually high-risk populations. Moreover, differences in genetic ancestry, environment, and lifestyle could further limit the transferability of genetic insights from European studies to underrepresented and high-risk populations.[70–72] This calls for immediate measures to address the genomic imbalance of studies in diverse populations.[64] Furthermore, genomic research in underrepresented populations is essential for mitigating future inequality in genomic medicine of pregnancy outcomes.[70]

In addition, there are significant advantages of increasing diversity in genomic research, including identifying novel associations with population-enriched variants, fine-mapping causal variants, improving genetic risk prediction accuracy for all populations (particularly underrepresented populations), and understanding shared versus unique genetic and environmental risk factors.[70,73] One clear example of population-enriched clinically important variants is APOL1 gene variations and pre-eclampsia, which is identified only in populations with African ancestry.[74,75]

Racism and social injustice have gained increased attention recently as fundamental contributors to health disparities, including adverse pregnancy outcomes such as PTB and low birth weight.[76,77] The impact of chronic stress associated with trans-generational racism on health requires a substantial reorientation of societal voices and leadership well beyond the healthcare system. These efforts are growing in number and impact as evidenced by prioritizing diversity, equity, and inclusion globally. Incorporating social determinants of health in electronic medical record dashboards and research databases will guide care providers in individualizing healthcare and researchers in analyzing the social factors integrated with other covariates. This will especially be powerful as broad areas of biological factors can simultaneously be assessed and intervened.[78,79] Tracking and incorporating these factors into preventive strategies has considerable supportive evidence for impacting population-attributable risk for PTB.[80] Further, some of the genetic regions that are associated with PTB risk might be targets for epigenetic and post-transcriptional regulations that arise from consequences of structural racism, social injustice, and adverse environmental exposures including infection.[81]

To help correct the lack of diversity in genomic research and to mitigate future inequality in genomic medicine, there is an urgent need for structural, organizational, and policy changes that ensure the intentional hiring of diverse researchers by institutes, allow researchers to form genuine partnerships with communities, enhance community engagement and participation in genomic studies among minority groups, encourage the funders to set up strategic funding schemes that promote research of underrepresented populations, and enact policies that create conducive environments for sustainable, diverse genomic studies of high-risk and marginalized populations.[64,82–84]

Large multiethnic GWA studies, such as the Population Architecture through Genomics and Environment study,[85] have illustrated the benefits of including diverse populations in genomic research. Similarly, community-based genomic initiatives, like the All of Us Research Program (https://allofus.nih.gov/), emphasize the urgent need to involve underrepresented groups. Despite these efforts, there is still a critical gap in specifically addressing disparities in pregnancy health. Addressing this gap, several recent studies focusing on underrepresented groups have been launched, with support from organizations like the Bill & Melinda Gates Foundation, the National Institutes of Health, the Burroughs Wellcome Fund, and the March of Dimes. These studies aim to enhance diversity in genomic research related to pregnancy outcomes, promising to yield novel genomic discoveries and benefit those most affected by adverse pregnancy outcomes.

Addressing Heterogeneity in Preterm Birth Etiology: Calling for an Integrative Approach

Despite its simple clinical definition, PTB is a syndrome with many causes.[86] Many pathologic processes can initiate the premature onset of labor. A broad spectrum of biological, psychosocial, behavioral, and environmental factors may influence the risk of PTB, and their effects may vary in individual cases.[87] This heterogeneity makes the prediction and management of PTB extremely challenging.

Large genomic studies can potentially uncover many genetic variants statistically associated with gestation duration or PTB. However, uncovering the biological mechanisms that link these genetic differences to the final phenotypic expression remains difficult. To bridge this gap, it is crucial to also explore relevant cellular and intermediate physiologic phenotypes that may have more direct connections with PTB. In addition, although identified genetic risk variants influence the baseline genetic predisposition to PTB, there may be stronger and immediate internal or environmental risk factors, when acting upon different genetic backgrounds can significantly modify an individual's risk and ultimately trigger premature labor. Answering these questions requires an integrative approach that goes beyond genomics to also including more refined phenotyping and multi-omics studies at different levels.

Many prospective birth cohort studies, such as the Avon Longitudinal Study of Parents and Children,[88] Born in Bradford,[89] the Generation R Study,[90] Alliance for Maternal and Newborn Health Improvement,[91] the Global Alliance to Prevent Prematurity and Stillbirth,[92] and Boston Birth Cohort,[93] have implemented comprehensive longitudinal deep phenotyping and established biobanks for a wide range of maternal and fetal biospecimens. These initiatives, when combined with cutting-edge omics technologies and innovative analytical methodologies, provide new opportunities for better prediction and understanding of PTB and related adverse pregnancy outcomes.[94,95]

SUMMARY

This review underscores the advances in genomic research that have begun to illuminate the intricate genetic factors that underpin gestational timing and the risk of PTB. Through genomic analyses at 3 different levels in mother–child pairs, studies have identified key genetic variants associated with gestational duration and PTB and revealed potential causal relationships and genetic architecture of diverse pregnancy-related phenotypes. Post-GWAS functional studies have further elucidated molecular mechanisms and biological pathways. Moreover, the review also highlighted the critical need for increasing diversity in genomic research to address disparities in PTB across different populations and to ensure that the benefits of genomic medicine extend to all, especially those most at risk. It calls for an integrative approach that combines genomics with refined phenotyping and other omics to fully capture the complexity of PTB. While significant challenges remain, the ongoing efforts to unravel the genetic basis of PTB and to incorporate comprehensive, multiomics, and socially aware research approaches represent vital steps toward better understanding, prediction, and prevention of PTB. These endeavors promise to advance our scientific understanding and pave the way for more personalized and equitable healthcare solutions for PTB.

DISCLOSURE

The authors declare no conflict of interest.

FUNDING

This work is supported by the Eunice Kennedy Shriver National Institute Of Child Health & Human Development of the National Institutes of Health under Award Number R01HD101669, the Bill & Melinda Gates Foundation (Investment ID: INV-037516), the Burroughs Wellcome Fund (Grant 10172896), and the March of Dimes Prematurity Research Center Ohio Collaborative.

Best Practices

What is the current practice for preterm birth?

Current genomic research on preterm birth (PTB) is primarily focused on identifying genetic variants associated with the condition. Through large-scale genomic studies involving both mothers and infants, numerous variants with significant associations have been identified, providing new insights into the biology of PTB. However, a notable limitation is that the majority of these studies have been conducted within European populations.

What changes in current practice are likely to improve outcomes?

Genomic analyses specifically designed for pregnancy outcomes, such as treating the mother–child pair as a single analytical unit, offer new opportunities to distinguish between maternal and fetal genetic influences on PTB. Conducting genomic studies at various levels could enhance our understanding of the causal relationships and shed light on the genetic architecture underlying PTB. In addition, there is an urgent need to expand diversity in genomic research on PTB. Incorporating deep phenotyping and multi-omics analyses is essential to understand the complex etiology of PTB.

REFERENCES

1. Perin J, Mulick A, Yeung D, et al. Global, regional, and national causes of under-5 mortality in 2000–19: an updated systematic analysis with implications for the Sustainable Development Goals. Lancet Child Adolesc Health 2022;6(2):106–15.
2. Ohuma EO, Moller AB, Bradley E, et al. National, regional, and global estimates of preterm birth in 2020, with trends from 2010: a systematic analysis. Lancet 2023;402(10409):1261–71.
3. Pennell CE, Jacobsson B, Williams SM, et al. Genetic epidemiologic studies of preterm birth: guidelines for research. AJOG 2007;196(2):107–18.
4. Blencowe H, Cousens S, Chou D, et al. Born too soon: the global epidemiology of 15 million preterm births. Reprod Health 2013;10(S1):S2.
5. Adams MM, Elam-Evans LD, Wilson HG, et al. Rates of and factors associated with recurrence of preterm delivery. JAMA 2000;283(12):1591.
6. Svensson AC, Sandin S, Cnattingius S, et al. Maternal effects for preterm birth: a genetic epidemiologic study of 630,000 families. Am J Epidemiol 2009;170(11):1365–72.
7. Boyd HA, Poulsen G, Wohlfahrt J, et al. Maternal contributions to preterm delivery. Am J Epidemiol 2009;170(11):1358–64.
8. Plunkett J, Feitosa MF, Trusgnich M, et al. Mother's genome or maternally-inherited genes acting in the fetus influence gestational age in familial preterm birth. Hum Hered 2009;68(3):209–19.
9. York TP, Eaves LJ, Lichtenstein P, et al. Fetal and maternal genes' influence on gestational age in a quantitative genetic analysis of 244,000 Swedish births. Am J Epidemiol 2013;178(4):543–50.
10. Bezold KY, Karjalainen MK, Hallman M, et al. The genomics of preterm birth: from animal models to human studies. Genome Med 2013;5(4):34.
11. York TP, Eaves LJ, Neale MC, et al. The contribution of genetic and environmental factors to the duration of pregnancy. AJOG 2014;210(5):398–405.
12. Sheikh IA, Ahmad E, Jamal MS, et al. Spontaneous preterm birth and single nucleotide gene polymorphisms: a recent update. BMC Genom 2016;17(S9):759.

13. Zhang G, Srivastava A, Bacelis J, et al. Genetic studies of gestational duration and preterm birth. Best Pract Res Clin Obstet Gynaecol 2018;52:33–47.

14. Wadon M, Modi N, Wong HS, et al. Recent advances in the genetics of preterm birth. Ann Hum Genet 2020;84(3):205–13.

15. Bhattacharjee E, Maitra A. Spontaneous preterm birth: the underpinnings in the maternal and fetal genomes. NPJ Genom Med 2021;6(1):43.

16. Jain VG, Monangi N, Zhang G, et al. Genetics, epigenetics, and transcriptomics of preterm birth. Am J Rep Immunol 2022;88(4):e13600.

17. Dauengauer-Kirlienė S, Domarkienė I, Pilypienė I, et al. Causes of preterm birth: genetic factors in preterm birth and preterm infant phenotypes. J Obstet Gynaecol 2023;49(3):781–93.

18. Mead EC, Wang CA, Phung J, et al. The role of genetics in preterm birth. Reprod Sci 2023;30(12):3410–27.

19. Committee Opinion No 700. Methods for Estimating the due date. Obstet Gynecol 2017;129(5):e150–4.

20. Altman DG, Royston P. The cost of dichotomising continuous variables. BMJ 2006;332(7549):1080–1.

21. Juodakis J, Ytterberg K, Flatley C, et al. Time-varying effects are common in genetic control of gestational duration. Hum Mol Genet 2023;32(14):2399–407.

22. Zhang G, Bacelis J, Lengyel C, et al. Assessing the causal relationship of maternal height on birth size and gestational age at birth: a mendelian randomization analysis. PLoS Med 2015;12(8):e1001865.

23. Warrington NM, Freathy RM, Neale MC, et al. Using structural equation modelling to jointly estimate maternal and fetal effects on birth weight in the UK Biobank. Int J Epidemiol 2018;47(4):1229–41.

24. Warrington NM, Beaumont RN, Horikoshi M, et al. Maternal and fetal genetic effects on birth weight and their relevance to cardio-metabolic risk factors. Nat Genet 2019;51(5):804–14.

25. McCarthy MI, Abecasis GR, Cardon LR, et al. Genome-wide association studies for complex traits: consensus, uncertainty and challenges. Nat Rev Genet 2008; 9(5):356–69.

26. Monangi NK, Brockway HM, House M, et al. The genetics of preterm birth: progress and promise. Semin Perinatol 2015;39(8):574–83.

27. Visscher PM, Wray NR, Zhang Q, et al. 10 Years of GWAS discovery: biology, function, and translation. Am J Hum Genet 2017;101(1):5–22.

28. Zhang G, Feenstra B, Bacelis J, et al. Genetic associations with gestational duration and spontaneous preterm birth. N Engl J Med 2017;377(12):1156–67.

29. Solé-Navais P, Flatley C, Steinthorsdottir V, et al. Genetic effects on the timing of parturition and links to fetal birth weight. Nat Genet 2023;55(4):559–67.

30. Wolf JB, Brodie ED. The coadaptation of parental and offspring characters. Evolution 1998;52(2):299–308.

31. Pasanen A, Karjalainen MK, FinnGen, et al. Meta-analysis of genome-wide association studies of gestational duration and spontaneous preterm birth identifies new maternal risk loci. In: Lynch VJ, editor. PLoS Genet 2023;19(10):e1010982.

32. Liu X, Helenius D, Skotte L, et al. Variants in the fetal genome near proinflammatory cytokine genes on 2q13 associate with gestational duration. Nat Commun 2019;10(1):3927.

33. Tiensuu H, Haapalainen AM, Karjalainen MK, et al. Risk of spontaneous preterm birth and fetal growth associates with fetal SLIT2. Barsh GS. PLoS Genet 2019; 15(6):e1008107.

34. Pavlicev M, McDonough-Goldstein CE, Zupan AM, et al. A SNP affects Wnt4 expression in endometrial stroma, with antagonistic implications for pregnancy, endometriosis and reproductive cancers. bioRxiv 2022;2022:513653.

35. Zhou G, Holzman C, Heng YJ, et al. EBF1 gene mRNA levels in maternal blood and spontaneous preterm birth. Reprod Sci 2020;27(1):316–24.

36. Wang L, Rossi RM, Chen X, et al. A functional mechanism for a non-coding variant near AGTR2 associated with risk for preterm birth. BMC Med 2023; 21(1):258.

37. Sakabe NJ, Aneas I, Knoblauch N, et al. Transcriptome and regulatory maps of decidua-derived stromal cells inform gene discovery in preterm birth. Sci Adv 2020;6(49):eabc8696.

38. Gibson G. Rare and common variants: twenty arguments. Nat Rev Genet 2012; 13(2):135–45.

39. Zhang G. Genetic architecture of complex human traits: what have we learned from genome-wide association studies? Curr Genet Med Rep 2015;3(4):143–50.

40. Torkamani A, Wineinger NE, Topol EJ. The personal and clinical utility of polygenic risk scores. Nat Rev Genet 2018;19(9):581–90.

41. Abdellaoui A, Yengo L, Verweij KJH, et al. 15 years of GWAS discovery: realizing the promise. Am J Hum Genet 2023;110(2):179–94.

42. Davey Smith G, Hemani G. Mendelian randomization: genetic anchors for causal inference in epidemiological studies. Hum Mol Genet 2014;23(R1):R89–98.

43. Pingault JB, O'Reilly PF, Schoeler T, et al. Using genetic data to strengthen causal inference in observational research. Nat Rev Genet 2018;19(9):566–80.

44. Chen J, Bacelis J, Solé-Navais P, et al. Dissecting maternal and fetal genetic effects underlying the associations between maternal phenotypes, birth outcomes, and adult phenotypes: a mendelian-randomization and haplotype-based genetic score analysis in 10,734 mother–infant pairs. PLoS Med 2020;17(8):e1003305.

45. Juliusdottir T, Steinthorsdottir V, Stefansdottir L, et al. Distinction between the effects of parental and fetal genomes on fetal growth. Nat Genet 2021;53(8): 1135–42.

46. Beaumont RN, Flatley C, Vaudel M, et al. Genome-wide association study of placental weight identifies distinct and shared genetic influences between placental and fetal growth. Nat Genet 2023;55(11):1807–19.

47. Huang S, Liu S, Huang M, et al. The Born in Guangzhou Cohort Study enables generational genetic discoveries. Nature Published online January 2024;31. https://doi.org/10.1038/s41586-023-06988-4.

48. Hattersley AT, Tooke JE. The fetal insulin hypothesis: an alternative explanation of the association of low birth weight with diabetes and vascular disease. Lancet 1999;353(9166):1789–92.

49. Horikoshi M, Beaumont RN, Day FR, et al. Genome-wide associations for birth weight and correlations with adult disease. Nature 2016;538(7624):248–52.

50. Yang J, Zeng J, Goddard ME, et al. Concepts, estimation and interpretation of SNP-based heritability. Nat Genet 2017;49(9):1304–10.

51. Manolio TA, Collins FS, Cox NJ, et al. Finding the missing heritability of complex diseases. Nature 2009;461(7265):747–53.

52. Yang J, Benyamin B, McEvoy BP, et al. Common SNPs explain a large proportion of the heritability for human height. Nat Genet 2010;42(7):565–9.

53. Yang J, Lee SH, Goddard ME, et al. GCTA: a tool for genome-wide complex trait analysis. Am J Hum Genet 2011;88(1):76–82.

54. Bulik-Sullivan BK, Loh PR, Finucane HK, et al. LD Score regression distinguishes confounding from polygenicity in genome-wide association studies. Nat Genet 2015;47(3):291–5.

55. Srivastava AK, Juodakis J, Solé-Navais P, et al. Haplotype-based analysis distinguishes maternal-fetal genetic contribution to pregnancy-related outcomes. bioRxiv 2020;2020:079863.

56. Eaves LJ, Pourcain BS, Smith GD, et al. Resolving the effects of maternal and offspring genotype on dyadic outcomes in Genome Wide Complex Trait Analysis ("M-GCTA"). Behav Genet 2014;44(5):445–55.

57. Qiao Z, Zheng J, Helgeland Ø, et al. Introducing M-GCTA a software package to estimate maternal (or paternal) genetic effects on offspring phenotypes. Behav Genet 2020;50(1):51–66.

58. Van Rheenen W, Peyrot WJ, Schork AJ, et al. Genetic correlations of polygenic disease traits: from theory to practice. Nat Rev Genet 2019;20(10):567–81.

59. Hamilton BE, Martin JA, Osterman MJ. Births: provisional data for 2021. Vital statistics rapid release; no. 20. Hyattsville, MD: National Center for Health Statistics; 2022.

60. Braveman P, Dominguez TP, Burke W, et al. Explaining the black-white disparity in preterm birth: a consensus statement from a multi-disciplinary scientific work group convened by the March of dimes. Front Reprod Health 2021;3:684207.

61. Braveman P, Heck K, Dominguez TP, et al. African immigrants' favorable preterm birth rates challenge genetic etiology of the Black-White disparity in preterm birth. Front Public Health 2024;11:1321331.

62. Thoma ME, Drew LB, Hirai AH, et al. Black–White disparities in preterm birth: geographic, social, and health determinants. Am J Prevent Med 2019;57(5): 675–86.

63. Sadovsky Y, Mesiano S, Burton GJ, et al. Advancing human health in the decade ahead: pregnancy as a key window for discovery. AJOG 2020;223(3):312–21.

64. Hindorff LA, Bonham VL, Brody LC, et al. Prioritizing diversity in human genomics research. Nat Rev Genet 2018;19(3):175–85.

65. Zhang H, Baldwin DA, Bukowski RK, et al. A genome-wide association study of early spontaneous preterm delivery. Genet Epidemiol 2015;39(3):217–26.

66. Rappoport N, Toung J, Hadley D, et al. A genome-wide association study identifies only two ancestry specific variants associated with spontaneous preterm birth. Sci Rep 2018;8(1):226.

67. Bhattacharjee E, Thiruvengadam R, Ayushi, et al. Genetic variants associated with spontaneous preterm birth in women from India: a prospective cohort study. Lancet Reg Health - Southeast Asia 2023;14:100190.

68. Juvinao-Quintero DL, Sanchez SE, Workalemahu T, et al. Genetic association study of preterm birth and gestational age in a population-based case-control study in Peru. medRxiv 2023;2023:23298891.

69. Hong X, Hao K, Ji H, et al. Genome-wide approach identifies a novel gene-maternal pre-pregnancy BMI interaction on preterm birth. Nat Commun 2017; 8(1):15608.

70. Gurdasani D, Barroso I, Zeggini E, et al. Genomics of disease risk in globally diverse populations. Nat Rev Genet 2019;20(9):520–35.

71. Sirugo G, Williams SM, Tishkoff SA. The missing diversity in human genetic studies. Cell 2019;177(1):26–31.

72. Kamiza AB, Toure SM, Vujkovic M, et al. Transferability of genetic risk scores in African populations. Nat Med 2022;28(6):1163–6.

73. Martin AR, Stroud RE, Abebe T, et al. Increasing diversity in genomics requires investment in equitable partnerships and capacity building. Nat Genet 2022; 54(6):740–5.

74. Reidy KJ, Hjorten RC, Simpson CL, et al. Fetal—not maternal—APOL1 genotype associated with risk for preeclampsia in those with African ancestry. Am J Hum Genet 2018;103(3):367–76.

75. Osafo C, Thomford NE, Coleman J, et al. APOL1 genotype associated risk for preeclampsia in African populations: rationale and protocol design for studies in women of African ancestry in resource limited settings. In: Antonello VS, editor. PLoS One 2022;17(12):e0278115.

76. Slaughter-Acey JC, Sealy-Jefferson S, Helmkamp L, et al. Racism in the form of micro aggressions and the risk of preterm birth among black women. Ann Epidemiol 2016;26(1):7–13.e1.

77. Giurgescu C, Misra DP. Structural racism and maternal morbidity among Black women. West J Nurs Res 2022;44(1):3–4.

78. Cantor MN, Thorpe L. Integrating data on social determinants of health into electronic health records. Health Aff 2018;37(4):585–90.

79. Chen M, Tan X, Padman R. Social determinants of health in electronic health records and their impact on analysis and risk prediction: a systematic review. J Am Med Inform Assoc 2020;27(11):1764–73.

80. Lorch SA, Enlow E. The role of social determinants in explaining racial/ethnic disparities in perinatal outcomes. Pediatr Res 2016;79(1–2):141–7.

81. Collier A, ris Y, Ledyard R, et al. Racial and ethnic representation in epigenomic studies of preterm birth: a systematic review. Epigenomics 2021;13(21):1735–46.

82. Lee SSJ, Appelbaum PS, Chung WK. Challenges and potential solutions to health disparities in genomic medicine. Cell 2022;185(12):2007–10.

83. Khoury MJ, Bowen S, Dotson WD, et al. Health equity in the implementation of genomics and precision medicine: a public health imperative. Genet Med 2022;24(8):1630–9.

84. Fatumo S, Chikowore T, Choudhury A, et al. A roadmap to increase diversity in genomic studies. Nat Med 2022;28(2):243–50.

85. Wojcik GL, Graff M, Nishimura KK, et al. Genetic analyses of diverse populations improves discovery for complex traits. Nature 2019;570(7762):514–8.

86. Romero R, Dey SK, Fisher SJ. Preterm labor: one syndrome, many causes. Science 2014;345(6198):760–5.

87. Institute of Medicine (US). In: Behrman RE, Butler AS, editors. Committee on understanding premature birth and assuring healthy outcomes. Preterm birth: causes, consequences, and prevention. Washington (DC): National Academies Press (US); 2007.

88. Fraser A, Macdonald-Wallis C, Tilling K, et al. Cohort profile: the Avon longitudinal study of parents and children: ALSPAC mothers cohort. Int J Epidemiol 2013; 42(1):97–110.

89. Wright J, Small N, Raynor P, et al. Cohort profile: the Born in Bradford multi-ethnic family cohort study. Int J Epidemiol 2013;42(4):978–91.

90. Kooijman MN, Kruithof CJ, Van Duijn CM, et al. The Generation R Study: design and cohort update 2017. Eur J Epidemiol 2016;31(12):1243–64.

91. Aftab F, Ahmed S, Ali SM, et al. Cohort profile: the alliance for maternal and Newborn health improvement (AMANHI) biobanking study. Int J Epidemiol 2022;50(6):1780–1.

92. Gravett MG, Rubens CE, Global Alliance to Prevent Prematurity and Stillbirth Technical Team. A framework for strategic investments in research to reduce the global burden of preterm birth. AJOG 2012;207(5):368–73.
93. Pearson C, Bartell T, Wang G, et al. Boston Birth Cohort profile: rationale and study design. Precis Nutr 2022;1(2):e00011.
94. Espinosa CA, Khan W, Khanam R, et al. Multiomic signals associated with maternal epidemiological factors contributing to preterm birth in low- and middle-income countries. Sci Adv 2023;9(21):eade7692.
95. Moufarrej MN, Vorperian SK, Wong RJ, et al. Early prediction of preeclampsia in pregnancy with cell-free RNA. Nature 2022;602(7898):689–94.

Social Determinants of Premature Birth

Nana Matoba, MD, MPH[a],*, Christina Kim, MD[b],
Tonia Branche, MD, MPH[b], James W. Collins Jr, MD, MPH[b]

KEYWORDS

- Racial disparity • Structural racism • Hypothalamic-pituitary-adrenal axis
- Low birthweight • Nerve growth factor • Maternal and Child Health

KEY POINTS

- Social determinants of health have received increasing attention in public health, leading to increased understanding of how social factors individual and contextual—shape the health of the mother and infant.
- Racial differences in birth outcomes persist, with incomplete explanation for the widening disparity.

INTRODUCTION

Preterm birth rates in the United States continue to rise and reached 10.5% in 2021, the highest level reported since 2007.[1] The preterm birth rate contributes to the high infant mortality rate (IMR) seen in this country, which ranks far below other developed nations with 5.42 infant deaths per 1000 livebirths in 2020.[2] Striking within the preterm birth and IMRs is the racial disparity. Compared with White women, Black women have higher rates of preterm birth (14.8% vs 9.5%) and higher infant mortality (10.9 vs 4.3 per 1000 livebirths) rates. To understand these disparities, research has identified several explanations, including a range of socioeconomic factors that vary across races/ethnicities. These studies have primarily focused on individual-level factors, such as health-related behaviors. However, racial/ethnic differences in birth outcomes persist even after accounting for individual-level factors and fail to explain the persistent and widening Black–White disparity.[3,4]

Research today has shifted focus to contextual factors in both longitudinal and transgenerational perspectives. Here, we highlighted the social determinants of

[a] Division of Neonatology, Rady Children's Hospital San Diego, Department of Pediatrics, University of California San Diego, 3020 Children's Way, MC 5008, San Diego, CA 92123, USA;
[b] Division of Neonatology, Ann & Robert H. Lurie Children's Hospital of Chicago, Department of Pediatrics, Northwestern University, 225 East Chicago Avenue, Box #45, Chicago, IL 60611, USA
* Corresponding author.
E-mail address: nmatoba@rchsd.org

Clin Perinatol 51 (2024) 331–343
https://doi.org/10.1016/j.clp.2024.02.002   perinatology.theclinics.com

preterm birth, with special attention to the social experiences among Black women in this country that are likely attributed to structural racism and discrimination throughout life.

MATERNAL NATIVITY

Birthweight (BW) is a commonly used proxy for gestational maturity. Using 15 years of Illinois vital records, we found that the overall BW distributions for infants of US-born White women and African-born women were almost identical, with US-born Black women's infants comprising a distinctly different population, weighing hundreds of grams less.[5] US-born Black women also experienced higher rates of very low birthweight (VLBW, <1500 g) than either White or African-born women and independent of traditional individual-level confounders.[5] Using the same transgenerational dataset, we found that recent European immigrants to the United States gave birth to girls of similar BW to girls born to established European American (White) families. These girls grew up to have daughters whose average BW was higher than their own.[6] In stark contrast, Black African and Caribbean immigrants gave birth to girls who were heavier than girls born into established Black American families. Most striking is that these first-generation US-born Black women had daughters whose BWs were lower on average than their own weights at birth. These findings provide strong evidence that the Black African women's experience of living in this country quickly confers reproductive disadvantage in a process partly explained by the concepts of weathering and allostatic load.

WEATHERING, ALLOSTATIC LOAD, AND LIFE-COURSE MODEL

Weathering is a hypothesis proposed by Geronimus[7] to account for early health deterioration among Black people in this country. It posits that they experience early health deterioration as a consequence of the cumulative impact of repeated experiences with social or economic adversity and political marginalization. On a physiologic level, health is affected by persistent coping with stressors[8] inherent in living in a society that disadvantages Blacks and lead to the accumulation of disproportionate physiologic deterioration at early ages. This accelerated aging hypothesis, or weathering, is seen in the deterioration in reproductive health over the childbearing years among Black women.[7]

Building on this idea, McEwen and colleagues[9] developed the concept of allostatic load, or the cumulative wear-and-tear on the body's systems owing to repeated adaptations to stressors. Although the biological mechanisms remain unclear, it has been proposed that chronic exposure to stress results in elevated and exaggerated hypothalamic-pituitary-adrenal axis (HPA) activity and worn-out axis due to the loss of feedback inhibition and downregulation of glucocorticoid receptors.[10]

These concepts have been synthesized into the life-course perspective proposed by Lu and colleagues[11] to provide a longitudinal and integrative approach for research, practice, and policy toward reducing disparities in birth outcomes. In this model, disparities in birth outcomes are viewed as consequences of different trajectories set forth by early life experiences, as well as the cumulative allostatic load over life.

EDUCATION

Low levels of maternal education have been associated with adverse birth outcomes but with different impact between races. In a statewide study of California births, maternal education was shown to have different effects on preterm birth rates on different races/ethnicities.[12] In general, favorable socioeconomic characteristics were associated with lower preterm birth rates among White but not Black women. Notably, within the most socioeconomically disadvantaged subgroups, there was no significant Black–White disparity in preterm birth rates. Among high school graduates, Black women were still at higher risk for preterm birth compared with White high school graduates (odds ratio [OR] 1.63; 95% confidence interval [CI] 1.29, 2.05). In contrast, among the most disadvantaged Black and White women who were poor, had not completed high school, whose infants' fathers were unemployed, and/or who lived in high-poverty census tracts, there was no significant racial disparity in preterm birth rates before or after adjustment for relevant confounders.

The risk for preterm birth among the least-educated and most-educated women has diverged over time.[13] In a population study of women giving birth between 1989 and 2006 in Michigan, preterm birth risk among women with less than 12 years of education increased marginally over time, compared with more educated women, whose preterm birth risk increased substantially in the same period. While the proportion of women completing a college degree or greater increased from 19.5% in 1989 to 34.0% in 2006, preterm birth risk was higher among the most-educated women in 2006 (7.2%) than the most-educated women in 1989 (4.6%). In the same period, preterm birth rate did not change appreciably among the least-educated women (10.5%–10.0%).

ADULTHOOD RESIDENTIAL ENVIRONMENT

Hypothesized mechanisms through which neighborhood environments may influence birth outcomes include social factors, availability of resources, and physical attributes.[14] Studies have shown that these measures of economic deprivation are associated with low birthweight (LBW) and preterm birth.[3,15]

Neighborhood poverty is a risk factor for preterm birth in both White and Black races,[16,17] but the impact appears to differ between the races. Geocoding census tract-level average household income, residence in a wealthier tract (>US$30,000/y median income) was associated with a reduced risk of preterm birth for Black (OR 0.59; 95% CI 0.36, 0.96) but not among White women in North Carolina in 1995 to 2000.[18] Similarly, Pickett and colleagues[19] have shown that for Black women, living in a neighborhood with either a high or low median household income was associated with an increased risk of preterm delivery; this association was not seen among White women.

The effect of neighborhood socioeconomics appears to cross generations. In the Dutch Famine cohort, maternal grandmother's exposure to social deprivation and extreme caloric restrictions were negatively associated with infant BW, independent of maternal factors.[20] The concept of transgenerational effect of neighborhood poverty is particularly important for Blacks, a group exposed to urban impoverishment over generations. In the Illinois transgenerational dataset, as maternal grandmothers' residential neighborhood income deteriorated during pregnancy, rates of LBW rose.[21] The OR for infant LBW for maternal grandmother's residence in poverty, compared with an affluent neighborhood, was 1.3 (95% CI 1.1, 1.4), adjusted for the mother's residential environment.

Beyond cross-sectional studies, histories of neighborhood poverty have been examined, in order to examine the changing dynamics of economic, social, and political forces that shape neighborhood environments.[22] In Californian neighborhoods across 2003 to 2009, using the Neighborhood Change Database (1970–2000), longitudinal trajectories of poverty were examined with preterm birth rates and showed that areas with long-term high poverty had increased odds of preterm birth compared with long-term low poverty.

POLICE KILLINGS AND POLICE PRESENCE

Disproportionate police killing of Blacks has regained national attention since the demises of George Floyd, Breonna Taylor, and more. In the United States, Blacks are 3 times more likely to be killed by police than Whites and 1.3 times more likely to be unarmed.[23] Using the Mapping Police Violence database from 2013 to 2018, states with more police killings of unarmed Black men had higher Black–White preterm disparities compared with states having fewer killings.[24]

High police presence are aggressive attempts by law enforcement to maintain order and have led to disproportionate high police presence in majority low-income and Black neighborhoods.[25] In a study in Minneapolis in 2016,[26] the odds of preterm birth for pregnant women living in a neighborhood with high police presence were significantly higher compared with the odds of their racial counterparts in a low-presence neighborhood for White (OR 1.9; 95% CI 1.9, 2.0), for US-born Black (OR 2.0; 95% CI 1.8, 2.2), and foreign-born Black individuals (OR 1.1; 95% CI 1.0, 1.2). Geospatial analyses revealed that the higher the proportion of Black residents in the neighborhood, the greater were the number of police incident reports.

PARENTAL INCARCERATION

The US incarcerates more of its population than any other country in the world,[27] but neighborhood rates of incarceration rates are highly variable. Emerging literature shows that communities with the highest rates of parental incarceration tend to be the most racially and socioeconomically disadvantaged.[28] Black and Latinx children are 7.5 and 2.5 times, respectively, more likely to have an incarcerated parent than White children.[28]

Few studies have examined the relationship between LBW, preterm birth, and parental incarceration. The results are mixed, with some reporting higher rates of preterm birth and LBW and others reporting no differences. Walker and colleagues[29] reported that infants born to women incarcerated during pregnancy had an increased likelihood of LBW and preterm compared with controls. Similarly, Dowell and colleagues[30] have found that maternal imprisonment before or during pregnancy was associated with LBW after adjustment for pregnancy risks. In Western Australia, they have also reported an association with infant mortality,[30] where infants whose mothers were incarcerated up to 5 years before birth or within their first year were over 2.2 times as likely to die within the first year compared with infants with mothers with no corrections record.

REDLINING

Redlining is an example of structural racism and is defined as the systemic implementation of racially based mortgage discrimination initiated by lending institutions in the 1930s, when neighborhoods were classified by their perceived level of lending risk and areas deemed "hazardous" were marked with a red line on a map, where banks would not invest.[31,32] Although redlining is no longer legal, the consequence of residential segregation continues to define a broad range of unequal resources including education, employment, housing, and health care.[33]

A growing body of literature has associated historical redlining with contemporary preterm birth, confirming its harmful consequences nearly a century later. Krieger and colleagues[34] have conceptualized the lasting inequities of historical redlining on the built environment, wealth acquisition, and segregation leading to inequities of pre-term birth risk. The association between historical redlining with differential access to critical determinants of health has also been described by Mehdipanah and colleagues.[35] We have previously reported that redlining was a modest risk factor for pre-term birth in Chicago, with higher rates among Black women living in redlined areas (18.5%) compared with Black women living in nonredlined areas (17.1%), with an adjusted OR of 1.08 (95% CI 1.03, 1.14).[36]

EARLY-LIFE RESIDENTIAL ENVIRONMENT

Using the Illinois transgenerational dataset, it was shown that Black mothers' upward economic mobility from early life impoverishment was associated with a decreased risk of preterm birth and infant mortality compared with those with lifelong residence in impoverished neighborhoods. These Black mothers had a preterm birth rate of 18.7%; those who with upward economic mobility had lower preterm birth rates. Formerly impoverished Black women who experienced even small or modest upward economic mobility by adulthood had lower rates of preterm birth than those with lifelong residence in impoverished neighborhoods. Women with upward mobility from early impoverished to affluent neighborhoods had the lowest preterm birth risk. It can be speculated that even relatively small improvement in the economic environment of Black women across the life course may translate into beneficial birth outcomes.

In contrast, downward economic mobility among White urban upper class-born women was associated with an increased risk of preterm birth. Among Chicago-born upper class (defined by early-life residence in affluent neighborhoods), those who did not experience downward economic mobility by the time of delivery had a preterm birth rate of 5.4%. Women who experienced slight, moderate, or extreme downward economic mobility had preterm birth rates of 6.5% (relative risk [RR] 1.2; 95% CI 1.0, 4.0), 8.5% (RR 1.6; 95% CI 1.3, 1.9), and 10.1% (RR 1.9; 95% CI 1.3, 2.6), respectively. Maternal downward economic mobility was associated with increased prevalence of biologic, medical, and behavioral risk factors.

Among former LBW women, downward economic mobility was strongly associated with increased risk of preterm birth, with an OR of 2.4 (95% CI 1.1, 5.3) among former LBW, and an OR of 1.1 (95% CI 1.0, 1.1) among nonformer-LBW women, compared with those with lifelong upper-class status. Notably, preterm birth rates did not decrease among former LBW impoverished-born Black women who experienced up-ward economic mobility in their life course. This pattern of transgenerational LBW transmission suggests intrauterine programming of reproductive health, a process called fetal programming.

LBW has been used as proxy of aberrant fetal programming. Stress from impover-ishment among former LBW mothers is suspected to result in stress hormones pass-ing into the fetal circulation during critical periods of neuroendocrine and HPA axis development, resulting in fetal growth restriction as measured by LBW. This could then lead to a female infant with a higher stress reactivity later in life that places her at greater risk for preterm labor in her pregnancy.[37]

Fetal programming acts at the level of the DNA in a phenomenon of epigenetics. Emerging epigenetic literature shows that prenatal maternal stress could lead to changes in DNA methylation. Maternal depressive symptoms in the third trimester have been associated with increased methylation of the nerve growth factor (NGF) binding site in the NR3C1 gene, which codes for the glucocorticoid receptor, playing a key role in the HPA axis functioning.[38] Methylation levels of NR3C1 were also found to be higher in 10 to 19 year old children whose mothers experienced partner violence before, during, and after pregnancy.[39]

RACISM

Maternal exposure to racism—interpersonal, structural, and institutional—is recognized as an influence on birth outcomes. An increasing body of literature has shown that Black women's exposure to interpersonal racism is a risk factor for poor health outcomes.[40,41] Interpersonal racism refers to the racial prejudice that leads to differential assumptions about abilities, motives, and intentions of others according to race.[42] In a study in Chicago, Black mothers who delivered VLBW preterm infants were twice as likely to report experiencing interpersonal racial discrimination during their lifetime than Black mothers who delivered normal BW infants at term.[43] The questions pertained to experiences consisted of racial discrimination at work, getting a job, at school, getting medical care, and getting service at a restaurant or store,[44] during pregnancy, or in their lifetime. The magnitude of the association between exposure to racial discrimination and VLBW infant was strongest in the "finding a job" and "at place of employment" categories.

In contrast, structural racism is a systemic and unequal distribution of resources based on race, which results in disparities in wealth, income, education, criminal justice, employment, housing, and access to health care. Through historical and persistent discriminatory policies and practices, structural racism has resulted in the concentration of poverty and segregated neighborhoods. By determining access to educational and employment opportunities, segregation has been a key mechanism by which racial inequality has been created and reinforced.[45] These areas lack health-promoting resources, socioeconomic opportunities, access to quality and timely health care, health literacy, disposable income, and social capital[34] and are associated with adverse maternal pregnancy morbidities.[46]

Implicit and explicit bias in medical care settings is another pathway through which structural racism influences birth outcomes. Black women are often given less attention and dismissed when expressing concerns about their well-being, with examples of Black women whose health has been compromised because of medical provider bias, regardless of their socioeconomic status.[47,48]

FATHERS

Paternal involvement has long been recognized as contributing to child development and health, but it also appears to impact birth outcomes. Historically, marital status was used as a surrogate indicator of paternal involvement, but marital status is not an accurate indicator of paternal involvement, as a spectrum of involvement exists between married and unmarried status.

Today, a major proxy of paternal involvement is paternal acknowledgment on the birth certificate with the naming of a father's first and/or last name. Using this definition, Ngui and colleagues[49] have reported that paternal noninvolvement was a risk factor for LBW across all racial/ethnic groups in Milwaukee. Using national vital records, DeSisto and colleagues[50] found that a father's noninvolvement contributed to a significant proportion of the excess preterm birth rate among US-born Black (vs foreign-born Black or US-born White women).

Paternal acknowledgment is also associated with neonatal and infant mortality and with racial/ethnic disparity. Using birth records in Florida, Alio and colleagues[51] showed that neonatal mortality rate of infants born to women with absent fathers was nearly 4 times that of their counterparts with involved fathers. The disparity existed between racial/ethnic groups as well as within each racial/ethnic group. Compared with White women with involved fathers, Black women with involved fathers had a 2 fold increased risk of infant mortality, whereas infants born to Black women with absent fathers had 7 times higher risk of infant mortality.

Paternal acknowledgment likely affects pregnancy outcomes by promoting healthy maternal behaviors, improving access to early prenatal care, reducing smoking, and providing emotional and financial support[52] that mitigates the effects of stress on risks of adverse birth outcomes. Such support has been associated with lower occurrence of maternal depression and increased preparedness around birth and birth complications.[52,53]

Despite emerging research, barriers remain regarding research on the fathers' role in birth outcomes leading to public health improvements. One challenge is the lack of paternal data available for research. To date, birth certificates remain the primary source of data for measuring a fathers' presence or absence, but the data are frequently incomplete and vary by state. Alio and colleagues[54] have outlined recommendations and policy priorities to address paternal involvement during pregnancy, including equitable paternity leave, elimination of marriage as a tax and public assistance penalty, integration of fatherhood initiatives in Maternal and Child Health programs, support of low-income fathers through employment training, father inclusion in family planning services, and expansion of birth data collection.

JOB STRAIN

In the United States, employed pregnant women today are working later into their pregnancies, in contrast to trends in Europe toward more liberal maternity leave. As such, conditions and stress at the workplace are studied for their possible contribution to birth outcomes, but with inconsistent results. Several observational studies have found an association between working conditions and preterm birth and LBW,[55] while other studies seem to contradict this association.[56]

In general, participation in the workforce itself does not appear to be detrimental to pregnancy and is actually associated with reduced preterm birth rates, since women in the workforce generally have more favorable sociodemographic profiles as well as social support and medical insurance.[57] Rather, certain working conditions could represent potential risk factors to adverse birth outcomes through psychosocial stress. These include long working hours, high physical workloads, prolonged standing, and psychosocial job strain.

Job strain is defined as response to jobs that have both high demands (fast pace and high levels of expectations) and low control (the command the worker has over the use of his/her abilities and the way in which work is accomplished). This job strain has been associated with preterm birth and LBW,[58,59] although not all studies support this association.[60]

An association was shown in a study of 1988 to 1991 births in North Carolina through telephone interviews 6 months after delivery.[57] Questions were asked about job demand, workload, responsibility, job decision latitude, creativity, control over pace, and content. Women employed at high-strain jobs during most of their pregnancies had a higher risk (OR 1.4; 95% CI 0.9, 2.2) of delivering a preterm infant than those working only at low-strain jobs. Women who worked at high-strain jobs for less than 30 weeks did not have an elevated risk (OR 1.1; 95% CI 0.7, 1.8), nor did those with high-strain work in third trimester. The associations were somewhat more consistently associated with preterm delivery among Black women, with the population attributable risk of job strain on preterm delivery at 9%.[57]

In contrast, a large study of Danish women did not show statistically significant association between job strain and birth outcomes.[60] Among women who worked at least 30 hours per week in the first trimester, birth outcomes were compared between those with relaxed (low demand, high control), active (high demand, high control), passive (low demands and low control), and high-strain (high demands, low control) jobs, but none of the findings were statistically significant.

The applicability of these associations to public health policy has been controversial because the magnitude of most of the associations is relatively modest, and the evidence is interpreted differently by various policy makers.[61] Although the magnitude of the associations remains small across most studies, working conditions are modifiable risk factors for adverse birth outcomes. At present, the National Institute for Occupational Safety and Health recommends a more restrictive policy on lifting during pregnancy than guidelines previously advocated by the American Medical Association.[62]

TERM INFANT MORTALITY

Many of the social determinants for preterm birth are also factors of term infant mortality. IMR for term infants is driven by the postneonatal period (29–365 days) when the impact of social and environmental factors is presumed to be the highest.[63] As in preterm births/deaths, race and racism are significant influencers of the term IMR. While the overall IMR in the United States has decreased in recent decades, the decline is narrower for Black infants whose IMR remains 2 to 3 times higher than IMR for White infants,[64,65] and the disparity is widened in the postneonatal period.[65]

A maternal nativity disparity exists in that the term IMR for infants born to US-born White, Black, and Mexican American mothers is higher than that of infants of foreign-born mothers independent of individual risk factors.[66] Across all races, other than congenital malformations, most term infant deaths in the postneonatal period are due to sudden unexpected infant death, specifically sudden infant death syndrome (SIDS).[67] Black term infants die from SIDS at a higher rate than White and Latinx infants.[67] The risk of SIDS is influenced by infant sleeping environment, which is affected by household resources and availability of family support.[68,69]

In addition, the risk of term IMR is higher with increasing poverty and in areas further from metropolitan areas.[70] Systemic policies that have disproportionately negatively affected the Black population contribute to the increased risk of mortality for Black term infants.[71] Even without prematurity as a risk factor, social determinants strongly influence the risk of death among Black infants.

CHALLENGES IN ELIMINATING DISPARITIES OF SOCIAL DETERMINANTS

Social determinants of health have received increasing attention in public health, leading to increased understanding of how social factors—individual and contextual—shape health of the mother and infant. An increasing focus has contributed to examining the determinants of racial and other disparities in birth outcomes.

Current gaps[72] in this research include pathways, biological mechanisms, and interventions to address social factors to improve birth outcomes and reduce disparities. Challenges include learning the complexity in the relationship between upstream social factors and birth outcomes that take over long periods and over generations. We also face limited ability to measure structural racism and social factors besides crude measures of income, wealth, and education from existing public data that do not fully capture a woman's lifelong context such as childhood experiences and lifelong racial discrimination.

Finally, the role of racism in birth outcomes is increasingly recognized, and there is consensus today among researchers that "race" is a social construct. However, there should be caution, as Braveman and colleagues[73] advise, in using the term "race" itself, as it reinforces notions of inherent biological differences based on physical appearance, or skin color. As emphasized in their report, we need to continue research among categories of people who differ in how they are perceived and treated, but using the term "race" itself is an obstacle to dismantling racism.

DISCLOSURE

The authors have no commercial or financial conflicts of interest, or funding sources for this article.

Best Practices

What is the current practice for studying social determinants of preterm birth?

Social determinants of health and health effects of structural racism are receiving increasing attention in public health.

What changes in current practice are likely to improve outcomes?

Improving the ability to measure factors that capture a woman's lifelong context such as childhood experiences and lifelong racial discrimination.

Pearls/Pitfalls at the point-of-care:

We need to accept that race is not a biological category, but a socially constructed concept. We need to continue research among categories of people who differ in how they are perceived and treated; however, using the term "race" itself may be an obstacle to dismantling racism.

Major Recommendations:

Bridging the gap in research by examining ecological pathways, biological mechanisms, and interventions to address social determinants of preterm birth and reduce disparities therein.

Bibliographic Source(s):

Braveman P, Egerter S, Williams DR. The social determinants of health: coming of age. Annu Rev Public Health 2011;32:381-98.

Braveman P, Parker Dominguez T. Abandon "race." Focus on racism. Front Public Health 2021;9:689,462.

REFERENCES

1. Osterman MJK, Hamilton BE, Martin JA, et al. Births: final data for 2021. Natl Vital Stat Rep 2023;72(1):1–53.
2. Kochanek KD, Murphy SL, Xu J, et al. Deaths: final data for 2020. Natl Vital Stat Rep 2023;72(10):1–92.
3. Collins JW Jr, David RJ. The differential effect of traditional risk factors on infant birthweight among blacks and whites in Chicago. Am J Public Health 1990;80(6): 679–81.
4. Sheehan TJ, Gregorio DI. Low birth weight in relation to the interval between pregnancies. N Engl J Med 1995;333(6):386–7.
5. Collins JW Jr, Wu SY, David RJ. Differing intergenerational birth weights among the descendants of US-born and foreign-born Whites and African Americans in Illinois. Am J Epidemiol 2002;155(3):210–6.

6. David RJ, Collins JW Jr. Differing birth weight among infants of U.S.-born blacks, African-born blacks, and U.S.-born whites. N Engl J Med 1997;337(17):1209–14.

7. Geronimus AT. Black/white differences in the relationship of maternal age to birth-weight: a population-based test of the weathering hypothesis. Soc Sci Med 1996; 42(4):589–97.

8. McEwen BS. Protective and damaging effects of stress mediators. N Engl J Med 1998;338(3):171–9.

9. McEwen BS, Seeman T. Protective and damaging effects of mediators of stress. Elaborating and testing the concepts of allostasis and allostatic load. Ann N Y Acad Sci 1999;896:30–47.

10. Sapolsky RM. Social subordinance as a marker of hypercortisolism. Some unexpected subtleties. Ann N Y Acad Sci 1995;771:626–39.

11. Lu MC, Halfon N. Racial and ethnic disparities in birth outcomes: a life-course perspective. Matern Child Health J 2003;7(1):13–30.

12. Braveman PA, Heck K, Egerter S, et al. The role of socioeconomic factors in Black-White disparities in preterm birth. Am J Public Health 2015;105(4): 694–702.

13. El-Sayed AM, Galea S. Temporal changes in socioeconomic influences on health: maternal education and preterm birth. Am J Public Health 2012;102(9):1715–21.

14. Culhane JF, Elo IT. Neighborhood context and reproductive health. Am J Obstet Gynecol 2005;192(5 Suppl):S22–9.

15. Gould JB, LeRoy S. Socioeconomic status and low birth weight: a racial comparison. Pediatrics 1988;82(6):896–904.

16. O'Campo P, Burke JG, Culhane J, et al. Neighborhood deprivation and preterm birth among non-Hispanic Black and White women in eight geographic areas in the United States. Am J Epidemiol 2008;167(2):155–63.

17. Collins JW Jr, Simon DM, Jackson TA, et al. Advancing maternal age and infant birth weight among urban African Americans: the effect of neighborhood poverty. Ethn Dis 2006;16(1):180–6.

18. Kaufman JS, Dole N, Savitz DA, et al. Modeling community-level effects on preterm birth. Ann Epidemiol 2003;13(5):377–84.

19. Pickett KE, Ahern JE, Selvin S, et al. Neighborhood socioeconomic status, maternal race and preterm delivery: a case-control study. Ann Epidemiol 2002; 12(6):410–8.

20. Lumey LH, Stein AD. Offspring birth weights after maternal intrauterine undernutrition: a comparison within sibships. Am J Epidemiol 1997;146(10):810–9.

21. Collins JW Jr, David RJ, Rankin KM, et al. Transgenerational effect of neighborhood poverty on low birth weight among African Americans in Cook County, Illinois. Am J Epidemiol 2009;169(6):712–7.

22. Margerison-Zilko C, Cubbin C, Jun J, et al. Beyond the cross-sectional: neighborhood poverty histories and preterm birth. Am J Public Health 2015;105(6):1174–80.

23. Sinyangwe SMD, Packnett B. Mapping police violence. 2020. Available at: https://mappingpoliceviolence.org.

24. Yang N, Collins JW Jr, Burris HH. States with more killings of unarmed Black people have larger Black-White preterm birth disparities. J Perinatol 2021;41(2):358–9.

25. Tyler TRJJ, Mentovich A. The consequences of being an object of suspicion: potential pitfalls of proactive police contact. J Empir Leg Stud 2015;12(4):602–36.

26. Hardeman RR, Chantarat T, Smith ML, et al. Association of Residence in high-police contact neighborhoods with preterm birth among Black and White individuals in Minneapolis. JAMA Netw Open 2021;4(12):e2130290.

27. Wildeman C, Wang EA. Mass incarceration, public health, and widening inequality in the USA. Lancet 2017;389(10077):1464–74.
28. Glaze LE ML. Parents in prison and their minor children. Washington, DC: Bureau of Justice Ststistics Special Report); 2008.
29. Walker JR, Hilder L, Levy MH, et al. Pregnancy, prison and perinatal outcomes in New South Wales, Australia: a retrospective cohort study using linked health data. BMC Pregnancy Childbirth 2014;14:214.
30. Dowell CM, Mejia GC, Preen DB, et al. Low birth weight and maternal incarceration in pregnancy: a longitudinal linked data study of Western Australian infants. SSM Popul Health 2019;7:008.
31. Greer JL. Historic home mortgage redlining in Chicago. JIll State Hist Soc 2014; 107(2):204–33.
32. Rothstein R. The Color of Law: a forgotten history of how our government segregated America. New York, NY: Liveright; 2017.
33. Williams DR, Collins C. Racial residential segregation: a fundamental cause of racial disparities in health. Public Health Rep 2001;116(5):404–16.
34. Krieger N, Van Wye G, Huynh M, et al. Structural racism, historical redlining, and risk of preterm birth in New York city, 2013-2017. Am J Public Health 2020;110(7): 1046–53.
35. Mehdipanah R, McVay KR, Schulz AJ. Historic redlining practices and contemporary determinants of health in the Detroit Metropolitan area. Am J Public Health 2023;113(S1):S49–57.
36. Matoba N, Suprenant S, Rankin K, et al. Mortgage discrimination and preterm birth among African American women: an exploratory study. Health Place 2019;59:102193.
37. Merlot E, Couret D, Otten W. Prenatal stress, fetal imprinting and immunity. Brain Behav Immun 2008;22(1):42–51.
38. Oberlander TF, Weinberg J, Papsdorf M, et al. Prenatal exposure to maternal depression, neonatal methylation of human glucocorticoid receptor gene (NR3C1) and infant cortisol stress responses. Epigenetics 2008;3(2):97–106.
39. Radtke KM, Ruf M, Gunter HM, et al. Transgenerational impact of intimate partner violence on methylation in the promoter of the glucocorticoid receptor. Transl Psychiatry 2011;1(7):e21.
40. Collins JW Jr, David RJ, Handler A, et al. Very low birthweight in African American infants: the role of maternal exposure to interpersonal racial discrimination. Am J Public Health 2004;94(12):2132–8.
41. Mustillo S, Krieger N, Gunderson EP, et al. Self-reported experiences of racial discrimination and Black-White differences in preterm and low-birthweight deliveries: the CARDIA Study. Am J Public Health 2004;94(12):2125–31.
42. Jones CP. Levels of racism: a theoretic framework and a gardener's tale. Am J Public Health 2000;90(8):1212–5.
43. Collins JW Jr, David RJ, Symons R, et al. Low-income African-American mothers' perception of exposure to racial discrimination and infant birth weight. Epidemiology 2000;11(3):337–9.
44. McNeilly MD, Anderson NB, Armstead CA, et al. The perceived racism scale: a multidimensional assessment of the experience of white racism among African Americans. Ethn Dis 1996;6(1–2):154–66.
45. Massey DSNAD. American Apartheid: segregation and the making of the Underclass. Cambridge: Harvard University Press; 1993.

46. Gazmararian JA, Adams MM, Pamuk ER. Associations between measures of socioeconomic status and maternal health behavior. Am J Prev Med 1996;12(2): 108–15.

47. Sacks TK. Invisible Visits: Black Middle-class women in the American healthcare system. Oxford University Press; 2019.

48. Saluja B, Bryant Z. How implicit bias contributes to racial disparities in maternal morbidity and mortality in the United States. J Womens Health (Larchmt) 2021; 30(2):270–3.

49. Ngui E, Cortright A, Blair K. An investigation of paternity status and other factors associated with racial and ethnic disparities in birth outcomes in Milwaukee, Wisconsin. Matern Child Health J 2009;13(4):467–78.

50. DeSisto CL, Hirai AH, Collins JW Jr, et al. Deconstructing a disparity: explaining excess preterm birth among U.S.-born black women. Ann Epidemiol 2018;28(4): 225–30.

51. Alio AP, Mbah AK, Kornosky JL, et al. Assessing the impact of paternal involvement on racial/ethnic disparities in infant mortality rates. J Community Health 2011;36(1):63–8.

52. Mini FSJ, Saltzman J, Simione M, et al. Expectant fathers' social determinants of health in early pregnancy. Glob Pediatr Health 2020;7(2333794X20975628).

53. Cohen K, Capponi S, Nyamukapa M, et al. Partner involvement during pregnancy and maternal health behaviors. Matern Child Health J 2016;20(11):2291–8.

54. Alio AP, Bond MJ, Padilla YC, et al. Addressing policy barriers to paternal involvement during pregnancy. Matern Child Health J 2011;15(4):425–30.

55. Simpson JL. Are physical activity and employment related to preterm birth and low birth weight? Am J Obstet Gynecol 1993;168(4):1231–8.

56. Klebanoff MA, Shiono PH, Rhoads GG. Outcomes of pregnancy in a national sample of resident physicians. N Engl J Med 1990;323(15):1040–5.

57. Brett KM, Strogatz DS, Savitz DA. Employment, job strain, and preterm delivery among women in North Carolina. Am J Public Health 1997;87(2):199–204.

58. Croteau A, Marcoux S, Brisson C. Work activity in pregnancy, preventive measures, and the risk of preterm delivery. Am J Epidemiol 2007;166(8):951–65.

59. Oths KS, Dunn LL, Palmer NS. A prospective study of psychosocial job strain and birth outcomes. Epidemiology 2001;12(6):744–6.

60. Henriksen TB, Hedegaard M, Secher NJ. The relation between psychosocial job strain, and preterm delivery and low birthweight for gestational age. Int J Epidemiol 1994;23(4):764–74.

61. Mozurkewich E. Working conditions and pregnancy outcomes: an updated appraisal of the evidence. Am J Obstet Gynecol 2020;222(3):201–3.

62. MacDonald LA, Waters TR, Napolitano PG, et al. Clinical guidelines for occupational lifting in pregnancy: evidence summary and provisional recommendations. Am J Obstet Gynecol 2013;209(2):80–8.

63. Bairoliya N, Fink G. Causes of death and infant mortality rates among full-term births in the United States between 2010 and 2012: an observational study. PLoS Med 2018;15(3):e1002531.

64. Ely DM, Driscoll AK, Matthews TJ. Infant mortality by age at death in the United States, 2016. NCHS Data Brief 2018;(326):1–8.

65. Singh GK, Yu SM. Infant Mortality in the United States, 1915-2017: large social inequalities have persisted for over a century. Int J MCH AIDS 2019;8(1):19–31.

66. Collins JW Jr, Soskolne GR, Rankin KM, et al. Differing first year mortality rates of term births to White, African-American, and Mexican-American US-born and foreign-born mothers. Matern Child Health J 2013;17(10):1776–83.

67. Reddy UM, Bettegowda VR, Dias T, et al. Term pregnancy: a period of heterogeneous risk for infant mortality. Obstet Gynecol 2011;117(6):1279–87.
68. Parks SE, Erck Lambert AB, Hauck FR, et al. Explaining sudden unexpected infant deaths, 2011-2017. Pediatrics 2021;147(5). e2020035873.
69. Moon RY, Carlin RF. Hand I, Task force on sudden infant death syndrome, the Committee on Fetus and Newborn. Sleep-related infant deaths: updated 2022 recommendations for reducing infant deaths in the sleep environment. Pediatrics 2022;150(1). e2022059737.
70. Mohamoud YA, Kirby RS, Ehrenthal DB. Poverty, urban-rural classification and term infant mortality: a population-based multilevel analysis. BMC Pregnancy Childbirth 2019;19(1):40.
71. Acevedo-Garcia D, Noelke C, McArdle N, et al. Racial and ethnic inequities in children's neighborhoods: evidence from the New Child Opportunity Index 2.0. Health Aff 2020;39(10):1693–701.
72. Braveman P, Egerter S, Williams DR. The social determinants of health: coming of age. Annu Rev Public Health 2011;32:381–98.
73. Braveman P, Parker Dominguez T. Abandon "race." Focus on racism. Front Public Health 2021;9:689462.

Computational Approaches for Connecting Maternal Stress to Preterm Birth

Amin Mirzaei, MS[a], Bjarne C. Hiller, MS[a], Ina A. Stelzer, PhD[b],
Kristin Thiele, PhD[d], Yuqi Tan, PhD[c], Martin Becker, PhD[a],*

KEYWORDS

- Stress • Preterm birth • Machine learning • Artificial intelligence

KEY POINTS

- Multiple studies hint at a complex connection between maternal stress and preterm birth (PTB), with PTB being the predominant cause of neonatal deaths globally.
- Novel technologies allow the profiling of stress exposures and responses in unprecedented ways and open avenues like the integration of multiple aspects of stress, continuous monitoring, or biological multiomics profiling.
- Machine learning and artificial intelligence methods can help reveal the underlying processes of stress and PTB but are currently not used to their full potential.

INTRODUCTION

Preterm birth (PTB), that is, a delivery before the 37th week of gestation, is the predominant cause of neonatal deaths,[1] and it can lead to severe long-term complications for mother and child.[2,3] Approximately 1 in 10 babies is born prematurely in the United States, incurring societal costs estimated at US$25.2 billion in 2016.[4] While the mortality rate of children aged under 5 years has significantly declined since 1990, the worldwide rate of PTB has, however, only been reduced slightly over the last decade, 13.4 million estimated in 2020,[1] urging for the development of effective and accessible interventions.

[a] Department of Computer Science and Electrical Engineering, Institute for Visual and Analytic Computing, Universität Rostock, Albert-Einstein-Straße 22, 18059 Rostock, Germany; [b] Department of Pathology, University of California San Diego, GPL/CMM-West, 9500 Gilman Drive, La Jolla, CA 92093, USA; [c] Department of Microbiology and Immunology, Stanford University School of Medicine, CSSR3220, 269 Campus Drive, Stanford, CA 94305, USA; [d] Division for Experimental Feto-Maternal Medicine, Department of Obstetrics and Fetal Medicine, University Medical Center Hamburg-Eppendorf, Center for Obstetrics and Pediatrics, Martinistrasse 52, 20246 Hamburg, Germany
* Corresponding author. Department of Computer Science and Electrical Engineering, Institut Visual and Analytic Computing, University of Rostock, Albert-Einstein-Straße 22, 18059 Rostock, Germany
E-mail address: martin.becker@uni-rostock.de

Clin Perinatol 51 (2024) 345–360
https://doi.org/10.1016/j.clp.2024.02.003
0095-5108/24/© 2024 Elsevier Inc. All rights reserved.
perinatology.theclinics.com

Various environmental, biological, and socioeconomic factors contribute to PTB, such as maternal health, genetics, lifestyle choices, socioeconomic conditions, environmental temperature, and, particularly, physiological and psychological stressors.[3] Although the association between prenatal stress and PTB has been examined in numerous studies,[5] the complexity and heterogeneity of stress perception and its consequences for maternal immune tolerance toward the fetus makes it difficult to gain a comprehensive understanding of functional links.[5] Therefore, to enable the process of introducing stress-lowering interventions into routine pregnancy care, an in-depth understanding of the connections between stress and PTB are urgently required.

The term "stress" lacks precision and a universal definition is difficult. Stress can be defined as an individual's perceived capacity to manage external demands,[6] which may lead to disturbances, irritations, and/or anxiety and contribute to impairments in mental and physical well-being. In this context, stress perception is personal and based on internal stressors related to a person's character and their own self-expectations, aspirations, and perfectionism as well as external stressors including various factors such as environmental noise or extreme temperatures, and personal financial problems or life-changing events.[7,8] Particularly, pregnant women face "pregnancy-specific stress" involving the health of their fetus and their own well-being, anxiety about labor, and concerns related to impending parenthood.[9] However, the impacts on mother and fetus strongly depend on the severity of the stressor, its duration, time point of exposure during gestation, a person's resilience, existing coping strategies,[10] and the availability of social support[11] demonstrating the high interindividual variabilities. Hence, a wide array of stress assessment tools is required to capture the multifaceted range of stress factors and susceptibility.[12,13]

The underlying processes of how stress affects biological systems in PTB are also complex. To ensure proper fetal growth and development, the maternal immune system actively adapts to the semiallogeneic fetus to establish and maintain immune tolerance.[14,15] This includes the adjustment of the immunologic processes,[16] which are highly vulnerable to disruption by environmental factors including prenatal stress. Stress responses are connected to the autonomic nervous system and the hypothalamic–pituitary–adrenal (HPA) axis, which can affect various biological pathways, including neuro-endocrine-immune balance. The associated increase in cortisol production due to prenatal stress can reduce progesterone (P4) production and consequently to the disruption of its immune suppressive capacity[17] leading to immune inflammation. In addition to this stress-induced neuro-endocrine-immune imbalance, the cardiovascular system (eg, changing the heart rate, blood pressure of mother and fetus), on the metabolic system (eg, release of glucose and fats to facilitate energy availability), as well as the behavioral patterns (eg, such as harmful behaviors like smoking) can also be impacted,[3,18] which all can further aggravate endocrine and immune system as well as other biological systems via indirect pathways.

The complex interaction between prenatal stress and PTB calls for a holistic approach incorporating a full characterization of physiological and psychological stressors and the study of underlying biological pathways. To this end, the use of validated questionnaires allows the evaluation of various factors across different psychometric domains, electronic health records (EHRs) store demographic information and patient history, and recent biotechnological advancements toward high-throughput, multiomics approaches enable the measurement of biological systems in a comprehensive, untargeted manner,[19] for example. Integrating these different modalities, advanced computational tools from the field of machine learning (ML) and artificial intelligence (AI) hold the potential to untangle and understand the underlying processes and risk factors for PTB. However, computational tools have only recently been employed to address PTB.[20–22] Here, we provide an overview of the current approaches that apply modern computational tools to study the association between stress and PTB. We also discuss how novel methods from the field of ML and AI can further enhance the study of stress and PTB. We believe that applying these methods can help shape the direction of future research in this domain. An overview of the content covered here is illustrated in **Fig. 1**.

METHODS AND MODALITIES FOR ASSESSING AND QUANTIFYING STRESS

Stress is typically assessed from 2 perspectives[23]: (1) *stressor exposures*, that is, discrete events with the potential to affect an individual's psychological or physiologic performance and (2) *stress responses*, which includes behavioral, cognitive, biological, and emotional reactions to stressors. The following sections cover common as well as ML-enabled methods for assessing stress.

Questionnaires for Measuring Stressor Exposures and Stress Responses

For the measurement of stressor exposures and stress responses, many different validated guidelines and tools exist, for example, as provided by the Stress Measurement Network.[12] This particularly includes questionnaires.

Negative life events, racism and discrimination,[24] lack of social support,[25] and domestic abuse[26] are examples of stressor exposures that are associated with PTB and measured using questionnaires. Questionnaires have also been utilized to collect surrogates for stressor exposures, such as sociodemographic data, social interaction, and lifestyle profiles. In the context of PTB, commonly studied sociodemographic factors include age, race, socioeconomic status, marital status, education, income, medical history, alcohol consumption, and smoking.[27]

In addition to measuring stressor exposures, questionnaires are also used to assess stressor responses of the mothers before, during, and after pregnancy. The Center for Epidemiological Studies Depression Scale, Prenatal Distress Questionnaire (PDQ), Pregnancy Specific Anxiety Measures, and the Perceived Stress Scale (PSS) are questionnaires used to measure stress responses, including depression, distress, anxiety, and perceived stress during pregnancy.[8]

Toward Objective Methods for Stress Response Measurements with Machine Learning

While using questionnaires to assess stress responses can be helpful to capture personalized and compound effects, their results can be highly subjective due to self-reporting of perceived stress and prone to questionnaire-specific limitations, such as method biases or variabilities between individuals.[23] Therefore, while potentially not covering the full spectrum of perceived stress,[28] the implementation of objective stress response measures, such as biological or physiological markers, may be useful.

For example, biomarkers can be employed to assess stress response on a systemic level. Cortisol in blood, salvia, and hair is a marker of short-term and long-term stresses and reflects prolonged HPA axis activity. Significantly different levels have been reported in mothers with term and PTBs in the third trimester.[29,30] Also, serum levels of various cytokines released from inflammatory pathways are indicative of stress responses, for example, interleukin-6.[31] At the same time, emerging high-throughput multiomics technologies enable unprecedented insights into stress responses and PTB by using ML methods,[32–34] demonstrating their potential to identify pathways connecting stress, biology, and PTB. However, measuring and evaluating

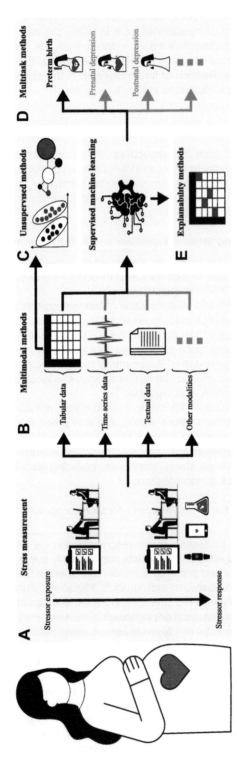

Fig. 1. Computational framework for analyzing the dynamic interplay between stress and PTB. (*A*) The image illustrates different assessment strategies to assess stress exposure and responses, yielding diverse modalities (*B*). These data types can be integrated by multimodal (*B*) multitask (*D*) ML models for a more holistic understanding of stress and PTB. (*C*) Similarly, unsupervised ML leverages identifies subgroups within across mothers and risk factors. (*E*) Explainability methods help understand complex ML methods.

biomarkers can be costly and time consuming and may be better suited for understanding underlying biological processes rather than for routine monitoring.

On the other hand, the Wearable Stress and Affect Detection dataset[35] illustrates more accessible and cost-effective tools that also enable long-term stress monitoring by ML. It incorporates a breadth of physiologic factors measured by wearable devices including blood volume, heart rate, electrical heart, skin, and muscle monitoring, respiration, body temperature, and physical activity, and uses ML methods to predict stress. Similarly, using ML, behavioral markers for stress can even be derived from social media comments, or even patterns from keyboard or mouse usage.[36,37] In the context of maternal stress, Bilal and colleagues,[38] collected a diverse dataset, incorporating questionnaire responses, mothers' voices, mobility metrics, smartphone usage patterns, data usage, and sleep patterns through a smartphone app designed to predict perinatal depression and PTB. Sarkar and colleagues[39] estimated cortisol levels, PSS, and PDQ stress scores of mothers from abdominal electrocardiograms (aECG), both using artificial neural networks. Finally, Ravindra and colleagues[40] employed a similar approach to predict gestational age at birth (GAB) from pregnant women's physical activity and sleep patterns, and indirectly established a connection between maternal stress and PTB.[41]

COMPUTATIONAL APPROACHES FOR UNDERSTANDING THE CONNECTION BETWEEN STRESS AND PRETERM BIRTH

The field of computational methods to study complex systems and their potential to be applied to stress and PTB is large. Here, we briefly review common univariable methods[42] (studying the connection between PTB and a single stress-related variable) as well as multivariable methods[43] (modeling the connection between PTB and multiple stress-related variables simultaneously). We then elaborate on ML methods that either have been applied in the context of stress and PTB or have the potential to significantly impact this domain. **Table 1** provides an overview of studies representative of applying the methods mentioned in this section.

Univariable and Multivariable Methods

Univariable analyses focus on the associations of each individual variable in a dataset (eg, anxiety level) to an outcome (eg, PTB). It can be used to study individual risk factors for PTB or to select variables for subsequent experiments or multivariable analyses.[44] Univariable associations measured by relative risks, odds ratios, or statistical tests have been used to identify potential stress-related risk factors related to PTB, including unintended pregnancy, lack of perceived social support, and pregnancy-related anxiety.[24,45]

In contrast to univariable methods, multivariable methods consider a combination of multiple explanatory variables simultaneously (eg, various stress and demographic factors) and assess their combined impact on the outcome—such as PTB or GAB.[46] While this collective approach may disregard individual effects of variables, the joint effects of factors such as stress-related variables, negative life events, racism and discrimination,[24] lack of social support,[25] and domestic abuse[26] have shown associations with PTB beyond univariable results. Common multivariable methods include linear regression, logistic regression, Poisson regression, and proportional hazard regression.[47] Note that such methods can be used to find multivariable relationships per se, or they can be used in predictive settings (eg, to estimate the risk of PTB in unseen patients).[47] However, particularly for predictive settings, ML methods can capture more complex relationships.[46]

Table 1
Overview of selected supervised and unsupervised computational methods utilized in analyzing stress and preterm birth. An "x" marks the covered aspects of the study.

Article, Year	Objective	Univariable	Multivariable	Supervised	Unsupervised	Multimodal	Multitask	Method	Data Description
Sarkar et al,[39] 2021	Classification: chronically stressed mothers vs controls; Regression: PSS, PDQ values, and maternal hair cortisol level	—	x	x	—	—	—	Deep learning	aECG data
Ravindra et al,[40] 2023	Regression: Gestational age	—	x	x	—	—	—	Deep learning	Wearable sensor data
Huang et al,[22] 2021	Classification: PTB	x	x	x	—	x	—	Lasso logistic regression, SVM	Cortisol and metabolites along with psychological questionnaires
Waynforth et al,[52] 2022	Classification: PTB	—	x	x	—	—	—	Random forest	Questionnaire-based data
Becker et al,[20] 2022	Classification: Pregnancy complication	x	x	x	—	x	x	Deep learning	Stress questionnaires and single-cell immune system data
Lee et al,[51] 2021	Classification: PTB	—	x	x	—	x	—	Random forest	Demographic, socioeconomic, particulate matter in air

Study	Task							Method	Data
Becker et al,[21] 2023	Classification: PTB	x	x	x	—	—	—	SVM	Chronic stress and psychosocial factors
García-Blanco et al,[53] 2017	Regression: Gestational age	—	x	x	—	x	—	Parametric survival model	Cortisol, α-amylase, age, parity
Vovsha et al,[54] 2014	Classification: PTB	—	x	x	—	x	—	SVM and logistic regression	Demographic, vaginal microbiota, cervical examination, and cervical and vaginal fetal fibronectin, questionnaire-based data
Maxson et al,[60] 2016	Subgroup analysis	—	x	x	x	—	—	k-means clustering	Psychosocial health measures
Molenaar et al,[80] 2023	Subgroup analysis	x	x	x	x	x	—	Latent class analysis	Self-reported data

The breadth of applicable methods from ML and AI to understand the connection between stress and PTB is shown.

Supervised Machine Learning Methods for Preterm Birth Prediction Based on Stress-Related Variables

To fully capture the multilayered network of interactions between stress and PTB, recent work moves toward methods from ML and AI, following similar trends in the general study of adverse pregnancy outcomes[48,49] allowing for nonlinear relationships. Predominantly, the methods employed in this context are supervised (see **Table 1**), aiming to establish relationships between stress and PTB and a multitude of variables simultaneously by leveraging labeled data to predict outcomes like PTB for unseen patients.

Multivariable machine learning

Many ML algorithms exist to predict an outcome like PTB from multiple variables simultaneously in a nonlinear manner. This includes, for example, methods like support vector machines (SVMs) to predict PTB from stress-related variables.[21] Other applicable methods include random forests, XGBoost, or artificial neural networks.[46] However, these methods work on tabular data only with a fixed set of variables per patient and a single outcome limiting their capabilities to capture a holistic picture of stress and PTB.

Multimodal machine learning

Multimodal ML considers multiple sources of information to predict outcomes.[50] This can be particularly useful when not only stress-related variables are of interest but also information from other modalities such as multiomics data and biomarkers like cortisol, cervical length, or selected EHR variables. Modern deep-learning methods can even directly integrate imaging or time series data with limited manual preprocessing.[50] In the context of stress and PTB, a particular use case may be integrating stress-related variables with imaging modalities such as transvaginal ultrasound. Rudimentary versions of multimodal modeling have been applied in studies concerning stress and PTB. For example, some articles combine different questionnaires to assess the psychological, parental health, social, demographic, economic, and behavioral risk factors of mothers and used SVMs or random forests to predict PTB.[21,51,52] Others incorporated more diverse modalities of measures such as cortisol, α-amylase level, various metabolites, vaginal microbiota, cervical examination, and cervical and vaginal fetal fibronectin, alongside subjective measures.[22,53,54] While such studies already demonstrate the potential of multimodal ML to simultaneously consider different aspects of stress, they do not yet fully exploit the capabilities of directly integrating diverse modalities such as imaging, text, or time series data. However, such approaches may hold the potential to better model and understand the complex cross talk among stress, various biological systems, and PTB.

Multitask machine learning

Pregnancy complications are rightly interrelated.[20,55] Thus, modeling multiple pregnancy complications together PTB can greatly improve the understanding of their interrelations as well as increase the predictive power of the model.[20] In this context, multitask models are designed to predict multiple outcomes.[56] While multitask learning has been employed in different studies related to pregnancy and child health,[57,58] it is not employed frequently for studying the connection between stress and PTB. Becker and colleagues[20] first used multitask neural networks to predict multiple outcomes simultaneously including early gestational age (as a proxy for PTB) as well as pre-eclampsia, superimposed pre-eclampsia, gestational diabetes, body mass index, diabetes, and hypertension based on an extensive set of stress variables assessed by questionnaires. The authors demonstrated that predicting GAB using a multitask ML approach can increase prediction power and help understand the relationship between pregnancy complications, compared to a single-task setup. This points toward the potential of multitask approaches to capture more intricate relationships of the underlying processes of adverse pregnancy outcomes like PTB and motivates a more holistic approach of studying the connection of stress and adverse pregnancy outcomes rather than isolating PTB.

Unsupervised Machine Learning Methods

Unsupervised ML methods, in contrast to supervised ML methods, have no knowledge about the modeled outcome (eg, PTB) and try to find hidden patterns in the data.[59] They can play an important role in stress and PTB studies by enabling the exploration of patterns within complex datasets.[49] Clustering, a fundamental unsupervised technique can categorize pregnancies into groups based on similar stress profiles, aiding in the discovery of patterns associated with pregnancy outcomes such as PTB. For example, the k-means algorithm has been used to discover clusters of stress resiliency (defined based on measures of paternal support, perceived stress, social support, depression, and self-efficacy) that were associated with different pregnancy-related complications including PTB.[60] Similarly, latent class analysis was used in multiple studies to divide a population of pregnant women into several subpopulations and then compare the rate of PTB in each subpopulation.[61,62]

Similar methods can be used to cluster stress-related variables to gain deeper insights into the relationships between various stress factors and how groups of similar stress-related variables are associated with PTB. For example, Becker and colleagues[21] clustered stress-related variables according to their correlation profiles using k-means clustering. They found prominent clusters of similar variables, like perceived pregnancy risk, health concerns, and emotional state, which were highly associated with PTB.

Overall, unsupervised learning, especially cluster analysis, enables the discovery of multidimensional stress-related phenotypes for PTB, potentially enabling more precise profiling and more effective stress interventions.

CONFOUNDING FACTORS AND CAUSALITY IN COMPUTATIONAL METHODS

By integrating increasingly complex data using ML and AI methods, particularly in predictive, that is, supervised, settings, unexpected confounders can cause misleading interpretations.[63] Similarly, the common focus of ML methods on predictive settings[64] promotes associative analyses and neglects causal connections.

Confounders

Premature contractions, or previous premature delivery, can be considered to influence stress and PTB simultaneously.[65] However, even if such confounding variables are excluded from the data, ML methods may pick up related signatures from other variables, for example, a combination of lifestyle factors or biological profiles.[66] Thus, accounting for such factors is essential, for example, by comparing the final results (eg, trained model for PTB prediction) with models derived from distinct subgroups of potential confounding factors[67] (eg, groups with and without previous premature delivery). Alternatively, propensity score matching is used to define case and control groups where the influence of potential confounding factors is limited by creating groups that are balanced in terms of observed covariates.[68] Studies employing ML methods tend to recognize potential issues with explicit as well as hidden confounding factors and list them as limitation.[20] However, novel studies applying ML needs to carefully consider confounding factors and appropriate counter measures due to the capability of ML to uncover hidden and potentially unintended patterns.[69,70]

Causality

The sensitivity of ML methods to confounders is rooted in their focus on predictive settings,[64] thus finding associations but not causal pathways. However, computational tools exist that allow testing hypothesized (causal inference) and discovering novel causal relationships (causal discovery).[71] The field of causal inference is concerned with testing whether 2 variables are related and assessing the impact of one on the other. For example, Harris and colleagues[72] found a causal association between a preconception maternal stress and offspring birth. However, such approaches for learning causal effects require hypothesizing causal structures. To address this, the field of causal discovery aims to learn such relations directly from the data. A wide variety of algorithms can address this issue.[71] For example, Mesner and colleagues[27] use the Peter–Clark algorithm to derive a causal graph illustrating the interactions between various stressors, demographic factors, and biomarkers in relation to different pregnancy outcomes, including PTB. While this shows the potential of causal discovery to understand the relation between risk factors and PTB and potentially derive novel interventions, neither computational causal inference nor causal discovery methods are common tools in this field.

INTERPRETABILITY AND EXPLAINABILITY OF MACHINE LEARNING MODELS

ML and, particularly, deep learning approaches often produce black box models, that is, even if an ML model accurately predicts PTB risk from a set of stress-related factors, it may not be clear which factors it used and how they were used to derive the risk. This can be a major hindrance in understanding the underlying processes. Some studies use univariable analysis as a surrogate for identifying candidates for the most influential stress-related variables associated with the PTB,[21] others use models that are inherently interpretable such as linear regression.[45] However, most state-of-the-art ML models like SVMs, gradient boosting machines, for example, XGBoost, and particularly deep learning models[73] remain opaque even to domain experts due to their high number of parameters. Although explainable AI (XAI) and interpretable ML are still active fields of research, there is already a wide arsenal of post hoc explanation methods available for these approaches.[74] This includes Shapley values, which originated from cooperative game theory to compute the contribution of each player in a coalition game. In the context of predicting PTB from EHR data, Shapley Additive Explanations (SHAP)[75] have been used to determine the individual contributions of clinical input features to PTB risk predictions,[76] allowing to identify the factors most relevant for the model's decision. Similarly, Ada and colleagues[77] used SHAP values to conclude that the number of consecutive stress minutes is highly predictive for the physiologic stress of the next day, and PSS has the most effect on the next day's perceived stress. Thus, despite the limitations of state-of-the-art XAI methods (eg, no integrated causal or effect modification discovery[55,62]), it is already possible to overcome the black box nature of ML models[74] to some extent to gain deeper insights into the connection between stress and PTB, potentially leading to the discovery of novel intervention methods.

DISCUSSION

The different aspects of stress exposure and response are hard to capture and isolate. Thus, studying the underlying processes of the relationship between stress and adverse pregnancy outcomes like PTB is a challenging task. However, novel technologies, for example, wearable sensors,[35] novel biomedical assays (eg, single-cell analysis),[20] or social media monitoring,[36] can give deeper insights by connecting objective observations to the more common subjective information collected by questionnaires.[13] However, the increasing amount and variety of data pose challenges on how to integrate and analyze this data to connect the captured stress-related patterns to PTB and from there derive accessible interventions. We believe that the quickly progressing development in the field of ML and AI can provide the tools to accomplish this.

While we have seen that ML, in general, is already applied in a significant number of studies relating stress to PTB, these studies currently do not exploit the full potential of available ML and artificial ML methods. For example, while some studies combine multiple modalities (eg, questionnaires and biomarkers), they are often limited to features that are manually crafted from more complex modalities[53] and do not employ full-fledged multimodal models.[50] The handcrafting process can severely limit the amount of information extracted from modalities such as time series data (eg, accelerometer data, heart rate, ECG, or even continuous questionnaires collected via smartphones)[38] compared with allowing ML methods access to the complete time series. Similarly, multitask learning is an established field in the ML community and has only recently been applied to study the connection between stress and PTB in order to gain a more holistic picture by jointly modeling a variety of adverse pregnancy outcomes.[20] Beyond these relatively straightforward applications, the first articles already point toward explicitly modeling joint connection of the pathway from stress over biology to adverse pregnancy outcomes[20] and motivate combining multimodal and multitask methods as applied in other disciplines.[78] Finally, novel developments like large language models, for example, ChatGPT, may help to better understand the complex connections in unstructured or even multimodal data.[79]

We have also pointed out the limitations of current ML models including their black box and ultimately associative nature. Current research is actively developing methods to mitigate these limitations including explainability as well as causal inference and discovery methods.[27,72,77] Particularly, the latter may allow to go beyond predictive settings ultimately leading to the development of novel interventions.

SUMMARY

Stress and PTB are tightly interwoven. We advocate a more holistic approach of studying this connection enabled by computational methods: One the one hand, by integrating not only commonly used subjective measurements of stressor exposures and stress responses, but also objective measures, for example, physiological as well as biological modalities. And on the other hand, by integrating PTB into the more holistic context of other adverse pregnancy outcomes, we believe that ML and AI methods have the potential to open novel avenues for studying the complex relationship of stress and ultimately yield novel, easily accessible interventions.

ACKNOWLEDGMENTS

AI technologies, including Grammarly (Grammarly, Inc., San Francisco, CA, USA) and ChatGPT (OpenAI, San Francisco, CA, USA), were exclusively used to enhance the language and readability of the article. This work was funded by the Federal Ministry of Education and Research (BMBF) (01IS22077) and the Free and Hanseatic City of Hamburg under the Excellence Strategy of the Federal Government and the Länder (Z5-V2-008: TN 2023 Preterm), as well as the National Institutes of Health (R00HD105016).

DISCLOSURE

The authors have nothing to disclose.

Best Practices

What is the current practice for employing computational methods to study the connection between stress and PTB?

- Many different measurement modalities are used to assess stressor exposures and stress responses and study its connection to PTB.
- Current methods are not exploiting the full potential of the quickly evolving fields of ML and AI.

What changes in current practice are likely to improve outcomes?

- ML and AI can unlock novel and more comprehensive profiling of stress responses, for example, through wearable devices or deep biological profiling.
- Multimodal and multitask ML may help to integrating multiple modalities for understanding the complex connections between stress and PTB as part of a more holistic view on adverse pregnancy outcomes.
- XAI methods can help to derive insights into otherwise black box ML methods to help identify novel stress-related interventions.

REFERENCES

1. Ohuma EO, Moller AB, Bradley E, et al. National, regional, and global estimates of preterm birth in 2020, with trends from 2010: a systematic analysis. Lancet 2023;402(10409):1261–71.
2. Henderson J, Carson C, Redshaw M. Impact of preterm birth on maternal well-being and women's perceptions of their baby: a population-based survey. BMJ Open 2016;6(10):e012676.
3. Institute of Medicine (US) Committee on Understanding Premature Birth and Assuring Healthy Outcomes. In: Behrman RE, Butler AS, editors. Preterm birth: Causes, consequences, and prevention. Washington, DC: National Academies Press (US); 2007.
4. Waitzman NJ, Jalali A, Grosse SD. Preterm birth lifetime costs in the United States in 2016: an update. Semin Perinatol 2021;45(3):151390.
5. Shapiro GD, Fraser WD, Frasch MG, et al. Psychosocial stress in pregnancy and preterm birth: associations and mechanisms. J Perinat Med 2013;41(6):631–45.
6. Selye H. The stress of life (Rev. ed.). New York, USA: McGraw Hill; 1978.
7. Witt WP, Cheng ER, Wisk LE, et al. Preterm birth in the United States: the impact of stressful life events prior to conception and maternal age. Am J Public Health 2014;104(S1):S73–80.
8. Staneva A, Bogossian F, Pritchard M, et al. The effects of maternal depression, anxiety, and perceived stress during pregnancy on preterm birth: a systematic review. Women Birth 2015;28(3):179–93.
9. Ibrahim SM, Lobel M. Conceptualization, measurement, and effects of pregnancy-specific stress: review of research using the original and revised Prenatal Distress Questionnaire. J Behav Med 2020;43(1):16–33.
10. Traylor CS, Johnson JD, Kimmel MC, et al. Effects of psychological stress on adverse pregnancy outcomes and nonpharmacologic approaches for reduction: an expert review. Am J Obstet Gynecol MFM 2020;2(4):100229.

11. Chen Z, Li Y, Chen J, et al. The mediating role of coping styles in the relationship between perceived social support and antenatal depression among pregnant women: a cross-sectional study. BMC Pregnancy Childbirth 2022;22(1):188.
12. Stress measurement network. University of California, san Francisco. Available at: https://www.stressmeasurement.org. [Accessed 8 September 2023].
13. Harville EW, Savitz DA, Dole N, et al. Stress questionnaires and stress biomarkers during pregnancy. J Womens Health 2009;18(9):1425–33.
14. Aghaeepour N, Ganio EA, Mcilwain D, et al. An immune clock of human pregnancy. Sci Immunol 2017;2(15):eaan2946.
15. Arck PC, Hecher K. Fetomaternal immune cross-talk and its consequences for maternal and offspring's health. Nat Med 2013;19(5):548–56.
16. Arruvito L, Giulianelli S, Flores AC, et al. NK cells expressing a progesterone receptor are susceptible to progesterone-induced apoptosis. J Immunol 2008; 180(8):5746–53.
17. Solano ME, Arck PC. Steroids, pregnancy and fetal development. Front Immunol 2019;10:3017.
18. Wadhwa PD, Culhane JF, Rauh V, et al. Stress and preterm birth: neuroendocrine, immune/inflammatory, and vascular mechanisms. Matern Child Health J 2001; 5(2):119–25.
19. Jehan F, Sazawal S, Baqui AH, et al. Multiomics characterization of preterm birth in low- and middle-income countries. JAMA Netw Open 2020;3(12):e2029655.
20. Becker M, Dai J, Chang AL, et al. Revealing the impact of lifestyle stressors on the risk of adverse pregnancy outcomes with multitask machine learning. Front Pediatr 2022;10:933266.
21. Becker M, Mayo JA, Phogat NK, et al. Deleterious and protective psychosocial and stress-related factors predict risk of spontaneous preterm birth. Am J Perinatol 2023;40(01):074–88.
22. Huang D, Liu Z, Liu X, et al. Stress and metabolomics for prediction of spontaneous preterm birth: a prospective nested case-control study in a tertiary hospital. Front Pediatr 2021;9:670382.
23. Epel ES, Crosswell AD, Mayer SE, et al. More than a feeling: a unified view of stress measurement for population science. Front Neuroendocrinol 2018;49: 146–69.
24. Dole N, Savitz DA, Hertz-Picciotto I, et al. Maternal stress and preterm birth. Am J Epidemiol 2003;157(1):14–24.
25. Hetherington E, Doktorchik C, Premji SS, et al. Preterm birth and social support during pregnancy: a systematic review and meta-analysis. Paediatr Perinat Epidemiol 2015;29(6):523–35.
26. Donovan B, Spracklen C, Schweizer M, et al. Intimate partner violence during pregnancy and the risk for adverse infant outcomes: a systematic review and meta-analysis. BJOG An Int J Obstet Gynaecol 2016;123(8):1289–99.
27. Mesner O, Davis A, Casman E, et al. Using graph learning to understand adverse pregnancy outcomes and stress pathways. PLoS One 2019;14(9):e0223319.
28. Dorsey A., Scherer E., Eckhoff R., et al., Measurement of human stress: a multidimensional approach, 2022, RIT Press, No. OP-0073-2206.
29. Giurgescu C. Are maternal cortisol levels related to preterm birth? J Obstet Gynecol Neonatal Nurs 2009;38(4):377–90.
30. Kim MY, Kim GU, Son HK. Hair cortisol concentrations as a biological marker of maternal prenatal stress: a systematic review. Int J Environ Res Public Health 2020;17(11):4002.

31. Coussons-Read ME, Lobel M, Carey JC, et al. The occurrence of preterm delivery is linked to pregnancy-specific distress and elevated inflammatory markers across gestation. Brain Behav Immun 2012;26(4):650–9.

32. Stelzer IA, Ghaemi MS, Han X, et al. Integrated trajectories of the maternal metabolome, proteome, and immunome predict labor onset. Sci Transl Med 2021; 13(592):eabd9898.

33. Espinosa CA, Khan W, Khanam R, et al. Multiomic signals associated with maternal epidemiological factors contributing to preterm birth in low- and middle-income countries. Sci Adv 2023;9(21):eade7692.

34. Ziegler LM, Fluriou-Servou A, Waag R, et al. Multiomic profiling of the acute stress response in the mouse hippocampus. Nat Commun 2022;13:1824.

35. Schmidt P, Reiss A, Duerichen R, et al. Introducing WESAD, a multimodal dataset for wearable stress and affect detection. Proceedings of the 20th ACM International Conference on Multimodal Interaction 2018;400–8.

36. Ahmed A, Aziz S, Toro CT, et al. Machine learning models to detect anxiety and depression through social media: a scoping review. Comput Methods Programs Biomed Update 2022;2:100066.

37. Naegelin M, Weibel RP, Kerr JI, et al. An interpretable machine learning approach to multimodal stress detection in a simulated office environment. J Biomed Inform 2023;139:104299.

38. Bilal AM, Fransson E, Bränn E, et al. Predicting perinatal health outcomes using smartphone-based digital phenotyping and machine learning in a prospective Swedish cohort (Mom2B): study protocol. BMJ Open 2022;12(4):e059033.

39. Sarkar P, Lobmaier S, Fabre B, et al. Detection of maternal and fetal stress from the electrocardiogram with self-supervised representation learning. Sci Rep 2021;11(1):24146.

40. Ravindra NG, Espinosa C, Berson E, et al. Deep representation learning identifies associations between physical activity and sleep patterns during pregnancy and prematurity. NPJ Digit Med 2023;6(1):1–16.

41. Padmaja B, Prasad VR, Sunitha KVN. A machine learning approach for stress detection using a wireless physical activity tracker. Int J Mach Learn Comput 2018;8(1):33–8.

42. Clayton D, Hills M. Statistical models in epidemiology. Oxford, England: Oxford University Press; 1993.

43. Rencher AC. A review of "methods of multivariate analysis, second edition.". IIE Trans 2005;37(11):1083–5.

44. Tanpradit K, Kaewkiattikun K. The effect of perceived stress during pregnancy on preterm birth. Int J Womens Health 2020;12:287–93.

45. Kramer MS, Lydon J, Séguin L, et al. Stress pathways to spontaneous preterm birth: the role of stressors, psychological distress, and stress hormones. Am J Epidemiol 2009;169(11):1319–26.

46. Sufriyana H, Husnayain A, Chen YL, et al. Comparison of multivariable logistic regression and other machine learning algorithms for prognostic prediction studies in pregnancy care: systematic review and meta-analysis. JMIR Med Inform 2020;8(11):e16503.

47. Schneider A, Hommel G, Blettner M. Linear regression analysis: part 14 of a series on evaluation of scientific publications. Dtsch Arztebl Int 2010;107(44): 776–82.

48. Włodarczyk T, Płotka S, Szczepański T, et al. Machine learning methods for preterm birth prediction: a review. Electronics 2021;10(5):586.

49. Espinosa C, Becker M, Marić I, et al. Data-driven modeling of pregnancy-related complications. Trends Mol Med 2021;27(8):762–76.

50. Kline A, Wang H, Li Y, et al. Multimodal machine learning in precision health: a scoping review. NPJ Digit Med 2022;5(1):1–14.

51. Lee KS, Kim HI, Kim HY, et al. Association of preterm birth with depression and particulate matter: machine learning analysis using national health insurance data. Diagnostics 2021;11(3):555.

52. Waynforth D. Identifying risk factors for premature birth in the UK Millennium Cohort using a random forest decision-tree approach. Reprod Med 2022;3(4): 320–33.

53. García-Blanco A, Diago V, Serrano De La Cruz V, et al. Can stress biomarkers predict preterm birth in women with threatened preterm labor? Psychoneuroendocrinology 2017;83:19–24.

54. Vovsha I., Rajan A., Salleb-Aouissi A., et al., Predicting preterm birth is not elusive: machine learning paves the way to individual wellness. In: AAAI Spring Symposia, 22 March 2014, Palo Alto, CA.

55. Shi P, Liu A, Yin X. Association between gestational weight gain in women with gestational diabetes mellitus and adverse pregnancy outcomes: a retrospective cohort study. BMC Pregnancy Childbirth 2021;21(1):508.

56. Ruder S. An overview of multi-task learning in deep neural networks. 2017. Available at: http://arxiv.org/abs/1706.05098. [Accessed 12 December 2023].

57. Francesco DD, Reiss JD, Roger J, et al. Data-driven longitudinal characterization of neonatal health and morbidity. Sci Transl Med 2023;15(683):eadc9854.

58. He L, Li H, Wang J, et al. A multi-task, multi-stage deep transfer learning model for early prediction of neurodevelopment in very preterm infants. Sci Rep 2020; 10(1):15072.

59. Celebi ME, Aydin K, editors. Unsupervised learning algorithms. Springer International Publishing; 2016. https://doi.org/10.1007/978-3-319-24211-8.

60. Maxson PJ, Edwards SE, Valentiner EM, et al. A Multidimensional approach to characterizing psychosocial health during pregnancy. Matern Child Health J 2016;20(6):1103–13.

61. Haviland MJ, YI Nillni, Cabral HJ, et al. Adverse psychosocial factors in pregnancy and preterm delivery. Paediatr Perinat Epidemiol 2021;35(5):519–29.

62. Hendryx M, Chojenta C, Byles JE. Latent class analysis of low birth weight and preterm delivery among Australian women. J Pediatr 2020;218:42–8.e1.

63. Skelly AC, Dettori JR, Brodt ED. Assessing bias: the importance of considering confounding. Evid-Based Spine-Care J 2012;3(1):9–12.

64. Mooney SJ, Keil AP, Westreich DJ. Thirteen questions about using machine learning in causal research (you won't believe the answer to number 10!). Am J Epidemiol 2021;190(8):1476–82.

65. Lilliecreutz C, Larén J, Sydsjö G, et al. Effect of maternal stress during pregnancy on the risk for preterm birth. BMC Pregnancy Childbirth 2016;16(1):5.

66. Mukherjee P, Shen TC, Liu J, et al. Confounding factors need to be accounted for in assessing bias by machine learning algorithms. Nat Med 2022;28(6):1159–60.

67. Pourhoseingholi MA, Baghestani AR, Vahedi M. How to control confounding effects by statistical analysis. Gastroenterol Hepatol Bed Bench 2012;5(2):79–83.

68. Rosenbaum PR, Rubin DB. The central role of the propensity score in observational studies for causal effects. Biometrika 1983;70(1):41–55.

69. Wyss R, Yanover C, El-Hay T, et al. Machine learning for improving high-dimensional proxy confounder adjustment in healthcare database studies: an

overview of the current literature. Pharmacoepidemiol Drug Saf 2022;31(9): 932–43.

70. Mathur MB, VanderWeele TJ. Methods to address confounding and other biases in meta-analyses: review and recommendations. Annu Rev Public Health 2022; 43(1):19–35.

71. Guo R, Cheng L, Li J, et al. A survey of learning causality with data: problems and methods. ACM Comput Surv 2021;53(4):1–37.

72. Harris ML, Hure AJ, Holliday E, et al. Association between preconception maternal stress and offspring birth weight: findings from an Australian longitudinal data linkage study. BMJ Open 2021;11(3):e041502.

73. Greener JG, Kandathil SM, Moffat L, et al. A guide to machine learning for biologists. Nat Rev Mol Cell Biol 2022;23(1):40–55.

74. Dwivedi R, Dave D, Naik H, et al. Explainable AI (XAI): core ideas, techniques, and solutions. ACM Comput Surv 2023;55(9):194, 1-194:33.

75. Lundberg S, Lee SI. A unified approach to interpreting model predictions. Published online November 24, 2017. https://doi.org/10.48550/arXiv.1705.07874.

76. Sterckx L, Vandewiele G, Dehaene I, et al. Clinical information extraction for preterm birth risk prediction. J Biomed Inform 2020;110:103544.

77. Ng A, Wei B, Jain J, et al. Predicting the next-day perceived and physiological stress of pregnant women by using machine learning and explainability: algorithm development and validation. JMIR MHealth Uhealth 2022;10(8):e33850.

78. Hu R., Singh A., UniT: multimodal multitask learning with a unified transformer. In: Proceedings of the IEEE/CVF International Conference on Computer Vision (ICCV) 2021:1439-1449. October 12, 2021. https://openaccess.thecvf.com/menu.

79. Yang X, Chen A, PourNejatian N, et al. A large language model for electronic health records. NPJ Digit Med 2022;5(1):1–9.

80. Molenaar JM, van der Meer L, Bertens LCM, et al. Defining vulnerability subgroups among pregnant women using pre-pregnancy information: a latent class analysis. Eur J Public Health 2023;33(1):25–34.

Ambient Environment and the Epidemiology of Preterm Birth

Gary M. Shaw, DrPH[a],*, David.J.X. Gonzalez, PhD[b],
Dana E. Goin, PhD[c], Kari A. Weber, PhD, MHS[d],
Amy M. Padula, PhD[e]

KEYWORDS

- Prematurity • Environment • Risk factors • Epidemiology
- Gene–environment interactions

KEY POINTS

- Environmental chemical and physical exposures have been associated with increased risks of preterm birth (PTB).
- Chemical and physical exposures during pregnancy may derive from air pollutants, water contaminants, and other sources in proximity to residential addresses.
- Numerous studies have examined the role of single environmental exposures in influencing PTB risk, but few studies have attempted to account for the complexities of multiple exposures — the exposome.
- Factors that modify risks of the exposome, including variations associated with the structural genome, epigenome, social stressors, and dietary factors, will be important to explore in the future.

INTRODUCTION

Preterm birth (PTB, delivery before 37 weeks of gestation) is associated with substantial morbidity and mortality with a global burden of greater than 15 million babies born preterm every year.[1,2] In the United States, PTB occurs in approximately 10% of all

[a] Epidemiology and Population Health, Obstetrics & Gynecology – Maternal Fetal Medicine, Department of Pediatrics, Stanford University School of Medicine, Center for Academic Medicine (CAM), 453 Quarry Road, Stanford, CA 94304, USA; [b] Division of Environmental Health Sciences, School of Public Health, University of California, 2121 Berkeley Way, CA 94720, USA; [c] Department of Epidemiology, Mailman School of Public Health, Columbia University, 722 West 168th Street, New York, NY 10032, USA; [d] Department of Epidemiology, Fay W. Boozman College of Public Health, University of Arkansas for Medical Sciences, 4301 West Markham Street, RAHN 6219, Rock, AR 72205, USA; [e] Department of Obstetrics, Gynecology and Reproductive Sciences, University of California San Francisco, 490 Illinois Street, #103N, San Francisco, CA 94158, USA
* Corresponding author.
E-mail address: gmshaw@stanford.edu

Clin Perinatol 51 (2024) 361–377
https://doi.org/10.1016/j.clp.2024.02.004
0095-5108/24/© 2024 Elsevier Inc. All rights reserved.

livebirths.[3,4] Frequency of PTB in the United States is higher than what is observed in other industrialized countries, for example, Canada (7%) and France (6%).[5] Despite medical advances, the frequency of PTB has increased in the United States for decades.[3] Part of the overall occurrence of PTB can be attributed to medical interventions to facilitate earlier delivery when there are complications endangering the health of the pregnant person or fetus. However, risk factors for the largest population burden of PTB, *spontaneous* PTB (sPTB), remain largely unexplained.

PTB is a complex phenomenon and not well understood as a singular condition defined simply by the arbitrary dichotomy of birth at less than 37 completed weeks of gestation (vs $\geq$37 weeks).[6] Our current etiologic understanding is somewhat hampered by the fact that no nonprimate experimental model exists that is sufficiently informative of the human condition of PTB. Thus, epidemiologic studies must be a critical part of our toolkit in solving the substantive problem of PTB. In experimental studies, the investigator has more "control" over the many exposures study subjects may encounter; whereas, in epidemiologic studies, the investigator is relegated to being an "observer" of what and how individuals in a study population are exposed to and affected by potential risk factors. In some instances, exposures may not be known or cannot be adequately controlled for. This may be a particular challenge to investigations involving environmental factors.

Our goal here is not to provide a comprehensive review of past epidemiologic work, but rather to capture the essence of the manifold environmental factors that have been observed to influence the risks of PTB. Although "environment" can be defined broadly as nongenetic in nature, the bulk of our focus will be on potential exposures associated with an individual's residential *ambient* environment and following with a brief overview of some of the other nongenetic risk factors such as demographic, substance use, nutritional, and stress studied for their association with PTB. These other nongenetic factors could be the subject of lengthy reviews on their own and are noted in brief here owing to their pertinence in the examination of risks associated with exposures in the ambient environment.

SELECT NONGENETIC FACTORS
Demographics

One of the strongest associations for PTB observed in the United States is the elevated risks of PTB that African American or Black women experience.[7,8] While Hispanics and Asians appear to have somewhat lowered risks of PTB relative to non-Hispanic Whites, African Americans have approximately double the risk of PTB compared with non-Hispanic Whites. This risk is approximately 3 fold for African Americans compared with non-Hispanic Whites for PTB before 28 weeks.[9] This Black–White risk disparity was comprehensively examined by a working group commissioned by the March of Dimes a few years ago.[7] The working group considered 33 hypothesized causes for their potential plausibility to contribute to the risk disparity and concluded *"Racism is a highly plausible, major upstream contributor to the Black-White disparity in PTB through multiple pathways and biological mechanisms."* Racism has been associated with numerous contributory risk factors, including socioeconomic disadvantage, chronic stress, and potentially harmful ambient environmental exposures.[10–12]

With respect to other demographic characteristics, younger maternal age (<20 years) and older maternal age (>35 years) have been associated with increased risk of PTB.[6] Multifetal pregnancy has been associated with increased PTB risk.[3] Increased risks of PTB have been observed for male offspring,[13] particularly those that occur before 28 weeks of gestation.[14]

Substance Use

Although cigarette smoking has been associated with several outcomes of pregnancy (eg, reduced birthweight), the association of cigarette smoking with PTB risk is modest and has not been consistently observed.[6] Similarly, the use of alcohol and caffeine has not revealed consistent associations with PTB.[6] The use of cocaine during pregnancy has shown consistent evidence of approximately a 2 fold increased risk of PTB.[6] Other substance use in pregnancy including opioids,[15] methamphetamines,[16] and cannabis[17] has been associated with increased PTB risk.

Nutrition

Dietary quality as well as specific nutrient intakes has been explored for their association with PTB, although consistent results have generally not been observed. Diets including more fruits, vegetables, whole grains, poultry, and fish have been associated with reduced PTB risk.[18] Some studies have reported the reduced risks of PTB associated with pre- and antenatal intake of folic acid.[19–22] An increased intake of iron, zinc, omega-3, omega-6, vitamin D, calcium, and magnesium[19,23] has been observed to decrease PTB risk. Higher levels of antioxidants such as carotenoids have been associated with a reduced risk of PTB.[24] Some findings indicate that probiotic dairy product intake may be associated with a reduced risk of PTB.[25] Other nutritional aspects that have been observed to increase the risk for PTB include both low and elevated prepregnancy body mass index.[26–28] Diabetes has also been associated with PTB risk.[29] Interestingly, recent findings have observed that PTB risk increases with elevated serum glucose levels during mid-pregnancy, but well short of levels seen in overt diabetes.[30]

Interpregnancy Interval

A short interpregnancy interval (IPI) (<6 months) between delivery of one pregnancy and conception of the next has been associated with adverse pregnancy outcomes, including PTB in numerous populations,[31–33] though it does not appear to contribute to the Black–White disparity in PTB risk.[34] The underlying explanation to a shortened IPI association is unknown with suggestions including potential confounding,[35] low nutrient levels such as lower folic acid,[36] and variation in microbiota taxa.[37]

Stress

Indicators of both biologic and psychosocial stress have been studied for their contributions to PTB risk.[38] Corticotrophin-releasing hormone, cortisol, other biomarkers of stress, as well as a variety of indicators of perceived stress (eg, life events) have been measured. Approaches employed thus far have produced what many investigators might conclude as being mixed results. A biomarker study that measured urinary catecholamines (dopamine, epinephrine, and norepinephrine), that is, biomarkers of stress, showed a 2- to 4-fold elevation for PTB among those with the highest urinary levels in mid-pregnancy.[39] A well-conducted Canadian study[40] investigated a sizable number of stress indicators and measures of psychological distress as predictors of sPTB. A woman's reported pregnancy-related anxiety (odds ratio = 1.8) was observed to be associated with PTB. The phenomenon of pregnancy-related anxiety has since been recapitulated as a PTB risk factor employing machine learning analytics.[41]

AMBIENT ENVIRONMENTAL FACTORS AND PRETERM BIRTH RISK

Here, we highlight aspects of the ambient environment that have been investigated for their influence on risk of PTB. By ambient, we definitionally focus on those aspects of the environment that are proximal to where a pregnant individual may reside. A discussion of possible occupational risks for PTB such as long working hours, shift work, physical labor, and chemical exposures is outside the ambit of this narrative, but an entry point into that literature can be found elsewhere.[42] Similarly, previous reviews have summarized associations between classes of environmental chemicals and PTB.[22]

Air Pollution

Air pollutants may be one of the most studied exposures associated with the ambient environment for risk of PTB. Most regularly monitored air pollutants (ie, nitrogen dioxide [NO_2], carbon monoxide, sulfur dioxide, ozone, and particulate matter) have been associated with PTB, but most consistent evidence for an association has been found with particulate matter with a diameter less than 2.5 μm ($PM_{2.5}$), which can penetrate the lung and enter the bloodstream. It has been estimated that 2.8 to 5.9 million PTBs may be associated with $PM_{2.5}$ exposure globally.[43] In a recent review, exposure to $PM_{2.5}$ was associated with an increased risk of PTB in 19 of 24 studies (79%).[44] A comprehensive review of air pollution and pregnancy outcomes found that exposure to $PM_{2.5}$ over the entire pregnancy was significantly associated with higher risk for PTB: the pooled odds ratio was a 1.24 per 10 μg/m^3 increase in $PM_{2.5}$ during the entire pregnancy.[45] High levels of $PM_{2.5}$ in the second trimester and at the end of pregnancy are the most critical periods[46] and associations are stronger for earlier PTB.[46] Notably, associations between air pollution and PTB have been stronger in neighborhoods with lower socioeconomic status (SES).[47]

Wildfires

Although there have been many studies on air pollution in general, the few studies on wildfire smoke and PTB had diverse methods and inconsistent results. A recent review[48] found 2 of 4 studies with evidence of associations between wildfire smoke and PTB. These studies have been conducted all over the world from wildfires in the western United States,[49,50] forest fires in South America,[51] and bushfires in Australia[52] with various exposure assessment methods. The largest study to date examined approximately 3 million births in California between 2006 and 2012 and found that each day of exposure to any wildfire smoke was associated with a 0.49% increase in risk of PTB.[50] Annual percentages of PTBs in California attributable to wildfire smoke between 2007 and 2012 ranged from 1.8% in 2011 to 6.3% in 2008, a high wildfire year.[50] The effect of stress due to the wildfire event has been associated with maternal mental health[53] and may be an additional pathway by which wildfires may affect PTB.

Greenspace

A recent area of study is proximity to greenspace and lowered risk of pregnancy outcomes.[54] Most studies that have explored PTB risk have employed the Normalized Difference Vegetation Index (NDVI), an index derived using remote sensing. The results have been inconsistent and have varied depending on the residential buffer used (ie, the concentric area around one's residential address used to determine greenspace exposure), environmental or socioeconomic factors that were adjusted for, and size of the study population. For example, one study of roughly 3 million births in Texas did not observe any associations between a higher residential NDVI in a 250 meter buffer and PTB after adjustment for individual and neighborhood factors.[55] A California study observed a decreased risk of selected subphenotypes of PTB (eg, <28 weeks of gestation) with higher residential NDVIs across all buffers (250, 500, 1000, and 2000 meters) with the strongest associations in the largest buffers.[56] These investigators also observed statistical interaction between NDVI and various measures of air pollution indicating the highest risk may be among those in areas with low residential greenspace and high air pollution.[56] Another California study observed an inverse association between more greenness and PTB risk in the largest examined residential buffers and after adjustment for certain air pollution measures, but not in the smaller residential buffers (50 meters).[57] A study in Rhode Island observed an association between NDVI and PTB birth, but it was attenuated after adjustment for SES.[58] A study in Pennsylvania adjusting for other environmental as well as demographic and clinical factors observed an inverse association between higher NDVI and PTB only in cities.[59] A study in Vancouver, Canada observed those in the highest quartile of residential NDVI within 100 meter buffers to have a lower odds of PTB compared with those in the lowest quartile and adjustment for other environmental factors such as air pollution, and noise did not meaningfully impact the associations.[60] Unraveling the beneficial mechanisms of greenspace to determine the most appropriate buffers and factors to adjust for may lead to more consistent associations.

Extreme Heat

An area of increasing focus, particularly due to climate change, has been the potential risks associated with heat waves. In a recent review, Dalugoda and colleagues[61] noted that 23 of 30 studies showed elevated temperatures to be associated with increased PTB risks. However, inferences from this body of work are challenged by the fact that extreme heat exposure has been variably defined based on temperature (eg, mean, maximum, or upper percentiles), duration at that temperature (eg, 2–7 days), and the investigated gestational timing of exposure. The biologic mechanisms that may underly an association between extreme heat and PTB risk are not well understood and will require further investigation. Although some studies have explored interactions between extreme heat and air pollutants, more efforts will be needed to determine the potential modifying influence one may have on the other. Interestingly, extreme heat exposure and PTB risk have recently been observed to be influenced by the levels of greenness and SES.[62] Of note, exposure to cold temperatures has also been associated with increased PTB risk.[63]

Oil and Gas Development

There is widespread residential exposure to oil and gas development in major petroleum producing countries such as the United States, where 17.6 million residents live within 1.6 km (1 mile) of active wells.[64] Numerous studies have investigated the association between PTB and proximity to such wells using data from the United States and Canada.[59,65–74] Drilling and operating oil and gas wells is associated with air pollutant emissions, water contamination, soil contamination, and noise pollution.[75] Researchers have observed elevated concentrations of pollutants known to be associated with PTB risk, such as $PM_{2.5}$, ozone, and being downwind of new and active wells.[76] Consequently, researchers working in this area have used proximity to wells as a metric for the complex mixture of physical and psychosocial stressors associated with oil and gas production.[77]

Most of the epidemiologic studies have reported positive associations between higher PTB risk and exposures to oil and gas development during gestation.[59,67,68,72,73,78,79] Four studies did not observe an association between exposures to oil and gas development and PTB risk,[66,70,71,74] and another study using data from Colorado found an inverse association between exposure to oil and gas development and PTB risk.[69] Most of these studies investigated exposures to unconventional (ie, hydraulically fractured) or conventional oil and gas wells. One study investigated exposures to natural gas flaring, where excess gas is combusted in situ, and found significantly higher PTB risk for those exposed during pregnancy.[65] More work is needed to investigate specific etiologic pathways by which exposures to oil and gas development confer risk of PTB.[77]

Pesticides

Several pesticides are known reproductive toxicants.[80] Despite this evidence and substantial concern from the public about potential reproductive risks, relatively few studies have investigated potential associations between exposures to specific pesticides and most reproductive outcomes including PTB. Suggested potential mechanisms for an association between pesticide exposures and PTB have included placental compromise with downstream alterations in nutrient transfer,[81] elevated oxidative stress,[82] and hormonal dysfunction.[83] The few studies that have explored this broad question of various pesticide compounds and PTB have observed inconsistent results.[84–89] Not unlike other environmental epidemiology studies, studies involving pesticide exposures have been limited by the exposure assessment used, the study design employed as well as small study population size, each of these limitations serving to challenge clear inferences to be drawn. Measures of exposure have included individual-level estimations such as serum measures of dichlorodiphenyldichloroethylene (DDE)[90] or chlordecone,[91] ecologic-level estimations such as county-level pesticide use,[86,92] and residential addresses of individuals and their proximity to pesticide applications.[93] Serum levels of dichlorodiphenyltrichloroethane (DDT)/DDE have been associated with increased PTB risks but not in all studies particularly in more recent studies where serum levels have been decreasing.[84]

Of note, a recent study in a highly agricultural region of California examined associations between a woman's residential proximity to agriculture-related pesticide applications during pregnancy and risk of sPTB[93] and preeclampsia (a major contributor to medically indicated PTB).[94] Despite a very large study population, consideration of narrowly defined phenotypes, and consideration of a variety of gestational exposure definitions such as chemical groups, specific chemicals, and number of pesticides, there was a notable lack of association between pesticide exposures and elevated risk of either sPTB or preeclampsia. Owing to some results showing decreased risks with exposures, the investigators speculated the possibility that unobserved early fetal loss hindered the ability to derive unbiased risk estimates. That is, pesticide exposures in pregnancies before 20 weeks, the earliest a birth would be identified in vital statistics files and before preeclampsia would be diagnosed, may selectively increase the odds of earlier losses in pregnancies destined to be preterm or preeclamptic and therefore not observable when only live birth data are used for the target study population.

Drinking Water Constituents

Other potential putative exposures in the environment such as water constituents have been investigated.[84,95] Previous studies have shown higher risk of PTB when there was worse overall drinking water quality or a violation of a maximum contaminant level for any contaminant in drinking water during pregnancy.[96] However, specific types of drinking water contamination (organic, inorganic, biological, and radiological[97]) are less studied and work that does exist shows inconsistent relationships. For example, organic contaminants include pharmaceuticals and personal care products, endocrine-disrupting chemicals, pesticides, and flame retardants[98] and can get into both surface and groundwater through leaking of industrial and domestic waste. Despite these broad categories, only atrazine (an herbicide) in drinking water has been well-studied with respect to PTB, but the results are inconsistent: one study showed a positive relationship[86] and others showed null or imprecise results.[99] Tri-halomethanes are formed when organic matter in the water interacts with the chlorine used to disinfect it. Some investigators have found modest associations of disinfection byproducts with the risk of PTB,[100] while others have not.[101] Inorganic contamination includes trace elements such as arsenic, barium, cadmium, lead, and vanadium. There is more evidence linking inorganic contaminants in drinking water with an increased risk of PTB, especially for arsenic[102] and nitrates.[103–106] Biological contamination can occur when there is an excess of algae, pathogenic bacteria, or viruses in the water. This is also usually a result of animal waste or industrial pollution entering the water source. Very little evidence exists regarding biological contamination of drinking water and risk of PTB. Radiological contamination occurs when radioactive minerals in the ground, such as radium and uranium, or radon gas, release radiation into the water. Only uranium in drinking water has been linked with an increased risk of PTB.[107] While evidence exists regarding maternal exposure to specific water contaminants during pregnancy, establishing drinking water as the source of exposure is difficult given the challenges in obtaining accurate exposure measurements.

Proximity to Point Source Emissions

Studies have observed modestly elevated PTB risks associated with residential proximity to petroleum industries[108,109] as well as to cement manufacturing[110] and electrical generation associated with coal emissions.[111] Residential proximity to waste sites has also been explored for associations with PTB. Potential exposure to waste site contamination varies based on what materials have been disposed of at the particular landfill. The limited studies of this potential hazard have generally showed null or small increased PTB risks.[84]

Residential exposures to concentrated animal feeding operations (CAFOs) (facilities that confine animals at high densities for prolonged periods of time) have been associated with decreased birthweight and shortened gestational time with closer distance between maternal residential address and poultry.[112]

Residential proximity to aircraft noise has been observed to increase PTB risk and that risk may be further amplified with exposures to traffic-related air pollutants.[113] Other sources of noise such as traffic on roads have also been observed to be associated with PTB risk.[114] Noise has been hypothesized to biologically increase stress.[115]

Other Environmental Exposures

Environmental-related exposures to various chemicals and risk of PTB have been explored. Elevated PTB risks associated with maternal exposures to lead have been observed. Exposures as measured in blood to lead and arsenic were recently observed to increase the risk of preeclampsia with inverse modifying influences from manganese.[116] Studies of exposures to polychlorinated biphenyls have generally not observed elevated PTB risks.[84]

Perfluoroalkyl and polyfluoroalkyl substances (PFAS) are extremely persistent chemicals in the environment based on their widespread usage to enable nonstick, waterproof, and stain-resistant coatings to a variety of consumer products, including cookware, food packaging, clothing, carpeting, cosmetics, and textiles. Exposures to these chemicals have been associated with shorter gestational length.[117,118]

Polycyclic aromatic hydrocarbons (PAHs), contaminants produced from combustion of fossil fuels and other sources, have been associated with an increased risk of PTB.[46,119]

Owing to their reproductive toxicity, endocrine disrupting chemicals have been investigated for possible increased PTB risk. Two broad chemical groupings most studied are phthalates and phenols. Interestingly, Chin and colleagues[120] observed that higher urinary concentrations of low molecular weight phthalates increased gestational length, whereas higher concentrations of higher molecular weight phthalates decreased gestational length. Recently, Zhang and colleagues[121] observed that combined levels as measured in urine of phthalates and phenols (bisphenol specifically) preconceptionally in both men and women were associated with an increased risk of PTB.

GENOMIC–ENVIRONMENT INTERACTIONS

Host susceptibility plays a role in PTB risk, evidenced, for example, by familial aggregation (mothers, sisters, and daughters share risks) and by variability across population subgroups and an individual's response to stressors and infections. Several genome-wide investigations have identified genetic variants that contribute to a modest proportion of the incidence of PTB. There are numerous gaps in our understanding of the genetic contributions to PTB — many of which have been nicely discussed by Jain and colleagues[122] One particular gap that will be important to fill is the need for more investigation of potential gene–environment interactions on risk of PTB. Such studies will better define possible at-risk loci as well as better define environmental exposure parameters that result in risk.

An overall pattern of results where various exposures, demographic factors, and genetic variants seem to insufficiently account for differences in disease risk, has led many to posit that individual *epigenetic* variability may underly etiology. DNA methylation is one of the most studied components of epigenesis. Variations in DNA methylation can be influenced by environmental exposures such as air pollutants, cigarette smoking, and stress associated with social context.[123–125]

Investigations have explored epigenetics and PTB.[122,126] In general, the extant literature indicates that findings are supportive for an association between epigenetics and PTB. Evidence of differential susceptibility to the air pollutants NO_2 and ozone via methylation changes (in placental and cord blood tissues) has been observed by Ladd-Acosta and colleagues.[125] Furthermore, an association has been reported between social support and alterations in DNA methylation on risk of PTB.[123] In their study population of the Boston Birth Cohort of 250 African American mothers, Surkan and colleagues[123] observed that the absence of support from the baby's father was associated with maternal DNA methylation changes in selected genes and a lack of support from family and friends was associated with maternal DNA hypermethylation on multiple genes. This study provides intriguing results suggesting biological embedding of social support during pregnancy on maternal DNA methylation. That group has also demonstrated an association between smoking during pregnancy, alterations in DNA methylation, and fetal development.[124]

Given that variations in DNA methylation can be altered by environmental exposures such as air pollution, individual behaviors, and social context, further investigation of these variations may reveal differences in PTB susceptibility. Such susceptibility may have resisted identification by studies that have simply examined exposures or genes alone, due to the lack of precision and accuracy of measurements and to unmeasured interactions between and within domains of exposure[127] indicated that studying epigenetic phenomena analytically can be informative for both in utero and transgenerational effects. Thus, it is known that epigenetic changes may be heritable as well as potentially reversible — with the former offering a possible explanation for observations from large epidemiologic studies that women are at higher risk for PTBs if they themselves were born preterm[128] and with the latter construct of reversibility offers opportunities for future prevention strategies.

FUTURE DIRECTIONS

As the above narrative shows, numerous studies have examined the role of single environmental exposures in influencing PTB risk, but few studies attempt to account for the complexities of multiple exposures — the exposome. Pregnant women are exposed to numerous environmental chemicals, psychosocial stressors, and variations in social constructs associated with the communities in which they live. A better understanding of the complexities of multiple exposures will facilitate etiologic discovery as well as provide evidence for policies and public health interventions.[129] Stingone and colleagues have suggested that to facilitate these efforts will require an interdisciplinary approach employing epidemiology, data science, and biomarker-based data collection that will combine to identify proximal biologic factors for PTB risk. As an illustration, being a race other than White, of lower SES, and residing in geographic areas with higher indices of social vulnerability have been associated with higher risks of PTB.[130] The cumulative impacts and potential interactions between elevated exposures to chemical and psychosocial stressors need to be explored further given that we have limited understanding of the extent to which prenatal exposures to environmental exposures and psychosocial stress act, independently and jointly, to contribute to PTB.

Factors that further modify the risks of the exposome will be important to explore in the future. Such factors can clearly include variations associated with the structural genome, epigenome, social stressors, and dietary factors. With respect to dietary influences on risk,[131] Eaves and Fry in their accompanying editorial of the study by Borghese and colleagues[116] where manganese was observed to inversely modify (antagonize) preeclampsia risk, suggested that dietary supplements that are known to contribute to detoxification pathways might be explored for their risk lowering impact. PTB risk associated with blood lead levels has been observed to be higher in women who also had lower blood levels of vitamin D.[132] Another recent example derives from Zhang and colleagues[117] in their study of adverse pregnancy outcomes and gestational exposures to perfluoroalkyl and PFAS, where they observed associations with earlier gestational age at delivery only among women whose prenatal dietary folate intake or plasma folate concentration was in the lowest quartile range. Low folate levels along with low intakes of low vitamins A, C, and E and carotene have been observed to modify the risk downward for PTB among women exposed to PAHs.[119] As Jardel and colleagues[133] recently observed, such studies have revealed a complex interplay between gestational diet and gestational timing of exposure to a particular air pollutant, on PTB risk, and therefore require substantial study populations to be informative.

PTB does not have a simple nor likely single etiology. PTB is a complex phenomenon and not well understood as a singular condition being defined only by the arbitrary dichotomy of birth of less than 37 completed weeks of gestation (vs $\geq$37 weeks).[6] This classification has been argued to be too simplistic for etiologic studies owing to the heterogeneity that has been observed with this outcome.[134] Indeed, finer phenotypic classifications have been suggested based on gestational timing such as less than 28 weeks, extremely preterm; 28 to 31 weeks, very preterm; and 32 to 36 weeks, moderately preterm weeks gestation,[135] or by sPTB versus medically indicated PTB. A very large proportion of the research between PTB and ambient environment has not fully considered these finer phenotypic definitions. There are indeed opportunities for substantial improvement going forward.

There is a growing understanding that PTB and other reproductive events have their etiologic roots in complex genomic–environment interactions. Thus, a concomitant consideration of biologic, genetic, behavioral, social, and our ambient environmental exposures as risk factors is fundamental to unraveling the complex etiologies of PTB.

DISCLOSURE

The authors have nothing to disclose.

Best Practices

What is the current practice for preterm birth?

There is no known best practice for the prevention for preterm birth.

What changes in current practice are likely to improve outcomes?

More studies on the complexities of exposures in the ambient environment will inform policy efforts to reduce potentially harmful exposures during pregnancy.

Bibliographic Sources

Stingone JA, Triantafillou S, Larsen A, et al. Interdisciplinary data science to advance environmental health research and improve birth outcomes. Environ Res 2021;197:111,019.

REFERENCES

1. Howson CP, Kinney MV, Lawn JE, editors. March of Dimes, PMNCH, Save the children, world health organization. Born too soon: the global action report on preterm birth. Geneva: World Health Organization; 2012.
2. Walani SR. Global burden of preterm birth. Int J Gynaecol Obstet 2020; 150(1):31–3.
3. Goldenberg RL, Culhane JF, Iams JD, et al. Epidemiology and causes of preterm birth. Lancet 2008;371(9606):75–84.
4. Frey HA, Klebanoff MA. The epidemiology, etiology, and costs of preterm birth. Semin Fetal Neonatal Med 2016;21(2):68–73.
5. Blondel B, Kogan MD, Alexander GR, et al. The impact of the increasing number of multiple births on the rates of preterm birth and low birthweight: an international study. Am J Publ Health 2002;92(8):1323–30.
6. Behrman R, Butler A. Institute of Medicine (US) Committee on Understanding Premature Birth and Assuring Healthy Outcomes. Preterm birth: causes, consequences, and prevention. Washington, DC: National Academies Press; 2007.
7. Braveman P, Dominguez TP, Burke W, et al. Explaining the Black-White disparity in preterm birth: a consensus statement from a multi-disciplinary scientific work group convened by the March of Dimes. Front Reprod Health 2021;3:684207.
8. Chantarat T, Van Riper DC, Hardeman RR. Multidimensional structural racism predicts birth outcomes for Black and White Minnesotans. Health Serv Res 2022;57(3):448–57.
9. Martin JA, Kung HC, Mathews TJ, et al. Annual summary of vital statistics: 2006. Pediatrics 2008;121(4):788–801.
10. Bailey ZD, Krieger N, Agenor M, et al. Structural racism and health inequities in the USA: evidence and interventions. Lancet 2017;389(10077):1453–63.
11. Clark R, Anderson NB, Clark VR, et al. Racism as a stressor for African Americans. A biopsychosocial model. Am Psychol 1999;54(10):805–16.
12. Howe CJ, Bailey ZD, Raifman JR, et al. Recommendations for using causal diagrams to study racial health disparities. Am J Epidemiol 2022;191(12):1981–9.

13. Murphy DJ. Epidemiology and environmental factors in preterm labour. Best Pract Res Clin Obstet Gynaecol 2007;21(5):773–89.

14. Shaw GM, Mayo JA, Eisenberg ML, et al. Male-to-female ratios, race/ethnicity, and spontaneous preterm birth among 11 million California infants. Am J Perinatol 2021;38(7):683–9.

15. Prasad M, Jones M. Medical complications of opioid use disorder in pregnancy. Semin Perinatol 2019;43(3):162–7.

16. Gorman MC, Orme KS, Nguyen NT, et al. Outcomes in pregnancies complicated by methamphetamine use. Am J Obstet Gynecol 2014;211(4):429 e1–e7.

17. Hayatbakhsh MR, Flenady VJ, Gibbons KS, et al. Birth outcomes associated with cannabis use before and during pregnancy. Pediatr Res 2012;71(2):215–9.

18. Kibret KT, Chojenta C, Gresham E, et al. Maternal dietary patterns and risk of adverse pregnancy (hypertensive disorders of pregnancy and gestational diabetes mellitus) and birth (preterm birth and low birth weight) outcomes: a systematic review and meta-analysis. Public Health Nutr 2018;22(3):1–15.

19. Best KP, Gomersall J, Makrides M. Prenatal nutritional strategies to reduce the risk of preterm birth. Ann Nutr Metab 2020;76(Suppl 3):31–9.

20. Cui Y, Liao M, Xu A, et al. Association of maternal pre-pregnancy dietary intake with adverse maternal and neonatal outcomes: a systematic review and meta-analysis of prospective studies. Crit Rev Food Sci Nutr 2023;63(19):3430–51.

21. Li B, Zhang X, Peng X, et al. Folic acid and risk of preterm birth: a meta-analysis. Front Neurosci 2019;13:1284.

22. Wu Y, Wang J, Wei Y, et al. Maternal exposure to endocrine disrupting chemicals (EDCs) and preterm birth: a systematic review, meta-analysis, and meta-regression analysis. Environ Pollut 2022;292(Pt A):118264.

23. Dunlop AL, Kramer MR, Hogue CJ, et al. Racial disparities in preterm birth: an overview of the potential role of nutrient deficiencies. Acta Obstet Gynecol Scand 2011;90(12):1332–41.

24. Kramer MS, Kahn SR, Platt RW, et al. Antioxidant vitamins, long-chain fatty acids, and spontaneous preterm birth. Epidemiology 2009;20(5):707–13.

25. Myhre R, Brantsaeter AL, Myking S, et al. Intake of probiotic food and risk of spontaneous preterm delivery. Am J Clin Nutr 2011;93(1):151–7.

26. Cnattingius S, Villamor E, Johansson S, et al. Maternal obesity and risk of preterm delivery. JAMA 2013;309(22):2362–70.

27. Mayo JA, Stevenson DK, Shaw GM. Population-based associations between maternal pre-pregnancy body mass index and spontaneous and medically indicated preterm birth using restricted cubic splines in California. Ann Epidemiol 2022;72:65–73.

28. Shaw GM, Wise PH, Mayo J, et al. Maternal prepregnancy body mass index and risk of spontaneous preterm birth. Paediatr Perinat Epidemiol 2014;28(4):302–11.

29. Chu SY, Kim SY, Lau J, et al. Maternal obesity and risk of stillbirth: a metaanalysis. Am J Obstet Gynecol 2007;197(3):223–8.

30. Liang R, Panelli DM, Stevenson DK, et al. Associations between pregnancy glucose measurements and risk of preterm birth: a retrospective cohort study of commercially insured women in the United States from 2003 to 2021. Ann Epidemiol 2023;81:31–39 e19.

31. Marinovich ML, Regan AK, Gissler M, et al. Associations between interpregnancy interval and preterm birth by previous preterm birth status in four high-income countries: a cohort study. BJOG 2021;128(7):1134–43.

32. Shachar BZ, Mayo JA, Lyell DJ, et al. Interpregnancy interval after live birth or pregnancy termination and estimated risk of preterm birth: a retrospective cohort study. BJOG 2016;123(12):2009–17.

33. Tessema GA, Marinovich ML, Haberg SE, et al. Interpregnancy intervals and adverse birth outcomes in high-income countries: an international cohort study. PLoS One 2021;16(7):e0255000.

34. Lonhart JA, Mayo JA, Padula AM, et al. Short interpregnancy interval as a risk factor for preterm birth in non-Hispanic Black and White women in California. J Perinatol 2019;39(9):1175–81.

35. Klebanoff MA. Interpregnancy interval and pregnancy outcomes: causal or not? Obstet Gynecol 2017;129(3):405–7.

36. Tanigawa K, Ikehara S, Cui M, et al. Association between interpregnancy interval and risk of preterm birth and its modification by folate intake: the Japan Environment and Children's Study. J Epidemiol 2023;33(3):113–9.

37. Costello EK, DiGiulio DB, Robaczewska A, et al. Abrupt perturbation and delayed recovery of the vaginal ecosystem following childbirth. Nat Commun 2023;14(1):4141.

38. Dunkel Schetter C. Psychological science on pregnancy: stress processes, biopsychosocial models, and emerging research issues. Annu Rev Psychol 2011; 62:531–58.

39. Holzman C, Senagore P, Tian Y, et al. Maternal catecholamine levels in midpregnancy and risk of preterm delivery. Am J Epidemiol 2009;170(8):1014–24.

40. Kramer MS, Lydon J, Seguin L, et al. Stress pathways to spontaneous preterm birth: the role of stressors, psychological distress, and stress hormones. Am J Epidemiol 2009;169(11):1319–26.

41. Becker M, Mayo JA, Phogat NK, et al. Deleterious and protective psychosocial and stress-related factors predict risk of spontaneous preterm birth. Am J Perinatol 2023;40(1):74–88.

42. Corchero-Falcon MDR, Gomez-Salgado J, Garcia-Iglesias JJ, et al. Risk factors for working pregnant women and potential adverse consequences of exposure: a systematic review. Int J Public Health 2023;68:1605655.

43. Ghosh R, Causey K, Burkart K, et al. Ambient and household PM2.5 pollution and adverse perinatal outcomes: a meta-regression and analysis of attributable global burden for 204 countries and territories. PLoS Med 2021;18(9):e1003718.

44. Bekkar B, Pacheco S, Basu R, et al. Association of air pollution and heat exposure with preterm birth, low birth weight, and stillbirth in the US: a systematic review. JAMA Netw Open 2020;3(6):e208243.

45. Liu XX, Fan SJ, Luo YN, et al. Global, regional, and national burden of preterm birth attributable to ambient and household PM(2.5) from 1990 to 2019: worsening or improving? Sci Total Environ 2023;871:161975.

46. Padula AM, Noth EM, Hammond SK, et al. Exposure to airborne polycyclic aromatic hydrocarbons during pregnancy and risk of preterm birth. Environ Res 2014;135:221–6.

47. Mekonnen A, Alemnew W, Abebe Z, et al. Adherence to iron with folic acid supplementation among pregnant women attending antenatal care in public health centers in Simada District, Northwest Ethiopia: using health belief model perspective. Patient Prefer Adherence 2021;15:843–51.

48. Amjad S, Chojecki D, Osornio-Vargas A, et al. Wildfire exposure during pregnancy and the risk of adverse birth outcomes: a systematic review. Environ Int 2021;156:106644.

49. Abdo M, Ward I, O'Dell K, et al. Impact of wildfire smoke on adverse pregnancy outcomes in Colorado, 2007-2015. Int J Environ Res Publ Health 2019;16(19): 3720.

50. Heft-Neal S, Driscoll A, Yang W, et al. Associations between wildfire smoke exposure during pregnancy and risk of preterm birth in California. Environ Res 2022;203:111872.

51. Requia WJ, Kill E, Papatheodorou S, et al. Prenatal exposure to wildfire-related air pollution and birth defects in Brazil. J Expo Sci Environ Epidemiol 2022;32(4): 596–603.

52. O'Donnell MH, Behie AM. Effects of wildfire disaster exposure on male birth weight in an Australian population. Evol Med Public Health 2015;2015(1): 344–54.

53. Verstraeten BSE, Elgbeili G, Hyde A, et al. Maternal mental health after a wildfire: effects of social support in the Fort McMurray Wood Buffalo Study. Can J Psychiatr 2021;66(8):710–8.

54. Weber KA, Yang W, Carmichael SL, et al. Assessing associations between residential proximity to greenspace and birth defects in the National Birth Defects Prevention Study. Environ Res 2023;216(Pt 3):114760.

55. Cusack L, Larkin A, Carozza S, et al. Associations between residential greenness and birth outcomes across Texas. Environ Res 2017;152:88–95.

56. Sun Y, Sheridan P, Laurent O, et al. Associations between green space and preterm birth: windows of susceptibility and interaction with air pollution. Environ Int 2020;142:105804.

57. Laurent O, Wu J, Li L, et al. Green spaces and pregnancy outcomes in Southern California. Health Place 2013;24:190–5.

58. Glazer KB, Eliot MN, Danilack VA, et al. Residential green space and birth outcomes in a coastal setting. Environ Res 2018;163:97–107.

59. Casey JA, James P, Rudolph KE, et al. Greenness and birth outcomes in a range of Pennsylvania communities. Int J Environ Res Publ Health 2016; 13(3):311.

60. Hystad P, Davies HW, Frank L, et al. Residential greenness and birth outcomes: evaluating the influence of spatially correlated built-environment factors. Environ Health Perspect 2014;122(10):1095–102.

61. Dalugoda Y, Kuppa J, Phung H, et al. Effect of elevated ambient temperature on maternal, foetal, and neonatal outcomes: a scoping review. Int J Environ Res Publ Health 2022;19(3):1771.

62. Son JY, Choi HM, Miranda ML, et al. Exposure to heat during pregnancy and preterm birth in North Carolina: main effect and disparities by residential greenness, urbanicity, and socioeconomic status. Environ Res 2022;204(Pt C): 112315.

63. Wang Q, Yin L, Wu H, et al. Effects of gestational ambient extreme temperature exposures on the risk of preterm birth in China: a sibling-matched study based on a multi-center prospective cohort. Sci Total Environ 2023;887:164135.

64. Czolowski ED, Santoro RL, Srebotnjak T, et al. Toward consistent methodology to quantify populations in proximity to oil and gas development: a National Spatial Analysis and Review. Environ Health Perspect 2017;125(8):086004.

65. Cushing LJ, Vavra-Musser K, Chau K, et al. Flaring from unconventional oil and gas development and birth outcomes in the Eagle Ford Shale in South Texas. Environ Health Perspect 2020;128(7):77003.

66. Erickson CL, Barron IG, Zapata I. The effects of hydraulic fracturing activities on birth outcomes are evident in a non-individualized county-wide aggregate data sample from Colorado. J Public Health Res 2021;11(1):2551.

67. Gonzalez DJX, Sherris AR, Yang W, et al. Oil and gas production and spontaneous preterm birth in the San Joaquin Valley, CA: a case-control study. Environ Epidemiol 2020;4(4):e099.

68. Hill EL. Shale gas development and infant health: evidence from Pennsylvania. J Health Econ 2018;61:134–50.

69. McKenzie LM, Guo R, Witter RZ, et al. Birth outcomes and maternal residential proximity to natural gas development in rural Colorado. Environ Health Perspect 2014;122(4):412–7.

70. Tran KV, Casey JA, Cushing LJ, et al. Residential proximity to oil and gas development and birth outcomes in California: a retrospective cohort study of 2006-2015 births. Environ Health Perspect 2020;128(6):67001.

71. Tran KV, Casey JA, Cushing LJ, et al. Residential proximity to hydraulically fractured oil and gas wells and adverse birth outcomes in urban and rural communities in California (2006-2015). Environ Epidemiol 2021;5(6):e172.

72. Walker Whitworth K, Kaye Marshall A, Symanski E. Drilling and production activity related to unconventional gas development and severity of preterm birth. Environ Health Perspect 2018;126(3):037006.

73. Whitworth KW, Marshall AK, Symanski E. Maternal residential proximity to unconventional gas development and perinatal outcomes among a diverse urban population in Texas. PLoS One 2017;12(7):e0180966.

74. Stacy SL, Brink LL, Larkin JC, et al. Perinatal outcomes and unconventional natural gas operations in Southwest Pennsylvania. PLoS One 2015;10(6): e0126425.

75. Adgate JL, Goldstein BD, McKenzie LM. Potential public health hazards, exposures and health effects from unconventional natural gas development. Environ Sci Technol 2014;48(15):8307–20.

76. Gonzalez DJX, Francis CK, Shaw GM, et al. Upstream oil and gas production and ambient air pollution in California. Sci Total Environ 2022;806(Pt 1):150298.

77. Deziel NC, Clark CJ, Casey JA, et al. Assessing exposure to unconventional oil and gas development: strengths, challenges, and implications for epidemiologic research. Curr Environ Health Rep 2022;9(3):436–50.

78. Cairncross ZF, Couloigner I, Ryan MC, et al. Association between residential proximity to hydraulic fracturing sites and adverse birth outcomes. JAMA Pediatr 2022;176(6):585–92.

79. Caron-Beaudoin E, Whyte KP, Bouchard MF, et al. Volatile organic compounds (VOCs) in indoor air and tap water samples in residences of pregnant women living in an area of unconventional natural gas operations: findings from the EXPERIVA study. Sci Total Environ 2022;805:150242.

80. Shepherd TH. Catalog of teratogenic agents (Shepherd's Catalog) last updated through Micromedex 2009. 8th edition. Baltimore: John Hopkins University Press; 1995.

81. Acosta-Maldonado B, Sanchez-Ramirez B, Reza-Lopez S, et al. Effects of exposure to pesticides during pregnancy on placental maturity and weight of newborns: a cross-sectional pilot study in women from the Chihuahua State, Mexico. Hum Exp Toxicol 2009;28(8):451–9.

82. Pathak R, Suke SG, Ahmed T, et al. Organochlorine pesticide residue levels and oxidative stress in preterm delivery cases. Hum Exp Toxicol 2010;29(5):351–8.

83. Windham GC, Lee D, Mitchell P, et al. Exposure to organochlorine compounds and effects on ovarian function. Epidemiology 2005;16(2):182–90.

84. Wigle DT, Arbuckle TE, Turner MC, et al. Epidemiologic evidence of relationships between reproductive and child health outcomes and environmental chemical contaminants. J Toxicol Environ Health B Crit Rev 2008;11(5–6): 373–517.

85. Shirangi A, Nieuwenhuijsen M, Vienneau D, et al. Living near agricultural pesticide applications and the risk of adverse reproductive outcomes: a review of the literature. Paediatr Perinat Epidemiol 2011;25(2):172–91.

86. Rinsky JL, Hopenhayn C, Golla V, et al. Atrazine exposure in public drinking water and preterm birth. Publ Health Rep 2012;127(1):72–80.

87. Harley KG, Huen K, Aguilar Schall R, et al. Association of organophosphate pesticide exposure and paraoxonase with birth outcome in Mexican-American women. PLoS One 2011;6(8):e23923.

88. Stillerman KP, Mattison DR, Giudice LC, et al. Environmental exposures and adverse pregnancy outcomes: a review of the science. Reprod Sci 2008; 15(7):631–50.

89. Willis WO, de Peyster A, Molgaard CA, et al. Pregnancy outcome among women exposed to pesticides through work or residence in an agricultural area. J Occup Med 1993;35(9):943–9.

90. Longnecker MP, Klebanoff MA, Zhou H, et al. Association between maternal serum concentration of the DDT metabolite DDE and preterm and small-for-gestational-age babies at birth. Lancet 2001;358(9276):110–4.

91. Kadhel P, Monfort C, Costet N, et al. Chlordecone exposure, length of gestation, and risk of preterm birth. Am J Epidemiol 2014;179(5):536–44.

92. Winchester P, Proctor C, Ying J. County-level pesticide use and risk of shortened gestation and preterm birth. Acta Paediatr 2016;105(3):e107–15.

93. Shaw GM, Yang W, Roberts EM, et al. Residential agricultural pesticide exposures and risks of spontaneous preterm birth. Epidemiology 2018;29(1):8–21.

94. Shaw GM, Yang W, Roberts EM, et al. Residential agricultural pesticide exposures and risks of preeclampsia. Environ Res 2018;164:546–55.

95. Ferguson KK, Chin HB. Environmental chemicals and preterm birth: biological mechanisms and the state of the science. Curr Epidemiol Rep 2017;4(1):56–71.

96. Currie J, Zivin JG, Meckel K, et al. Something in the water: contaminated drinking water and infant health. Can J Econ 2013;46(3):791–810.

97. Sharma S, Bhattacharya AJ. Drinking water contamination and treatment techniques. Appl Water Sci 2017;7(3):1043–67.

98. Capdeville MJ, Budzinski H. Trace-level analysis of organic contaminants in drinking waters and groundwaters. TrAC, Trends Anal Chem 2011;30(4): 586–606.

99. Ochoa-Acuna H, Frankenberger J, Hahn L, et al. Drinking-water herbicide exposure in Indiana and prevalence of small-for-gestational-age and preterm delivery. Environ Health Perspect 2009;117(10):1619–24.

100. Kumar S, Forand S, Babcock G, et al. Total trihalomethanes in public drinking water supply and birth outcomes: a cross-sectional study. Matern Child Health J 2014;18(4):996–1006.

101. Tardiff RG, Carson ML, Ginevan ME. Updated weight of evidence for an association between adverse reproductive and developmental effects and exposure to disinfection by-products. Regul Toxicol Pharmacol 2006;45(2):185–205.

102. Huang H, Woodruff TJ, Baer RJ, et al. Investigation of association between environmental and socioeconomic factors and preterm birth in California. Environ Int 2018;121(Pt 2):1066–78.

103. Lin L, St Clair S, Gamble GD, et al. Nitrate contamination in drinking water and adverse reproductive and birth outcomes: a systematic review and meta-analysis. Sci Rep 2023;13(1):563.

104. Young HA, Kolivras KN, Krometis LH, et al. Examining the association between safe drinking water act violations and adverse birth outcomes in Virginia. Environ Res 2023;218:114977.

105. Sherris AR, Baiocchi M, Fendorf S, et al. Nitrate in drinking water during pregnancy and spontaneous preterm birth: a retrospective within-mother analysis in California. Environ Health Perspect 2021;129(5):57001.

106. Coffman VR, Jensen AS, Trabjerg BB, et al. Prenatal exposure to nitrate from drinking water and markers of fetal growth restriction: a population-based study of nearly one million Danish-born children. Environ Health Perspect 2021;129(2): 27002.

107. Padula AM, Huang H, Baer RJ, et al. Environmental pollution and social factors as contributors to preterm birth in Fresno County. Environ Health 2018;17(1):70.

108. Lin MC, Chiu HF, Yu HS, et al. Increased risk of preterm delivery in areas with air pollution from a petroleum refinery plant in Taiwan. J Toxicol Environ Health 2001;64(8):637–44.

109. Tsai SS, Yu HS, Liu CC, et al. Increased incidence of preterm delivery in mothers residing in an industrialized area in Taiwan. J Toxicol Environ Health 2003; 66(11):987–94.

110. Yang CY, Chang CC, Tsai SS, et al. Preterm delivery among people living around Portland cement plants. Environ Res 2003;92(1):64–8.

111. Tsai SS, Yu HS, Chang CC, et al. Increased risk of preterm delivery in women residing near thermal power plants in Taiwan. Arch Environ Health 2004;59(9): 478–83.

112. Mendrinos A, Ramesh B, Ruktanonchai CW, et al. Poultry concentrated animal-feeding operations on the Eastern Shore, Virginia, and geospatial associations with adverse birth outcomes. Healthcare (Basel) 2022;10(10):2016.

113. Wing SE, Larson TV, Hudda N, et al. Aircraft noise and vehicle traffic-related air pollution interact to affect preterm birth risk in Los Angeles, California. Sci Total Environ 2022;829:154678.

114. Sun J, Yang R, Xian H, et al. Association between maternal family history of hypertension and preterm birth: modification by noise exposure and multivitamin intake. J Matern Fetal Neonatal Med 2022;35(26):10458–65.

115. Basner M, Babisch W, Davis A, et al. Auditory and non-auditory effects of noise on health. Lancet 2014;383(9925):1325–32.

116. Borghese MM, Fisher M, Ashley-Martin J, et al. Individual, independent, and joint associations of toxic metals and manganese on hypertensive disorders of pregnancy: results from the MIREC Canadian pregnancy cohort. Environ Health Perspect 2023;131(4):47014.

117. Zhang Y, Mustieles V, Sun Q, et al. Association of early pregnancy perfluoroalkyl and polyfluoroalkyl substance exposure with birth outcomes. JAMA Netw Open 2023;6(5):e2314934.

118. Meng Q, Inoue K, Ritz B, et al. Prenatal exposure to perfluoroalkyl substances and birth outcomes; an updated analysis from the Danish National Birth Cohort. Int J Environ Res Publ Health 2018;15(9):1832.

119. Zhao N, Wu W, Cui S, et al. Effects of benzo[a]pyrene-DNA adducts, dietary vitamins, folate, and carotene intakes on preterm birth: a nested case-control study from the birth cohort in China. Environ Health 2022;21(1):48.

120. Chin HB, Jukic AM, Wilcox AJ, et al. Association of urinary concentrations of early pregnancy phthalate metabolites and bisphenol A with length of gestation. Environ Health 2019;18(1):80.

121. Zhang Y, Mustieles V, Williams PL, et al. Parental preconception exposure to phenol and phthalate mixtures and the risk of preterm birth. Environ Int 2021; 151:106440.

122. Jain VG, Monangi N, Zhang G, et al. Genetics, epigenetics, and transcriptomics of preterm birth. Am J Reprod Immunol 2022;88(4):e13600.

123. Surkan PJ, Hong X, Zhang B, et al. Can social support during pregnancy affect maternal DNA methylation? Findings from a cohort of African-Americans. Pediatr Res 2020;88(1):131–8.

124. Xu R, Hong X, Zhang B, et al. DNA methylation mediates the effect of maternal smoking on offspring birthweight: a birth cohort study of multi-ethnic US mother-newborn pairs. Clin Epigenet 2021;13(1):47.

125. Ladd-Acosta C, Feinberg JI, Brown SC, et al. Epigenetic marks of prenatal air pollution exposure found in multiple tissues relevant for child health. Environ Int 2019;126:363–76.

126. Park B, Khanam R, Vinayachandran V, et al. Epigenetic biomarkers and preterm birth. Environ Epigenet 2020;6(1):dvaa005.

127. Saenen ND, Martens DS, Neven KY, et al. Air pollution-induced placental alterations: an interplay of oxidative stress, epigenetics, and the aging phenotype? Clin Epigenet 2019;11(1):124.

128. Klebanoff MA, Schulsinger C, Mednick BR, et al. Preterm and small-for-gestational-age birth across generations. Am J Obstet Gynecol 1997;176(3): 521–6.

129. Stingone JA, Triantafillou S, Larsen A, et al. Interdisciplinary data science to advance environmental health research and improve birth outcomes. Environ Res 2021;197:111019.

130. Givens M, Teal EN, Patel V, et al. Preterm birth among pregnant women living in areas with high social vulnerability. Am J Obstet Gynecol MFM 2021;3(5): 100414.

131. Eaves LA, Fry RC. Invited perspective: toxic metals and hypertensive disorders of pregnancy. Environ Health Perspect 2023;131(4):41303.

132. Fisher M, Marro L, Arbuckle TE, et al. Association between toxic metals, vitamin D and preterm birth in the maternal-infant research on environmental chemicals study. Paediatr Perinat Epidemiol 2023;37(5):447–57.

133. Jardel H, Martin CL, Hoyo C, et al. Interplay of gestational parent exposure to ambient air pollution and diet characteristics on preterm birth. BMC Publ Health 2023;23(1):822.

134. Zhang J, Savitz DA. Duration of Gestation and Timing of Birth. New York: Oxford University Press; 2011.

135. McElrath TF, Hecht JL, Dammann O, et al. Pregnancy disorders that lead to delivery before the 28th week of gestation: an epidemiologic approach to classification. Am J Epidemiol 2008;168(9):980–9.

Predicting Preterm Birth Using Cell-Free Ribonucleic Acid

Alison D. Cowan, MD, MSCR[a],*, Morten Rasmussen, PhD[b],
Maneesh Jain, PhD[c], Rachel M. Tribe, PhD[d]

KEYWORDS

- Cell-free RNA • Transcriptomics • Screening model • Etiology
- Spontaneous preterm birth • Preterm prelabor rupture of membranes
- Cervical insufficiency

KEY POINTS

- Spontaneous preterm birth (sPTB) is the leading cause of perinatal mortality.
- Interventions for the primary prevention of sPTB are limited today, in part because the underlying causes of sPTB are inadequately understood.
- Cell-free ribonucleic acid is dynamic and may reflect both cell turnover and gene expression; as such, it may provide insights into the underlying pathophysiology of sPTB.

INTRODUCTION

Preterm birth (PTB) is the leading cause of perinatal mortality in the United States and globally, impacting an estimated 14 million pregnancies annually and leading to an estimated 900,000 deaths per year.[1] An estimated 70% of PTBs are spontaneous and are preceded by either preterm labor (PTL) or preterm prelabor rupture of membranes (PPROM).[2] PTB rates vary by region and country, and the United States accounted for an estimated 10.4% in 2022.[3]

Given the burden of the disease in the United States and globally, substantial resources have been devoted to a better understanding of its underlying causes and potential strategies for its prevention. Despite these efforts, the overall PTB rate has remained stagnant globally in recent years.[1] In addition, 1 of the only prophylactic

[a] Department of Medical Affairs, Mirvie, Inc., 651 Gateway Boulevard, Suite 1200, South San Francisco, CA 94080, USA; [b] Department of Research and Development, Mirvie, Inc., 651 Gateway Boulevard, Suite 1200, South San Francisco, CA 94080, USA; [c] Mirvie, Inc., 651 Gateway Boulevard, Suite 1200, South San Francisco, CA 94080, USA; [d] Department of Women and Children's Health, School of Life Course and Population Sciences, King's College London, St. Thomas's Hospital Campus, Westminster Bridge Road, London SE1 7EH, UK
* Corresponding author. 651 Gateway Boulevard, Suite 1200, South San Francisco, CA 94080.
E-mail address: research@mirvie.com

Clin Perinatol 51 (2024) 379–389
https://doi.org/10.1016/j.clp.2024.02.008
0095-5108/24/© 2024 Elsevier Inc. All rights reserved.

interventions for spontaneous PTB (sPTB), 17-hydroxyprogesterone, was removed from the market in the United States after follow-up data showed a lack of efficacy in preventing sPTB, leaving vaginal progesterone as the sole pharmacologic intervention available.[4]

Indeed, efforts to develop novel effective interventions to prevent sPTB have been hampered by a limited ability to predict it early enough in pregnancy and distinguish between its subtypes. While there have been familial and genetic associations identified for sPTB,[5,6] its underlying causes are multifactorial and remain incompletely understood, with environmental and other factors appearing to play significant roles. sPTB is associated with a variety of clinical, demographic, and environmental risk factors including prior PTB, multifetal pregnancies, race, nutrition, and smoking. In addition, it has also been associated with factors related to inflammation, including gingivitis and subclinical as well as clinically recognized infection.[2] Among the clinical risk factors, a prior history of sPTB is most strongly associated with sPTB, with an approximately 2.5-fold increase in risk.[7] However, the majority of sPTBs occur in individuals without identifiable risk factors, and conversely, many individuals who appear to have risk factors nevertheless go on to deliver at term.[8] Thus, without more effective strategies to predict sPTB, many individuals who might stand to benefit from preventive measures are not identified. Similarly, many individuals who are identified as being at risk for sPTB experience unnecessary and potentially harmful interventions, such as bed rest and steroid administration.[8]

Attempts at effective prediction of sPTB have, unfortunately, seen mixed results to date. Cervical length (CL) remains the most predictive clinical metric, with an inverse relationship observed between CL and sPTB.[9] However, it is not sufficiently clinically predictive as a screening tool, failing to identify many who go on to deliver preterm and likewise identifying many "at risk" individuals who go on to have term deliveries.[9] Quantitative fetal fibronectin (fFN) has been evaluated as a potential biomarker both alone and in combination with CL and is used in the United Kingdom and Europe via the QUiPP app to risk-stratify high-risk asymptomatic individuals and those with threatened PTL,[10] but is not available in the United States. CL measurements alone can also be used with QUiPP and may be useful for clinical management of the same conditions. However, there remains a significant unmet need in the prediction of sPTB for asymptomatic individuals who lack preexisting obstetric risk factors.

Thus, novel approaches to better understand this complex and heterogeneous process are urgently needed. In recent years, cell-free ribonucleic acid (cfRNA) of the entire transcriptome has emerged as a promising new technology to aid in the identification of individuals at risk for sPTB. As in the case of cell-free deoxyribonucleic acid (cfDNA) in pregnancy, detectable fragments of cfRNA exist in maternal plasma that originate from the fetus, placenta, and the pregnant individual (**Fig. 1**). To date, cfRNA from maternal whole blood and plasma has demonstrated its potential uses across a variety of antenatal conditions. In evaluating normal pregnancies, cfRNA signatures have shown predictable patterns across gestation that correlate to known periods in fetal organogenesis.[11–13] These predictable observations have enabled the estimation of gestational age based on cfRNA expression that is comparable in accuracy to second-trimester ultrasound.[11,13] In addition, cfRNA expression patterns have been shown to predict preeclampsia and fetal growth restriction.[11,14–16]

In contrast to the static nature of fetal cfDNA (helpful in the screening for fetal aneuploidy), cfRNA expression is dynamic and may reflect both cell turnover and gene expression at a given point in time.[17] Thus, cfRNA may be uniquely suited to assessing heterogeneous and dynamic conditions such as sPTB. Here, the authors review the available evidence for the prediction of sPTB using cfRNA, and assess the current state of the evidence, challenges, and future directions.

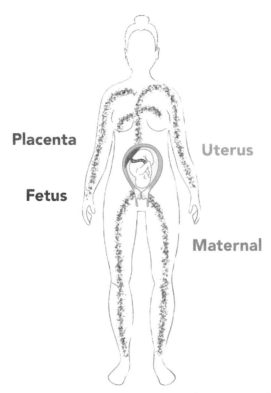

Fig. 1. Circulating cell-free RNA can originate from the fetus, uterus, placenta, and other maternal sources.

DISCUSSION

Prediction of sPTB can be thought of in at least 2 clinically relevant categories: the first relates to prediction of sPTB when individuals are already symptomatic; and the second relates to prediction of sPTB in asymptomatic patients, preferably early in pregnancy, as this would enable improved surveillance and potentially therapeutic interventions in pregnancies identified as at risk.

The first group of symptomatic individuals, that is, those with "threatened" PTL, is clinically relevant because patients often present with symptoms of PTL, yet it can be difficult to clinically distinguish between true PTL and threatened labor that is not destined to result in imminent or preterm delivery. Improved methods to distinguish between these outcomes in symptomatic individuals could aid in the decision-making related to the provision of steroids and tocolytics, an important question of timing given the limited window of benefit that has been demonstrated for fetuses exposed to steroids for anticipated preterm delivery and the fact that steroid administration is limited to a maximum of 2 courses in clinical practice.[18]

CELL-FREE RIBONUCLEIC ACID AND SPONTANEOUS PRETERM BIRTH IN THREATENED PRETERM LABOR: INFLAMMATORY AND IMMUNE PATHWAYS PREDOMINATE

Several investigators have evaluated whether there are appreciable differences in the pregnancy transcriptomes detectable in maternal blood, in addition to other tissues including placental tissue, chorion, amnion, decidua, cord blood, and myometrium, in order to gain insights into the pathophysiology of sPTB as compared with a term delivery. Chim and colleagues[19] investigated the placentas of 10 pregnancies complicated by sPTB compared to 10 spontaneous term deliveries to identify 36 transcripts that were differentially expressed in individuals with sPTB. Using that information, the investigators noted pathways involving ribonucleic acid (RNA) stabilization, extracellular matrix binding, and the acute inflammatory response were all altered in pregnancies complicated by sPTB. They further postulated that genes that would be upregulated and expressed more than *PLAC4*, a placental gene that was known to be detectable in maternal plasma, may be detectable in maternal plasma, and they found that *1LRL1* messenger RNA (mRNA) was detected in 6/10 women with spontaneous preterm labor (sPTL) who delivered preterm, and only in 1 of 27 samples at matched gestational weeks collected from women without PTL. As *1LRL1* is implicated in inflammatory pathways, this lends some support to the notion that sPTB is an inflammatory process, albeit with a limited sample size.

Similarly, Bukowski and colleagues[20] investigated a group undergoing cesarean delivery in 4 clinical scenarios in order to better elucidate the transcriptomics signature for sPTL. They evaluated women experiencing sPTL (n = 8), non-labor PTB (n = 10), term labor (n = 7), and term without labor (n = 10), with the preterm pregnancies ranging from 24 to 34 weeks and term pregnancies ranging from 39 to 41^{+6} weeks of gestation. The investigators evaluated transcriptomics data from a variety of sample types, including maternal whole blood, chorion, amnion, placenta, decidua, fetal blood, and myometrium from both the fundus and lower uterine segments, finding that the largest differences in expression were observed in decidua, chorion, and amnion, with progressively lower expression differences for other tissues, the lowest being for maternal blood. Differentially expressed transcripts demonstrated enrichment in genes involved in infection, inflammation, and immune response, with the investigators postulating that normal term pregnancy is characterized by the suppression of chemokines and cytokines, and that with the onset of labor, withdrawal of chemokine suppression leads to term labor, with PTL characterized by activation of multiple pathways in the immune system. However, despite these insights, predictive capability based on the differential gene expression observed in these 4 groups did not perform well in distinguishing between the 4 clinical groups, with only 42% of patients correctly classified overall.

Additional studies in symptomatic patients have similarly identified perturbations in pathways related to inflammation and immune response. Heng and colleagues[21] identified disruptions in cytokine and cytokine-related/chemokine-related genes and their related transcriptional factors in patients with threatened PTL who went on to have an sPTB within 48 hours (n = 48) compared with those who did not, along with pathways related to metabolic processes, response to stress, and signal transduction. They created a genes-only model that performed modestly, with an area under the curve (AUC) of 0.733, demonstrating improvement with the addition of clinical factors and fFN to 0.926, reporting a sensitivity of 91.7% and a specificity of 88.0%. Notably, 27 of 106 controls nevertheless went on to have a preterm delivery which was greater than 48 hours from presentation.

Paquette and colleagues[22] evaluated maternal whole blood transcriptome in symptomatic patients with threatened PTL and sPTB at 24 to 34 weeks (n = 20), and compared them to estimated gestational age (EGA)–matched term-delivery controls (n = 30), evaluating genes demonstrating differential expression in both whole blood and peripheral monocytes, finding 39 positively associated with sPTB, many of which were associated with inflammation, including *CXCL3, CXCL8, IL1B, IL18 R,* and *IL1R2.* *ADAMTS2,* a gene for a matrix metalloproteinase involved in blood vessel homeostasis, placental angiogenesis, and "reproductive diseases" was identified as the most differentially expressed gene, suggesting potential additional pathways involved in addition to inflammation.

CELL-FREE RIBONUCLEIC ACID, PRETERM PRELABOR RUPTURE OF MEMBRANES, AND PREDICTION OF CHORIOAMNIONITIS

While the identification of threatened PTL destined to result in sPTB is 1 important clinical need, also of interest is an assessment to determine which women presenting with PPROM are most likely to have concomitant chorioamnionitis. Clinicians lack a sensitive, noninvasive, and specific tool to identify individuals at highest risk of infection, relying on maternal fever and additional clinical factors to guide the presumptive diagnosis of suspected intraamniotic infection, which generally can only be confirmed after delivery.[23,24] Often, by the time chorioamnionitis is clinically evident, substantial maternal and fetal morbidity have already occurred. Thus, given that PPROM poses a scenario in which expectant management up to 36 weeks' gestation may be undertaken in appropriate circumstances, it would be helpful to better discern which patients are most likely to develop chorioamnionitis, as suspected intraamniotic infection is an indication for delivery.[25]

One study undertook a targeted investigation of genes identified in maternal blood based on those previously reported to be differentially expressed in PPROM, chorioamnionitis, and sPTB, and also performed a larger polymerase chain reaction (PCR) array for inflammatory cytokines, identifying 1 gene, *IL1B,* that was differentially expressed in individuals with PPROM and chorioamnionitis versus those without, and validated in a population confirming increased expression in patients with chorioamnionitis and PPROM compared with controls.[26] This study provides intriguing early evidence that there may be detectable cfRNA in blood indicative of chorioamnionitis, which could one day have potential clinical application in noninvasively assessing the risk for intraamniotic infection if validated in future studies.

CELL-FREE RIBONUCLEIC ACID FOR THE PREDICTION OF SPONTANEOUS PRETERM BIRTH IN ASYMPTOMATIC INDIVIDUALS: MULTIPLE POTENTIAL PATHWAYS IDENTIFIED

In addition to the evaluation of symptomatic individuals, clinicians have long sought a predictor of PTB in asymptomatic individuals, particularly for women who have no apparent obstetric risk factors. As in the case of threatened PTL, it has been equally if not more challenging to identify predictors of sPTB before symptoms occur. As in the case of symptomatic threatened PTL, qualitative fFN has been evaluated as a potential predictor of PTL in asymptomatic patients, but its positive predictive value is poor, and use in asymptomatic individuals in the United States is not recommended.[24,27] While the QUiPP offers a more sophisticated option in Europe[10] and elsewhere, there is still a need for a less invasive biomarker test (ie, blood based rather than requiring swabs taken by a clinical examination requiring a speculum). cfRNA isolated from maternal blood therefore presents a potential opportunity to noninvasively identify changes in gene expression that predate symptoms. With the complex etiology of PTB, having a dynamic marker that could potentially differentiate signal between subtypes of PTB could open the door to new precision therapeutics for prevention, an area in which innovation is urgently needed.

EVIDENCE SUGGESTING INFLAMMATION PRECEDES SYMPTOMS IN SPONTANEOUS PRETERM BIRTH

Heng and colleagues[28] continued their investigations of cfRNA to predict sPTB in an asymptomatic population of 51 sPTBs and 114 term controls, evaluating maternal whole blood between 17 and 23 weeks and again at 27 to 33 weeks to predict sPTBs. While no individual genes were significant at a false detection rate of 5%, inflammatory pathways were found to be upregulated at both timepoints, with involved pathways including leukocyte migration, lysosomes, nuclear factor kappa-light-chain-enhancer of activated B cells activation, cytokines and their receptors (eg, interleukin (IL)-1, IL-2, IL-6, interferon, IL-1 receptor, tumor necrosis factor receptor, C-C chemokine receptor type 3, C-X-C chemokine receptor type 4, and cluster of differentiation 40), and toll-like receptor and nucleotide oligomerization domain–like receptor signaling. sPTB deliveries also demonstrated lower RNA metabolism, RNA processing, and T-cell activation compared with term deliveries. As pregnancy progressed to the third trimester sampling point, sPTBs demonstrated increased cellular proliferation, cell migration signaling, extracellular matrix degradation involving lysosomes, and decreased cellular transcription. The investigators hypothesized that the increase in IL signaling observed may indicate leukocyte migration into gestational tissues as early as 18 weeks, which could accelerate cervical ripening and lead to increased oxytocin and prostaglandin production. Furthermore, they developed several models for prediction of sPTB, with the best-performing among them including 8 genes and clinical factors reaching an AUC of 0.841, with 65% sensitivity and 88% specificity. These findings still require robust validation in a larger study.

In another study, Ngo and colleagues[13] developed a model for prediction of sPTB using cfRNA in maternal plasma in symptomatic individuals with threatened PTL (n = 15), and subsequently validated it in an asymptomatic high-risk population (n = 23), with an AUC of 0.81. While including small numbers overall, this study provided encouraging early data with a reasonably high performance demonstrated in an entirely separate validation population, differing geographically and temporally from the discovery cohort. In addition, while discovery was performed in a symptomatic cohort, the validation cohort was asymptomatic, and demonstrated the predictive capability of cfRNA up to 2 months preceding delivery. While different specific genes were identified than in prior investigations, genes implicated in inflammatory pathways were again observed (*DAPP1* and *RGS18*), in addition to several other genes implicated in labor and development.

EVIDENCE SUGGESTING THE ROLE OF DYSFUNCTIONAL MYOMETRIAL QUIESCENCE IN SPONTANEOUS PRETERM BIRTH

Recently, Weiner and colleagues[29–31] have published a series of investigations in asymptomatic high-risk individuals with a focus on extremely PTB at ≤32 weeks. First, in a discovery cohort of individuals at high risk for sPTB without other comorbidities, they evaluated maternal plasma samples collected from asymptomatic individuals at 22 to 24 weeks' gestation to identify differentially expressed mRNA and microRNA.[29] They noted that none of the several hundred differentially expressed genes had previously been associated with pregnancy, with pathway analysis revealing genes implicated in hypertension and neurologic/neurobehavioral manifestations ranking highest in the analysis. In order to better assess the potential biological relevance of the genes identified, the group performed in silico analysis with the identified differentially expressed genes and a set of known myometrial genes that have been demonstrated to have differential regulation in women with sPTB ≤32 weeks. The in silico analysis revealed no genes in common between the 2 groups, but did identify 5 cfRNAs (*PSME2, NAMPT, APOA1, APOA4,* and *Hsa-Let7g*) that interacted with 7 known preterm initiator genes; this interaction was the basis for selecting the 5 cfRNAs for further evaluation. In a small validation of asymptomatic individuals at 16 to 19 weeks' EGA with sPTB ≤32 weeks (n = 40) compared to term spontaneous deliveries (n = 20), 4 of the 5 genes were found to be significantly associated with extremely PTBs. Follow-up investigations to further validate these findings demonstrated a significant association between PSME2 and HSA-Let7g and sPTB ≤32 weeks, as well as a significant association between PSME2 and sPTB less than 37 weeks.[30] Modeling with the associated genes demonstrated moderate performance for extremely PTBs with an AUC of 0.76 (95% confidence interval [CI]: 0.65, 0.87), improved to 0.83 (95% CI: 0.74, 0.92) with the addition of clinical factors, while a genes-only model of prediction of sPTB less than 37 weeks was not significant (AUC: 0.58; 95% CI: 0.50, 0.66) without the addition of clinical factors.

Finally, the same group studied whether it might be possible to predict sPTB in the first trimester using the same genes identified in their prior work.[31] In a population of 11 to 14 week nulliparous patients including 40 sPTBs ≤32 weeks and 20 term controls, the investigators identified 2 genes that were differentially expressed in the first trimester (APOA1 and PSME2), with the AUC including clinical factors reaching 0.79 (95% CI: 0.66, 0.91.)

In considering the underlying biological functions of these genes that had not previously been implicated in sPTBs, all appear to have the potential to increase intracellular calcium, which in turn can increase myometrial contractility as well as prostaglandin and oxytocin production. While they may play a role in the pathogenesis of sPTB, there were several women with high expression of all 5 identified genes and term delivery, causing the investigators to posit that the genes identified are unlikely to be the proximate cause of sPTB. However, they hypothesize that increased expression of the identified genes may predispose individuals to premature uterine contractility in the event of an inciting factor.

EVIDENCE FOR DIFFERING PATHWAYS IN SPONTANEOUS PRETERM BIRTH AT DIFFERENT GESTATIONAL AGES: METABOLIC VERSUS COLLAGEN AND EXTRACELLULAR MATRIX

Recently, Camunas-Soler and colleagues[32] published a study of asymptomatic high-risk individuals with plasma collected between 12 and 23[+6] weeks experiencing sPTB less than 35 weeks (n = 46) or very early sPTB less than 25 weeks (n = 16), compared with term controls (n = 194). In total, 25 transcripts were associated with sPTB, with notable differences emerging between individuals with very early versus later sPTB. While collagen and extracellular matrix genes were implicated in sPTB less than 35 weeks, with COL14A1 and ELN identified as significantly associated, insulinlike growth factor and amino acid metabolism were predominant in sPTB less than 25 weeks, with AC0010043.1, IGFBP2, and SH3GL3 identified. A genes-only model for the prediction of sPTB less than 35 weeks demonstrated an AUC of 0.80 (95 CI: 0.72, 0.87) and for sPTB less than 25 weeks, it demonstrated an AUC of 0.76 (95% CI: 0.63, 0.87). This work provides encouraging early evidence in a diverse population of the potential for identification of distinct biological subtypes of sPTBs based on delivery timing, which in turn may be associated with different underlying pathophysiology.

SUMMARY: CHALLENGES AND FUTURE DIRECTIONS

While the last decade has brought substantial new evidence related to pathways associated with sPTB (**Fig. 2**), the field remains nascent. Numerous studies in symptomatic individuals, along with several in asymptomatic individuals, point to the role of inflammation and the immune system in the pathogenesis of sPTB. However, the individual genes identified have not generally been reproducible between studies, the sample sizes have been small and not externally validated, and there has been substantial heterogeneity in study designs in terms of populations studied and tissue types, making it difficult to compare them. Rapid technological advancement in the field has introduced further complexity. The entry of RNA sequencing (RNA-Seq) allows for whole transcriptome analysis and the detection of subtler perturbations in gene expression as well as non-coding RNAs, low -bundance RNAs, alternative-spliced isoforms, and novel transcripts as compared to microarray or quantitative PCR. Such technological advancements have also contributed to interstudy heterogeneity, with older studies in addition to some present-day studies continuing to use microarray over RNA-Seq.[33]

There have been 2 meta-analyses undertaken using the National Institutes of Health (NIH) genomic database in order to try to better understand the sPTB signatures across studies. In the first, Vora and colleagues[34] aggregated the microarray data from 3 published studies,[20,21,28] identifying 210 differentially expressed genes, identifying a strong immune signature including 9 genes encoding secreted proteins, including *IL-1R1* and *TFPI*, which were overexpressed as early as the second trimester, making them potential targets for future biomarker predictors. Ran and colleagues[35] similarly aggregated data from 3 studies,[21,22,36] also confirming a strong immune signature, with the IL6 pathway notably increased in pregnancies with sPTB compared to term pregnancies, developing a model for prediction of sPTB based on the IL6 signature with an AUC of 0.761 overall. These studies illustrate the importance of transcriptomic databases to enable aggregation across studies and reanalyses, which may alter or reinforce prior conclusions given the benefit of increasingly large and diverse datasets.

While inflammatory and immune pathways have predominated in studies of symptomatic individuals, further study is needed in unselected diverse populations in order to further elucidate the potential genes implicated months in advance of symptoms, when the greatest potential for intervention exists. In addition, the

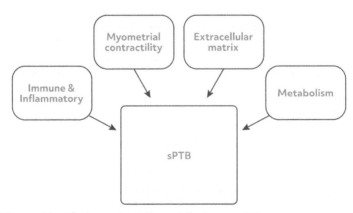

Fig. 2. Pathways identified as potentially contributing to sPTB.

identification of genes-driven subtypes of sPTBs would benefit from optimal clinical risk stratification. sPTB has varied clinical presentations that may have different underlying biologies, all of which could be masked if evaluated without clinically subtyping them into biologically relevant groupings. Potential clinically relevant subtypes of sPTBs could include simply evaluating sPTBs across the spectrum of EGAs at which delivery occurs, as initial evidence indicates the potential for different underlying cfRNA signatures at these different delivery gestational ages.[32] In addition, evaluating the cfRNA signatures across clinically distinct phenotypes of sPTBs, including PPROM, cervical insufficiency, and PTL, would be helpful to better understand whether their underlying pathophysiology shares common or distinct pathways. In practical terms, it would also be helpful to know whether cfRNA signatures can stratify for risk within pregnancies that have a prior poor obstetric history associated with mid-trimester loss and sPTB or inform who is more likely to develop a short cervix and subsequent PTL. While some have taken into account CL where available, suggesting potential improved prediction with combined CL and cfRNA signature,[30] none have yet systematically evaluated a mid-trimester CL in combination with the cfRNA signature to understand whether the 2 combined modalities could provide an improved screening modality compared with CL alone. Given the challenges inherent in studying rare diseases, identifying an optimal set of clinical factors to collect as "best practice" in omics studies including cfRNA would aid in future studies, along with continued aggregation of data enabled by the NIH genomic database.

Finally, future research must remain focused on the potential actionability of test results. While studies evaluating the extremes of sPTB may be illuminating, it is challenging to imagine how such models could be practically implemented in routine practice. For example, a model that predicts extremely preterm deliveries versus term deliveries is of limited utility unless it also provides meaningful information about the probability of delivery across the entire gestational age range. However, if a biomarker at any gestational age of interest elucidates unique and potentially treatable pathophysiologies, this could make even models constrained to narrower gestational age ranges clinically useful if they enable the development of precision therapeutics that address the underlying biological processes.

In conclusion, cfRNA signatures in the maternal circulation have the potential to identify biologically relevant subtypes of sPTBs, and could one day be used to predict and prevent sPTBs in asymptomatic individuals, and potentially aid in prognosis and management for individuals presenting with threatened PTL and PPROM. This would represent a meaningful and needed shift toward precision medicine in obstetrics, where we have historically lagged compared with other fields such as cardiology and oncology. Further research and validation of predictive models in large, unselected, geographically, and racially diverse populations will be a critical step toward establishing a clinically useful test.

ACKNOWLEDGMENTS

R.M. Tribe funded by Action Medical Research, United Kingdom, Borne Foundation, Rosetrees Trust, United Kingdom, and the KHP Centre for Translational Medicine

DISCLOSURE

A.D. Cowan, M. Rasmussen, and M. Jain are all employees of and hold equity in Mirvie, Inc.

REFERENCES

1. Ohuma EO, Moller A-B, Bradley E, et al. National, regional, and global estimates of preterm birth in 2020, with trends from 2010: a systematic analysis. Lancet 2023;402(10409):1261–71.
2. Goldenberg RL, Culhane JF, Iams JD, et al. Epidemiology and causes of preterm birth. Lancet 2008;371(9606):75–84.
3. 2023 March of Dimes Report card | March of Dimes. Available at: https://www.marchofdimes.org/report-card. [Accessed 25 January 2024].
4. Publications & Guidelines | SMFM.org - the Society for maternal-fetal medicine. Available at: https://www.smfm.org/publications/467-smfm-special-statement-response-to-the-food-and-drug-administrations-withdrawal-of-17-alpha-hydroxyprogesterone-caproate. [Accessed 20 October 2023].
5. Bhattacharjee E, Thiruvengadam R, Ayushi, et al. Genetic variants associated with spontaneous preterm birth in women from India: a prospective cohort study. Lancet Reg Health Southeast Asia 2023;14:100190.
6. Zhang G, Feenstra B, Bacelis J, et al. Genetic associations with gestational duration and spontaneous preterm birth. N Engl J Med 2017;377(12):1156–67.
7. Mercer BM, Goldenberg RL, Moawad AH, et al. The preterm prediction study: effect of gestational age and cause of preterm birth on subsequent obstetric outcome. National Institute of Child Health and Human Development Maternal-Fetal Medicine Units Network. Am J Obstet Gynecol 1999;181(5 Pt 1):1216–21.
8. Son M, Miller ES. Predicting preterm birth: cervical length and fetal fibronectin. Semin Perinatol 2017;41(8):445–51.
9. Grobman WA, Lai Y, Iams JD, et al. Prediction of spontaneous preterm birth among nulliparous women with a short cervix. J Ultrasound Med 2016;35(6):1293–7.
10. Watson HA, Seed PT, Carter J, et al. Development and validation of predictive models for QUiPP App v.2: tool for predicting preterm birth in asymptomatic high-risk women. Ultrasound Obstet Gynecol 2020;55(3):348–56.
11. Rasmussen M, Reddy M, Nolan R, et al. RNA profiles reveal signatures of future health and disease in pregnancy. Nature 2022;601(7893):422–7.
12. Koh W, Pan W, Gawad C, et al. Noninvasive in vivo monitoring of tissue-specific global gene expression in humans. Proc Natl Acad Sci USA 2014;111(20):7361–6.
13. Ngo TTM, Moufarrej MN, Rasmussen M-LH, et al. Noninvasive blood tests for fetal development predict gestational age and preterm delivery. Science 2018;360(6393):1133–6.
14. Moufarrej MN, Vorperian SK, Wong RJ, et al. Early prediction of preeclampsia in pregnancy with cell-free RNA. Nature 2022;602(7898):689–94.
15. Hannan NJ, Stock O, Spencer R, et al. Circulating mRNAs are differentially expressed in pregnancies with severe placental insufficiency and at high risk of stillbirth. BMC Med 2020;18(1):145.
16. Munchel S, Rohrback S, Randise-Hinchliff C, et al. Circulating transcripts in maternal blood reflect a molecular signature of early-onset preeclampsia. Sci Transl Med 2020;12(550):eaaz0131.
17. Moufarrej MN, Wong RJ, Shaw GM, et al. Investigating pregnancy and its complications using circulating cell-free RNA in women's blood during gestation. Front Pediatr 2020;8:605219.
18. American College of Obstetricians and Gynecologists' Committee on Practice Bulletins—Obstetrics. Practice Bulletin No. 171: Management of Preterm Labor. Obstet Gynecol 2016;128(4):e155–64.

19. Chim SSC, Lee WS, Ting YH, et al. Systematic identification of spontaneous preterm birth-associated RNA transcripts in maternal plasma. PLoS One 2012;7(4): e34328.
20. Bukowski R, Sadovsky Y, Goodarzi H, et al. Onset of human preterm and term birth is related to unique inflammatory transcriptome profiles at the maternal fetal interface. PeerJ 2017;5:e3685.
21. Heng YJ, Pennell CE, Chua HN, et al. Whole blood gene expression profile associated with spontaneous preterm birth in women with threatened preterm labor. PLoS One 2014;9(5):e96901.
22. Paquette AG, Shynlova O, Kibschull M, et al. Comparative analysis of gene expression in maternal peripheral blood and monocytes during spontaneous preterm labor. Am J Obstet Gynecol 2018;218(3):345.e1–30.
23. Committee Opinion No. 712: Intrapartum Management of Intraamniotic Infection. *Obstet Gynecol.* 130 (2), 2017, e95-e101.
24. Hall M, Hutter J, Suff N, et al. Antenatal diagnosis of chorioamnionitis: a review of the potential role of fetal and placental imaging. Prenat Diagn 2022;42(8):1049–58.
25. Siegler Y, Weiner Z, Solt I. ACOG Practice Bulletin No. 217: Prelabor Rupture of Membranes. Obstet Gynecol 2020;136(5):1061.
26. Stock O, Gordon L, Kapoor J, et al. Chorioamnionitis occurring in women with preterm rupture of the fetal membranes is associated with a dynamic increase in mRNAs coding cytokines in the maternal circulation. Reprod Sci 2015;22(7):852–9.
27. Prediction. Prevention of Spontaneous Preterm Birth: ACOG Practice Bulletin, Number 234. Obstet Gynecol 2021;138(2):e65–90.
28. Heng YJ, Pennell CE, McDonald SW, et al. Maternal whole blood gene expression at 18 and 28 weeks of gestation associated with spontaneous preterm birth in asymptomatic women. PLoS One 2016;11(6):e0155191.
29. Weiner CP, Dong Y, Zhou H, et al. Early pregnancy prediction of spontaneous preterm birth before 32 completed weeks of pregnancy using plasma RNA: transcriptome discovery and initial validation of an RNA panel of markers. BJOG 2021;128(11):1870–80.
30. Weiner CP, Cuckle H, Weiss ML, et al. Evaluation of a maternal plasma RNA panel predicting spontaneous preterm birth and its expansion to the prediction of preeclampsia. Diagnostics 2022;12(6):1327.
31. Weiner CP, Zhou H, Cuckle H, et al. Maternal plasma RNA in first trimester nullipara for the prediction of spontaneous preterm birth $\leq$ 32 weeks: validation study. Biomedicines 2023;11(4):1149.
32. Camunas-Soler J, Gee EPS, Reddy M, et al. Predictive RNA profiles for early and very early spontaneous preterm birth. Am J Obstet Gynecol 2022;227(1):72.e1–16.
33. Whitehead CL, Walker SP, Tong S. Measuring circulating placental RNAs to noninvasively assess the placental transcriptome and to predict pregnancy complications. Prenat Diagn 2016;36(11):997–1008.
34. Vora B, Wang A, Kosti I, et al. Meta-analysis of maternal and fetal transcriptomic data elucidates the role of adaptive and innate immunity in preterm birth. Front Immunol 2018;9:993.
35. Ran Y, Huang D, Yin N, et al. Predicting the risk of preterm birth throughout pregnancy based on a novel transcriptomic signature. Matern Fetal Med 2023;5(4): 213–22.
36. Tarca AL, Pataki BÁ, Romero R, et al. Crowdsourcing assessment of maternal blood multi-omics for predicting gestational age and preterm birth. Cell Rep Med 2021;2(6):100323.

Predicting Preterm Birth Using Proteomics

Ivana Marić, PhD[a],*, David K. Stevenson, MD[a],
Nima Aghaeepour, PhD[b,c], Brice Gaudillière, MD, PhD[b,c],
Ronald J. Wong, PhD[a], Martin S. Angst, MD[b]

KEYWORDS

- Preeclampsia • Proteome • Omics • Multiomics • Biomarkers • Biosignatures
- Composite signatures • Computation

KEY POINTS

- Numerous studies have revealed that proteins present in prenatal maternal samples are significantly associated with preterm birth (PTB) and preeclampsia (PE), thereby providing a compelling rationale for advanced proteomics research to derive sufficiently accurate biosignatures to support clinical decision-making in women at risk for PTB or PE.
- Current protein biomarker candidates possess insufficient or too restricted predictive power as they lack sufficient accuracy, reliability, and generalizability across diverse populations.
- The advancement of highly multiplexed and sensitive platforms simultaneously assessing a large array of proteins, advanced computational methods, and protocols combining proteomics data with other omics and clinical datasets holds considerable promise for uncovering predictive biosignatures with sufficient accuracy for their clinical use.

INTRODUCTION

The global prevalence of preterm birth (PTB) has remained mostly unchanged in the decade between 2010 (at 9.8%) and 2020 (at 9.9%), with approximately 13.4 million infants being born too early in 2020.[1] The rates remained the highest in South Asia and Sub-Saharan Africa where survival, especially for those born extremely preterm, is the lowest.[1] In the United States, the rates have also varied but only modestly: from 10.6% in 1990 to its peak of 12.8% in 2006 and back to 10.4% in 2022, resulting in 380,548 infants being born too early in 2020.[2,3]

[a] Division of Neonatal and Developmental Medicine, Department of Pediatrics, Stanford University School of Medicine, 453 Quarry Road, Palo Alto, CA 94304, USA; [b] Department of Anesthesiology, Perioperative and Pain Medicine, Stanford University School of Medicine, Grant Building, Office 276A, 300 Pasteur Drive, Stanford, CA 94305-5117, USA; [c] Division of Neonatal and Developmental Medicine, Department of Pediatrics, Stanford University School of Medicine, 300 Pasteur Drive, Grant S280, Stanford, CA 94305, USA
* Corresponding author.
E-mail address: ivanam@stanford.edu

Clin Perinatol 51 (2024) 391–409
https://doi.org/10.1016/j.clp.2024.02.011
0095-5108/24/© 2024 Elsevier Inc. All rights reserved.

Prematurity is an important risk factor for neonatal mortality and adverse infant outcomes such as sepsis, necrotizing enterocolitis, jaundice (hyperbilirubinemia), and neurodevelopmental delay. This persistent threat to a healthy pregnancy could be greatly reduced by the development of prediction tools that can identify—early in pregnancy and with high accuracy—women who are at risk. Once identified, these women could, for example, be offered a treatment, such as low-dose aspirin known to reduce the risk[4] and be closely followed until the delivery. In low-income settings, where efficient resource utilization is particularly critical, prediction tools could become crucial to save lives, allowing women at risk to be more efficiently triaged and monitored. Furthermore, identified biomarkers could lead to a better understanding of the biological pathways that are critical in the etiology of PTB, thereby guiding and improving prenatal care pathways.

Why the Proteome?

The complexity of PTB, both spontaneous and medically induced, and its various etiologies and associated risk factors pose a challenge to developing prediction tools and unveiling the etiologies of PTB.[5] High-throughput measurements covering the genome, transcriptome, proteome, metabolome, lipidome, or microbiome have enabled the collection of detailed omics measurements that reflect biological processes in human physiology and capture molecular differences caused by diseases. Various omics approaches have captured the dynamics of pregnancy[6,7] and its adverse outcomes, including PTB,[8] preeclampsia (PE),[9,10] and onset of labor.[11]

The genome is the fundamental code of DNA that determines an organism's capacity for expressing myriad of proteins, many of which are further modified after they have been translated from mRNA. These modifications include phosphorylation, glycosylation, ubiquitination, methylation, acetylation, oxidation, and nitrosylation. Protein translation is cell-dependent, time-dependent, and condition-dependent, and posttranslational modifications affect protein structure and function. While relevant, these processes are not the focus of this review.

The transcriptome reflects the active expression of genes. However, the biological consequences of gene expression are probably better understood when evaluating proteins, as not all transcripts result in protein synthesis, and posttranslational alterations of proteins (alternative splicing, which allows a single gene to code for multiple proteins) and abundance can be directly measured. Moreover, transcripts are more transient in the circulation, and their measurements can be more technically challenging.

The metabolome encompasses the complete set of small molecules in a biological system (including substrates, intermediates, and products of cellular metabolism more generally) and constitutes a more complex array of molecules than the proteome. Metabolites can serve as biomarkers and help identify pathways that are contributing to a particular phenotype as they are directly linked to cellular function. However, the complexities and the dynamic nature of the metabolome pose challenges requiring highly standardized collection and processing protocols to ensure reproducibility.

This review focuses on the discovery of proteomics signatures in plasma, sera, urine, or cervicovaginal fluid that might be useful for diagnosing or predicting various adverse pregnancy outcomes, such as spontaneous PTB or PE. The latter is a significant cause of PTB because early delivery may be indicated to protect the mother and/or the baby. Discovered signatures can be a reflection of early physiologic changes and underlying biology associated with PTB and therefore serve as potential predictive biomarkers. The proteome of amniotic fluid has been studied for the same purpose, but now access to this source is limited, as amniocentesis has become less common due to the introduction of noninvasive pregnancy tests. Thus, the proteome of amniotic fluid will not be discussed in detail. Importantly, there is ample evidence to suggest that the proteome represented in plasma, sera, and urine contains diagnostic and predictive information regarding the risk for PTB and PE. Moreover, combining proteomics approaches with other omics, some of them involving single cell proteomics measures (eg, single cell mass cytometry by time-of-flight [TOF] mass spectrometry [MS]) does improve its diagnostic and predictive value. The analysis of the proteome can also provide insight into the pathogenesis of PTB and PE, thereby revealing possible targets for intervention.

The proteome reflects both genetic and environmental influences, such as toxic chemicals in the environment, on a biological system and contains information that allows predicting pregnancy outcomes[12] including PTB[8] with typically better accuracy than other omics. However, the predictive power of proteomics signatures can be enhanced when integrated with other omics datasets (**Fig. 1**).[8,10] Numerous protein biomarker candidates have been reported for PTB.[8,13–30] These findings are encouraging and provide the basis for continued efforts aiming at the development of clinically useful tests for the early prediction of PTB and PE using a broadly available assay. Such efforts will need to address major challenges including the prospective validation of identified protein biomarker candidates and the demonstration of their robustness across diverse populations.

METHODS FOR PROTEOME ANALYSIS

Analytical methods to assess the proteome are classified as "targeted" and "untargeted." The primary objective of targeted approaches is to identify biomarker candidates in a predetermined set of proteins; whereas, untargeted approaches aim to identify proteins without predefining specific targets.[31] The major analytical platforms for targeted approaches use either antibodies or aptamers.[32,33] The scope of targeted approaches has dramatically changed during the last decade as current assays can be highly multiplexed, allowing for the simultaneous analysis of over 10,000 proteins in a given specimen. As such, targeted approaches, originally not suitable for relevant discovery work, are now commonly used to derive health-relevant biosignatures. Compared with untargeted approaches, they currently also provide higher sensitivity for the detection of low abundance proteins, particularly in sera and plasma. However, untargeted approaches have limitations. They may provide biased results as antibodies or aptamers against relevant proteins may not be included in the assay.[34] Additionally, different antibody-based or aptamer-based assays may provide incongruent results as the specificity and binding sites of used antibodies and aptamers can vary.[35] As such, validation of targeted proteomic results by an alternative assay is critically important when developing a predictive or diagnostic tool, or inferring relevant biology.

Untargeted approaches are anchored in MS, which measures the mass-to-charge ratio (m/z) of ionized analytes, thereby detecting the number of ions at each m/z value and mapping it to the *mass spectrum*.[36] MS methods include surface-enhanced laser desorption ionization (SELDI), matrix-assisted laser desorption ionization coupled with TOF, and gas chromatography MS or liquid chromatography MS (LC-MS).[37] Untargeted approaches overcome some of the limitations inherent to targeted approaches. A major advantage is their ability to identify proteins that were not initially thought of in an experimental context. In other words, untargeted approaches can protect against preconceived notions. They can also identify proteins that would be missed by antibodies or aptamers designed for their detection due to the posttranslational modifications of these proteins. As indicated earlier, a major limitation of untargeted approaches is

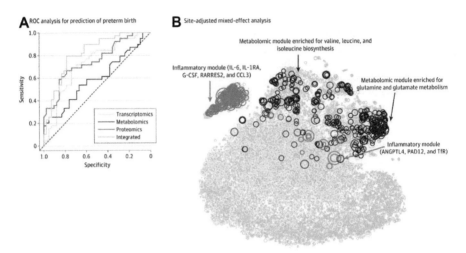

Fig. 1. Predictive modeling of PTB. (*A*) This receiver operating characteristic (ROC) curve analysis used each biological modality and the integrated approach. The mean area under the ROC (AUROC) curve and 95% CI for each modality were as follows: transcriptomics (AUROC; 0.73; 95% CI: 0.61, 0.83), metabolomics (AUROC: 0.59; 95% CI: 0.47, 0.72), proteomics (AUROC: 0.75; 95% CI: 0.64, 0.85), and integrated (AUROC: 0.83; 95% CI: 0.72, 0.91). (*B*) Circle size is proportional to −log10 (Wilcoxon) p-value for discrimination between term pregnancies and PTBs. Top features included an inflammatory module (which included interleukin 6 [IL-6]; IL-1 receptor antagonist [IL-1RA], a regulatory member of the IL-1 family whose expression is induced IL-1β under inflammatory conditions; granulocyte colony-stimulating factor [G-CSF]; retinoic acid receptor responder protein 2 [RARRES2]; chemokine ligand 3 [CCL3]; angiopoietin-like 4 [ANGPTL4]; protein-arginine deiminase type II [PADI2]; and transferrin receptor [TfR]) and a metabolomic module (which was enriched for glutamine and glutamate metabolism [Fisher test for pathway enrichment analysis $P < 4.4 \times 10^{-9}$] and valine, leucine, and isoleucine biosynthesis pathways [$P < 7.3 \times 10^{-6}$]). (*From* Jehan F, Sazawal S, Baqui AH, et al. Multiomics characterization of preterm birth in low- and middle-income countries. JAMA Netw Open 2020;3(12):e2029655.)

the detection of low abundance proteins as their representation on the *mass spectrum* may be masked by high abundance proteins.

Considering the advantages and disadvantages of targeted and untargeted approaches, they should be considered complementary methods. The selection of either or both approaches critically depends on a particular study design and rationale.

BIOLOGICAL COMPARTMENTS

The search for proteomics signatures predictive or diagnostic of PTB spans the analyses of specimens from different sources including tissue (eg, placenta), plasma, sera, urine, cervicovaginal fluid, amniotic fluid, and exosomes. The choice of the specimen source is ideally driven by a particular study question. However, access to tissue and the feasibility of sample collection often dictates the source. It is, therefore, not surprising that most investigations heavily rely on the collection of blood specimens. For blood specimens, proteomic analyses can be performed in either sera or plasma, which are processed differently. The question then arises whether the diagnostic or predictive power of proteomics signatures varies when derived in sera or plasma. Addressing this question requires the direct comparison of the predictive power of sera-derived and plasma-derived biosignatures using simultaneously collected samples. Such a study was recently performed using samples from 73 pregnant women and assaying over a thousand proteins to derive a signature predicting gestational age at the time of sampling.[38] The results demonstrated a significantly higher predictive power for a plasma-derived signature compared to a serum-derived signature. A likely explanation for this difference is that serum is subjected to the degradation of proteins while processed.

STATISTICAL ANALYSES

Statistical and computational analyses of proteomic data sets include both classic statistics methods and machine-learning approaches. Hypothesis-driven analyses testing associations between a few proteins and PTB can be addressed with classic hypothesis testing,[39] along with an adjustment for multiple comparisons to control for false discovery.[40] In contrast, finding the most predictive biomarkers among thousands of proteins requires the use of machine-learning methods. Most suitable for the analysis of these *high-dimensional* data sets, characterized by numerous measurements (features) and typically a smaller number of samples, are sparsity-promoting regression methods that select a small subset of the most informative features from all features. In principle, such analysis requires evaluating the predictive power of all possible feature subsets. However, in the case of high-dimensional data, the number of generated subsets is too large to allow for such evaluation. This challenge is addressed by introducing penalization schemes that remove features with poor predictive power, thereby selectively considering features with the highest predictive power.[41] Another challenge in a clinical setting is that computational algorithms for feature selection have to be trained in data sets obtained in relatively small cohorts. A consequence of a limited cohort size is that small perturbations in the data set can yield different model features. The limited reliability of feature selection is a well-recognized problem of stability in high-dimensional statistical inference.[42,43] In other words, there remains significant uncertainty regarding the choice of model features, if such models are derived in small cohorts. Advanced algorithms specifically addressing this problem include Stability selection,[44] Knockoffs-based,[45,46] bootstrap-enhanced Lasso (Bolasso),[47] and Stabl.[48] These novel approaches result in a sparse and reliable set of biomarkers. The stability selection method improves model robustness by using bootstrapping and selecting features that are chosen with the highest frequency, whereas the approach by Barber and Candès[45] and Candès and colleagues[46] introduces artificial features to separate random feature selection from the selection of truly informative features (ie, knockoffs). Stabl is the latest implementation of such an algorithm that integrates both approaches. Specifically, Stabl determines a feature frequency selection threshold based on data, by adding random features to the data set and allowing separating noise from signal. Truly informative features are selected more frequently during bootstrapping then the added random features. By using this approach, Stabl creates a sparse set of highly reliable features. The above approaches provide a high-impact advancement, as the cohort sizes of many clinical studies are too small to allow for meaningful analyses with deep-learning (DL) algorithms. However, when large datasets are available, complex patterns could potentially be discovered by DL algorithms, resulting in prediction with higher accuracy. A few studies have used DL for the discovery of predictive biosignatures in proteomics[49] and a multiomics data set.[50]

CLINICAL STUDIES

Numerous studies have examined the association between proteins in different biological compartments, most commonly sera or plasma, and PTB as well as PE resulting in PTB. These studies reported an array of proteins. Sentinel results are reviewed in this section and are listed in **Table 1**. A comprehensive list of omics biomarkers, including the proteome, has been published in a recent systematic review.[51]

The strong association between intrauterine infection and PTB suggests that the resulting inflammatory response is a main driver of PTB.[52] A hallmark of inflammation is the increase of cytokines including interleukin (IL)-1, IL-6, IL-8, and C-reactive protein (CRP).[53,54] Associations of different proinflammatory cytokines with PTB have been observed in multiple studies. For example, associations between IL-6 and PTB were shown in different biological compartments including amniotic fluid,[24] cervical fluid,[16,22] and sera.[18,28] Consistent with these reports is a recently published proteomics profile derived with aid of a machine-learning analysis and considering 1125 simultaneously measured plasma proteins. This profile included IL-6.[29] Further evidence highlighting the importance of inflammation in PTB are increased levels of CRP in amniotic fluid[15] and plasma,[28] and increased levels of IL-1β and IL-8, next to IL-6, in cervical fluid.[22]

A remarkably large study including 248 women with spontaneous PTB pregnancies examined the ratio of insulin-like growth factor-binding protein 4 (IBP4) and sex hormone-binding globulin (SHBG) in serum.[27] The cohort was split into discovery, verification, and validation subcohorts. In the validation cohort, the IBP4/SHBG ratio predicted spontaneous PTB with modest accuracy (area under the curve [AUC] = 0.67) when measured between 19 and 21 weeks of gestation, and with an increased accuracy (AUC = 0.75) after stratification by the body mass index (BMI). These findings were subsequently validated with an AUC = 0.67 considering the ratio and an AUC = 0.71 after BMI stratification.[23] A subsequent study in a cohort of 300 women from Bangladesh, Pakistan, and Tanzania validated this biomarker with lower accuracy (AUC = 0.64), which could be increased (AUC = 0.79) by adding endoglin, prolactin, and tetranectin to the prediction model.[20] These studies resulted in the development of a commercially available test for predicting the risk of PTB based on the IBP4/SHBG ratio.

Studies using an untargeted approach identified a number of proteins in sera[13,18,25] and plasma that were significantly associated with PTB.[8,21,29] For example, a study reporting a readout of 628 proteins in serum of 20 women using two-dimensional gel electrophoresis (2DE) and MS identified 30 proteins involved in immunologic, developmental, and metabolic processes.[13] Another study, using a targeted approach to measure 1012 proteins in plasma from 81 women[8] built a multivariate model to predict the risk of PTB. However, the model had moderate predictive power as evidenced by an AUC of 0.75.

Comparisons among studies[8,13,18,21,25,29] examining and reporting a wide array of protein candidates reveal limited overlap with some exceptions, one being IL-6. While divergent findings may partially be due to methodological differences, inconsistent findings likely reflect the heterogeneity of the studied cohorts and pathophysiologies underlying PTB. This view is supported by a recent investigation measuring over 1000 plasma proteins with the same analytical platform to predict the risk of PE in 2 demographically distinct cohorts of pregnant women.[14] Multivariate models derived separately in each cohort predicted the risk of PE with good accuracy in the respective cohort. However, either model failed to predict the risk of PE in the alternative cohort, emphasizing the need to study large and diverse cohorts to develop generalizable prediction models. While the proteins associated with PTB vary across studies,[8,13,18,21,25,29] pathway analysis points to important biology that likely drives the development of PTB including pathways relevant to inflammation[8,25,29] and angiogenesis.[13,18]

Table 1
Overview of studies on proteomic biomarkers for prediction of preterm birth

Study	Identified Biomarkers	Matrix	Size	When	Method
Targeted studies					
Massaro et al,[24] 2009	• IL-6	• Amniotic fluid	• 8 PTB • 92 Term	• 16–22 wk	• ELISA • $P < .05$
Manning et al,[22] 2019	• IL-1β • IL-8 • IL-6	• Cervical fluid	• 44 PTB • 90 Term • All with history of PTB or cervical surgery	• 22–24 wk	• Multiplex platform • ELISA • PCR • Bonferroni corr. ($P < .01$)
Goepfert et al,[16] 2001	• IL-6	• Cervical fluid	• 125 PTB • 125 Term	• 22–24$^{6/7}$ wk	• ELISA
Sorokin et al,[28] 2010	• IL-6 • CRP	• Sera	• 47 PTB (<32 wk) • 423 Term	• 24–32 wk	• ELISA • $P < .05$
Ghezzi et al,[15] 2002	• CRP	• Amniotic fluid	—	—	—
Wallenstein et al,[30] 2016	• sVEGFR-3 • sIL-2Rα • sTNFR1	• Sera	• 34 PTB • 34 Term • BMI > 30 kg/m²	• 15–20 wk	• Random forest: classification and regression trees
Saade et al,[27] 2016	• IBP4/SHBG ratio	• Sera	• 248 Spontaneous PTB	• 19–21 wk	—
Markenson et al,[23] 2020	• IBP4/SHBG ratio	—	—	—	—
Khanam et al,[20] 2022	• IBP4/SHBG ratio	—	• 300 Women	—	—
Untargeted studies					
D' Silva et al,[13] 2018	• 30, including 9 phosphoproteins, 11 glycoproteins • Pathways: blood coagulation, plasminogen activation, vitamin D metabolism, and angiogenesis	• Sera	• 10 PTB • 10 Term	• 11–13$^{+6/7}$ wk	• 2DE and MS

(continued on next page)

Table 1
(continued)

Study	Identified Biomarkers	Matrix	Size	When	Method
Gunko et al,[18] 2016	• 25 including IL-6, VEGFA • Pathways: angiogenesis, proteolysis, transcription, inflammation processes, binding, and transportation of various ligands	• Serum	• 10 PTB • 10 Term	• 16–17 wk	• MS • $P < .05$
Pereira et al,[25] 2010	• Pathways: complement/ coagulation cascade; inflammation/immune response; fetal-placental development; extracellular matrix proteins	• Serum (glycoproteome and peptidome)	• 48 Spontaneous PTB $\leq$ 33 wk • 62 PTB with GA $\geq$ 34 wk	• 20–33[6/7] wk	• $P < .05$
Jehan et al,[8] 2020	• An inflammatory module	• Plasma	• 39 PTB • 42 term	• Early pregnancy (median 13.6 wk)	• Targeted proteomics (1002) AUC: 0.75 95% CI: 0.64, 0.85
Tarca et al,[29] 2021	• PDE11 A • ITGA2B • IL-6 • ANGPT1 • MMP7 • ITGA2B • Vascular wall pathways, nervous system development, developmental biology, focal adhesion, VEGFA/VEGFR-2 signaling, and membrane trafficking pathways	• Plasma	• 62 Spontaneous PTB • 4 PPROM • 39 Term	• 17–23 wk • 27–33 wk	• Targeted plasma proteomics (1125) AUC: 0.76 95% CI: 0.72, 0.8

Study	Biomarkers/Pathways	Sample	Cohort	GA	Method
Lynch et al,[21] 2016	• Complement factors B and H • Coagulation factors IX and IX ab • Pathways: complement cascade, the immune system, and the clotting cascade	• Plasma	• 41 PTB • 88 Term	• 10–15 wk	• *Targeted* proteomics (1129)
Gudicha et al,[17] 2022	• SNAP25 GPI • PTPN11 • OLR1 • ENO1 • GAPDH • CHI3L1 • RETN • CSF3 • LCN2 • CXCL1 • CXCL8 • PGLYRP1 • LDHB • IL-6 • MMP8 • PRTN3	• Amniotic fluid	• 90 Women with a short cervix	—	• 1310 proteins measured using aptamer-based multiplex platform (SOMAmer)
Romero et al,[26] 2008	• 39 features identified	• Amniotic fluid	• 60 PTB • 59 Term	—	• SELDI
Hong et al,[19] 2020	• VEGFR-1 • Lipocalin-2 • Fc fragment of IgG binding protein	• Amniotic fluid	• 139	• 24–32$^{6/7}$ wk	• LC-MS • validation using ELISA

Abbreviations: 2DE, 2-dimensional gel electrophoresis; AUC, area under the curve; BMI, body mass index; CI, confidence interval; CRP, C-reactive protein; ELISA, enzyme-linked immunosorbent assay; IL, interleukin; LC, liquid chromatography; MS, mass spectrometry; PCR, polymerase chain reaction; PPROM, preterm premature rupture of membranes; SELDI, surface-enhanced laser desorption ionization.

From an interventional perspective, the established association between IL-1 and PTB is interesting, as it may offer a therapeutic approach by targeting IL-1. While several IL-1 antagonists have been approved for clinical use, none have been approved for the prevention of PTB.[55] One hindrance is that IL-1 antagonists have failed to prevent PTB in animal models.[56] Furthermore, there is a relevant risk that straight antagonism at the IL-receptor to decrease IL-1 binding, which has a role during labor, may interfere with normal delivery.[55] These obstacles may be overcome by further examining an IL-1R allosteric modulator, which has proven effective in mice.[57] However, from a drug development perspective, a significant challenge is the difficulty in conducting randomized clinical trials to evaluate therapeutic candidates, as the incidence of PTB is about 10%. Developing a reliable test for the early prediction of PTB would allow for an enriched trial design, greatly enhancing the feasibility of conducting interventional clinical studies.

Preeclampsia

While the pathophysiology of PE is not fully understood, placental ischemia likely plays a causal role.[58] Ischemia changes the level of circulating angiogenic and antiangiogenic factors, including decreases of angiogenic factors such as vascular endothelial growth factor (VEGF) and placental growth factor, and increases of antiangiogenic factors such as soluble VEGF receptor-1 (sVEGFR-1) or Soluble Fms-Like Tyrosine Kinase-1 (sFlt-1) and soluble endoglin (sEng).[59] Investigations focusing on biomarker discovery to predict PE indeed revealed changes in circulating angiogenic factors[60] with multiple studies showing increased sFlt-1 and decreased of PlGF levels.[61] However, neither of these biomarkers had shown sufficient predictive power when examined alone.[62,63] Importantly, examining the sFlt-1/PlGF ratio increased the prediction accuracy and is now used in clinical practice.[64–66] The use of the sFlt-1/PlGF ratio is recommended by the current National Institute for Health and Care Excellence guidelines.[67] They specifically suggest that a ratio greater than 38 is indicative for the short-term PE risk during the 24 to 36$^{6/7}$ weeks gestational period. The sFlt-1/PlGF ratio can be used in conjunction with clinical factors and uterine artery Doppler results to increase accuracy.[64] However, determining the sFlt-1/PlGF ratio is particularly useful in pregnancy after the 24th week, while clinical features suggestive of PE may already have manifested.[68] As such, the sFlt-1/PlGF ratio can viewed as diagnostic rather than a predictive tool. The search for proteomics signatures that can help predict PE early during pregnancy rather than diagnose it later during pregnancy remains a high-yield objective.[10] **Table 2** summarized the results of untargeted studies, which predominantly revealed angiogenic and inflammatory proteins associated with PE early and late in pregnancy.[69,70]

Increased levels of leptin in early and midpregnancy have been observed in pregnant women developing clinically overt PE later in pregnancy, if adjusted for maternal BMI.[10,71,72] Associations of PE with other potential biomarkers include plasma protein-A (PAPP-A)[73] and uric acid.[6] However, the predictive power of reported isolated proteins is poor. Instead, integrating these proteins in composite signatures can significantly improve predictive accuracy.[74,75] Specifically, first trimester screening information including maternal clinical factors, the uterine artery pulsatility index, the mean arterial pressure (MAP), and the maternal serum proteins PAPP-A and PlGF resulted in a 95% detection rate with a 10% false-positive rate.[74] A large subsequent study including over 35,000 women as a training cohort and over 25,000 women as a validation cohort confirmed the utility of the composite signature approach. First trimester screening of maternal factors, MAP, uterine artery pulsatility index, and PlGF resulted in an AUC greater than 95% for early-onset PE and greater than 80% for PE in general.[75] While

Table 2
Overview of studies on proteomic biomarkers for prediction of preeclampsia

Study	Identified Biomarkers	Matrix	Size	When	Method
Targeted studies					
Honigberg et al,[61] 2016	• sFlt-1 • PlGF		• 2355 Women	• 10 wk • 18 wk • 26 wk • 5 wk	• AUROC curve
Zeisler et al,[66] 2016	• sFlt-1/PlGF ratio	• Sera	• 500 Discovery • 550 Validation	• 24–36[6/7] wk	• Elecsys assays for sFlt-1 • Electrochemiluminescence immunoassay platform for PlGF
Levine et al,[65] 2006	• sEng • sFlt-1/PlGF ratio	• Sera	• 72 PTB PE • 120 Term PE • 120 Gestational hypertension • 120 SGA • 120 Controls	• 21–32 wk • 33–42 wk	• ELISA
Herraiz et al,[64] 2018	• sFlt-1/PlGF ratio	—	—	• 24–28 wk	—
Taylor et al,[72] 2015	• Leptin	• Sera	• 430 PE • 316 Controls	• 9–26 wk	• Generalized linear model
Untargeted studies					
Ouyang et al,[71] 2007	• Leptin	• Plasma	• 53 PE • 20 Controls	—	—
Chen et al,[70] 2022	• IGFBP4 • ITIH2-4	• Plasma	• 17 Early-onset PE • 18 Late-onset PE • 18 Controls	• At hospital admission for delivery	• Untargeted MS; 370 proteins • *Targeted* for validation
Maric et al,[10] 2022	• Leptin • VEGFA • SEL-L • SEL-E	• Plasma	• 17 PE • 16 Controls	• Longitudinally	• *Untargeted LC-MS (1305 proteins)*

(continued on next page)

Table 2
(continued)

Study	Identified Biomarkers	Matrix	Size	When	Method
Beernik et al,[69] 2022	• ApoD • SEL-L • Ficolin-2 • Serum amyloid A-1 • Fibrinogen beta chain • Cartilage acidic protein 1 • Mannan-binding lectin serine protease 1	• Sera	• 23 PE • 23 Controls	• 11 wk • 14 wk	• *Untargeted* LC-MS

Abbreviations: AUROC, area under the receiver operating characteristics curve; ELISA, enzyme-linked immunosorbent assay; LC, liquid chromatography; MS, mass spectrometry; SGA, small-for-gestational-age.

yielding high accuracy, these composite signatures require tests that are not conducted during routine prenatal care. As such, proteomic signatures composed of multiple proteins and derived by interrogating a large array of proteins with machine-learning methods do have the potential to advance the development of sufficiently accurate prediction models that may not require results of demanding clinical tests.[10]

FUTURE DIRECTIONS

Significant research efforts aiming to develop tests that predict PTB and PE before they become clinically manifest and point to underlying mechanisms have identified an array of biomarker candidates including genes, proteins, and metabolites. Yet, the development of predictive tools that are sufficiently accurate to be of clinical utility has been hindered by limited predictive power, missing or incomplete validation, restricted generalizability, and constrained clinical use as pointed out for the sFlt-1/ PIGF ratio. The development of highly multiplexed and sensitive platforms allowing for the simultaneous analysis of over 10,000 proteins holds the promise that predictive tests with higher accuracy will be developed in the future. Importantly, the derivation of predictive proteomics signatures will rely on advanced computational algorithms that adequately address the highly intercorrelated and redundant nature of the proteome. As important is the derivation of such signatures in large and diverse populations using designs that allow for cross validation and independent validation. It is conceivable that these investigations will reveal that accurate proteomic signatures vary for different demographic groups, subgroups of PTB and PE with different or only partially congruent underlying pathophysiology, and a particular clinical context including gestational age at the time of specimen sampling. Large-scale proteomics studies in diverse populations will also shed more light on the biology and pathways driving PTB and PE, which are incompletely understood. Such knowledge will facilitate the development of preventive and therapeutic interventions.

A highly promising approach to derive predictive tests of sufficient accuracy is the combination of proteomics with other omics, that is, the conduct of multiomics studies. The integration of information from various biological layers, including the genome, transcriptome, proteome, and immunome in midsized study cohorts has already revealed that multiomics models improve predictive power.[8] They also provide a more complete view of the biological process underlying PTB and PE and, as such, may be a powerful approach to improve disease diagnostics,[76] predictive accuracy,[8] and the understanding of interrelationships between different omics, thereby pointing to important pathophysiologic drivers of PTB and PE.[10] Various advanced computational methods exist for the integration of omics datasets, generally classified as early, late, or hybrid fusions.[77] Early-fusion approaches concatenate and use features from all omic sources to train and validate a predictive model. Late-fusion approaches first build predictive models for each omics dataset and then combine these predictions to build an integrated model. As noted previously, including the proteome in an integrative approach can greatly enhance the accuracy of an integrated model, as it offers superior accuracy on its one when compared with other omics.[8,10] A common approach when deriving integrated models is to assign more weight to the omics dataset that are particularly informative.[78] As such the proteome, likely being quite informative, will weigh heavily on the accuracy of the final model. Inclusion of the proteome should, therefore, be strongly considered when engaging in a multiomics approach.

One important limitation of multiomics models is that some relevant multiomics data may be difficult to obtain in a clinical setting. Multiomics biosignatures may, therefore, not directly translate into a simple predictive test. They may require substitution of parameters that cannot readily be measured, and such substitutions will require the simultaneous consideration of all available biological, demographic, and clinical data. The promise of this approach resides in the inherently redundant nature of these datasets.

In summary, PTB is a complex and diverse clinical syndrome influenced by a combination of genetic, biological, and environmental factors. The risk of PTB has been associated with maternal characteristics (eg, BMI),[79] comorbidities and medical history (eg, previous PTB, and family history of PTB),[80] and the interpregnancy interval.[81] Similarly, risks factors for PE include a history of PE, chronic hypertension, diabetes, kidney disease, obesity, and nulliparity.[82] These data are typically available from the electronic health records, an important source for improving risk assessment.[83] Integration of these clinical data with omics measurements, while challenging due to data heterogeneity and high-dimensionality, will be important to improve the accuracy of predicting and diagnosing PTB and PE.[10,84]

DISCLOSURE

The authors have nothing to disclose.

FUNDING

This work was supported, in part, by the Prematurity Research Fund, the March of Dimes Prematurity Research Center at Stanford University, the Charles B. and Ann L. Johnson Research Fund, the Christopher Hess Research Fund, the Providence Foundation Research Fund, the Roberts Foundation Research Fund, Bill and Melinda Gates Foundation, r35gm138353, and the Stanford Maternal and Child Health Research Institute.

Best Practices

What is the current practice for PTB?

Currently, there is no best practice for the prevention for PTB.

What changes in current practice are likely to improve outcomes?

Further studies are needed to establish a set of robust proteomic biomarkers and develop a predictive tool to identify women who would benefit from frequent clinical follow-up and medical interventions, including the preemptive treatment with low-dose aspirin, which reduces the risk of PTB.

Bibliographic Sources:

Magee LA, von Dadelszen P. Aspirin from early pregnancy to reduce preterm birth. Lancet Glob Health 2023;11(3):e314-e5.

REFERENCES

1. Ohuma EO, Moller AB, Bradley E, et al. National, regional, and global estimates of preterm birth in 2020, with trends from 2010: a systematic analysis. Lancet 2023;402(10409):1261–71.
2. Centers for Disease Control. Percentage of preterm births in the United States from 1990 to 2021 [Graph]. 2023. Available at: https://www.statista.com/statistics/276 075/us-preterm-birth-percentage/. [Accessed 9 January 2024].

3. March of Dimes. The 2023 March of Dimes Report Card. 2023. Available at: https://www.marchofdimes.org/report-card.

4. Magee LA, von Dadelszen P. Aspirin from early pregnancy to reduce preterm birth. Lancet Glob Health 2023;11(3):e314–5.

5. Romero R, Dey SK, Fisher SJ. Preterm labor: one syndrome, many causes. Science 2014;345(6198):760–5.

6. Aghaeepour N, Ganio EA, McIlwain D, et al. An immune clock of human pregnancy. Sci Immunol 2017;2(15):eaan2946.

7. Liang L, Rasmussen MH, Piening B, et al. Metabolic dynamics and prediction of gestational age and time to delivery in pregnant women. Cell 2020;181(7): 1680–1692 e15.

8. Jehan F, Sazawal S, Baqui AH, et al. Multiomics characterization of preterm birth in low- and middle-income countries. JAMA Netw Open 2020;3(12):e2029655.

9. Han X, Ghaemi MS, Ando K, et al. Differential dynamics of the maternal immune system in healthy pregnancy and preeclampsia. Front Immunol 2019;10:1305.

10. Marić I, Contrepois K, Moufarrej MN, et al. Early prediction and longitudinal modeling of preeclampsia from multiomics. Patterns (NY) 2022;3(12):100655.

11. Stelzer IA, Ghaemi MS, Han X, et al. Integrated trajectories of the maternal metabolome, proteome, and immunome predict labor onset. Sci Transl Med 2021; 13(592):eabd9898.

12. Aghaeepour N, Lehallier B, Baca Q, et al. A proteomic clock of human pregnancy. Am J Obstet Gynecol 2018;218(3):347 e1–e14.

13. D'Silva AM, Hyett JA, Coorssen JR. Proteomic analysis of first trimester maternal serum to identify candidate biomarkers potentially predictive of spontaneous preterm birth. J Proteomics 2018;178:31–42.

14. Ghaemi MS, Tarca AL, Romero R, et al. Proteomic signatures predict preeclampsia in individual cohorts but not across cohorts - implications for clinical biomarker studies. J Matern Fetal Neonatal Med 2022;35(25):5621–8.

15. Ghezzi F, Franchi M, Raio L, et al. Elevated amniotic fluid C-reactive protein at the time of genetic amniocentesis is a marker for preterm delivery. Am J Obstet Gynecol 2002;186(2):268–73.

16. Goepfert AR, Goldenberg RL, Andrews WW, et al. The preterm prediction study: association between cervical interleukin 6 concentration and spontaneous preterm birth. National Institute of Child health and human development maternal-fetal medicine units network. Am J Obstet Gynecol 2001;184(3):483–8.

17. Gudicha DW, Romero R, Gomez-Lopez N, et al. The amniotic fluid proteome predicts imminent preterm delivery in asymptomatic women with a short cervix. Sci Rep 2022;12(1):11781.

18. Gunko VO, Pogorelova TN, Linde VA. Proteomic profiling of the blood serum for prediction of premature delivery. Bull Exp Biol Med 2016;161(6):829–32.

19. Hong S, Lee JE, Kim YM, et al. Identifying potential biomarkers related to preterm delivery by proteomic analysis of amniotic fluid. Sci Rep 2020;10(1):19648.

20. Khanam R, Fleischer TC, Boghossian NS, et al. Performance of a validated spontaneous preterm delivery predictor in South Asian and Sub-Saharan African women: a nested case control study. J Matern Fetal Neonatal Med 2022; 35(25):8878–86.

21. Lynch AM, Wagner BD, Deterding RR, et al. The relationship of circulating proteins in early pregnancy with preterm birth. Am J Obstet Gynecol 2016;214(4): 517 e1–e8.

22. Manning R, James CP, Smith MC, et al. Predictive value of cervical cytokine, anti-microbial and microflora levels for pre-term birth in high-risk women. Sci Rep 2019;9(1):11246.

23. Markenson GR, Saade GR, Laurent LC, et al. Performance of a proteomic pre-term delivery predictor in a large independent prospective cohort. Am J Obstet Gynecol MFM 2020;2(3):100140.

24. Massaro G, Scaravilli G, Simeone S, et al. Interleukin-6 and Mycoplasma hominis as markers of preterm birth and related brain damage: our experience. J Matern Fetal Neonatal Med 2009;22(11):1063–7.

25. Pereira L, Reddy AP, Alexander AL, et al. Insights into the multifactorial nature of preterm birth: proteomic profiling of the maternal serum glycoproteome and maternal serum peptidome among women in preterm labor. Am J Obstet Gynecol 2010;202(6):555 e1–e10.

26. Romero R, Espinoza J, Rogers WT, et al. Proteomic analysis of amniotic fluid to identify women with preterm labor and intra-amniotic inflammation/infection: the use of a novel computational method to analyze mass spectrometric profiling. J Matern Fetal Neonatal Med 2008;21(6):367–88.

27. Saade GR, Boggess KA, Sullivan SA, et al. Development and validation of a spontaneous preterm delivery predictor in asymptomatic women. Am J Obstet Gynecol 2016;214(5):633 e1–e24.

28. Sorokin Y, Romero R, Mele L, et al. Maternal serum interleukin-6, C-reactive protein, and matrix metalloproteinase-9 concentrations as risk factors for preterm birth <32 weeks and adverse neonatal outcomes. Am J Perinatol 2010;27(8):631–40.

29. Tarca AL, Pataki BA, Romero R, et al. Crowdsourcing assessment of maternal blood multi-omics for predicting gestational age and preterm birth. Cell Rep Med 2021;2(6):100323.

30. Wallenstein MB, Jelliffe-Pawlowski LL, Yang W, et al. Inflammatory biomarkers and spontaneous preterm birth among obese women. J Matern Fetal Neonatal Med 2016;29(20):3317–22.

31. Sobsey CA, Ibrahim S, Richard VR, et al. Targeted and untargeted proteomics approaches in biomarker development. Proteomics 2020;20(9):e1900029.

32. Sun BB, Maranville JC, Peters JE, et al. Genomic atlas of the human plasma proteome. Nature 2018;558(7708):73–9.

33. Eldjarn GH, Ferkingstad E, Lund SH, et al. Large-scale plasma proteomics comparisons through genetics and disease associations. Nature 2023;622(7982): 348–58.

34. Edwards AM, Isserlin R, Bader GD, et al. Too many roads not taken. Nature 2011; 470(7333):163–5.

35. Method of the year 2012. Nat Methods 2013;10(1):1.

36. Aebersold R, Mann M. Mass spectrometry-based proteomics. Nature 2003; 422(6928):198–207.

37. Meuleman W, Engwegen JY, Gast MC, et al. Comparison of normalisation methods for surface-enhanced laser desorption and ionisation (SELDI) time-of-flight (TOF) mass spectrometry data. BMC Bioinf 2008;9:88.

38. Espinosa C, Ali SM, Khan W, et al. Comparative predictive power of serum vs plasma proteomic signatures in feto-maternal medicine. AJOG Glob Rep 2023; 3(3):100244.

39. Rice JA. Mathematical statistics and data analysis. 3rd edition. Belmont: Brooks/Cole; 2007.

40. Benjamini Y, Hochberg Y. Controlling the false discovery rate: a practical and powerful approach to multiple testing. J R Stat Soc Series B Stat Methodol 1995; 57(1):289–300.

41. Tibshirani R, Wainwright M, Hastie T. Statistical learning with sparsity: the Lasso and generalizations. New York: Chapman and Hall/CRC; 2015.

42. Yu B. Stability. Bernoulli 2013;19(4):1484–500.

43. Huan X, Caramanis C, Mannor S. Sparse algorithms are not stable: a no-free-lunch theorem. IEEE Trans Pattern Anal Mach Intell 2012;34(1):187–93.

44. Meinshausen N, Bühlmann P. Stability selection. J R Stat Soc Series B Stat Methodol 2010;72(4):417–73.

45. Barber RF, Candès EJ. Controlling the false discovery rate via knockoffs. Ann Statist 2015;43(5):2055–85.

46. Candès EJ, Fan Y, Janson L, et al. Panning for gold: 'Model-X' knockoffs for high dimensional controlled variable selection. J R Stat Soc Series B Stat Methodol 2018;80(3):551–77.

47. Bach FR. Bolasso: model consistent lasso estimation through the bootstrap. In: Proceedings of the 25th international conference on Machine learning, 2008; 33-40.

48. Hedou J, Marić I, Bellan G, et al. Discovery of sparse, reliable omic biomarkers with Stabl. Nat Biotechnol 2024. https://doi.org/10.1038/s41587-023-02033-x.

49. Hartman E, Scott AM, Karlsson C, et al. Interpreting biologically informed neural networks for enhanced proteomic biomarker discovery and pathway analysis. Nat Commun 2023;14(1):5359.

50. Leng D, Zheng L, Wen Y, et al. A benchmark study of deep learning-based multi-omics data fusion methods for cancer. Genome Biol 2022;23(1):171.

51. Gupta JK, Alfirevic A. Systematic review of preterm birth multi-omic biomarker studies. Expert Rev Mol Med 2022;24:1–24.

52. Romero R, Gomez R, Chaiworapongsa T, et al. The role of infection in preterm labour and delivery. Paediatr Perinat Epidemiol 2001;15(Suppl 2):41–56.

53. Pandey M, Chauhan M, Awasthi S. Interplay of cytokines in preterm birth. Indian J Med Res 2017;146(3):316–27.

54. Prairie E, Cote F, Tsakpinoglou M, et al. The determinant role of IL-6 in the establishment of inflammation leading to spontaneous preterm birth. Cytokine Growth Factor Rev 2021;59:118–30.

55. Nadeau-Vallee M, Obari D, Quiniou C, et al. A critical role of interleukin-1 in preterm labor. Cytokine Growth Factor Rev 2016;28:37–51.

56. Leitner K, Al Shammary M, McLane M, et al. IL-1 receptor blockade prevents fetal cortical brain injury but not preterm birth in a mouse model of inflammation-induced preterm birth and perinatal brain injury. Am J Reprod Immunol 2014; 71(5):418–26.

57. Dabouz R, Cheng CWH, Abram P, et al. An allosteric interleukin-1 receptor modulator mitigates inflammation and photoreceptor toxicity in a model of retinal degeneration. J Neuroinflammation 2020;17(1):359.

58. Dimitriadis E, Rolnik DL, Zhou W, et al. Pre-eclampsia. Nat Rev Dis Primers 2023; 9(1):8.

59. Romero R, Chaiworapongsa T. Preeclampsia: a link between trophoblast dysregulation and an antiangiogenic state. J Clin Invest 2013;123(7):2775–7.

60. Karumanchi SA. Angiogenic factors in preeclampsia: from diagnosis to therapy. Hypertension 2016;67(6):1072–9.

61. Honigberg MC, Cantonwine DE, Thomas AM, et al. Analysis of changes in maternal circulating angiogenic factors throughout pregnancy for the prediction of preeclampsia. J Perinatol 2016;36(3):172–7.

62. Danielli M, Thomas RC, Gillies CL, et al. Blood biomarkers to predict the onset of pre-eclampsia: a systematic review and meta-analysis. Heliyon 2022;8(11):e11226.

63. Widmer M, Cuesta C, Khan KS, et al. Accuracy of angiogenic biomarkers at ≦20weeks' gestation in predicting the risk of pre-eclampsia: a WHO multicentre study. Pregnancy Hypertens 2015;5(4):330–8.

64. Herraiz I, Simon E, Gomez-Arriaga PI, et al. Clinical implementation of the sFlt-1/PlGF ratio to identify preeclampsia and fetal growth restriction: a prospective cohort study. Pregnancy Hypertens 2018;13:279–85.

65. Levine RJ, Lam C, Qian C, et al. Soluble endoglin and other circulating antiangiogenic factors in preeclampsia. N Engl J Med 2006;355(10):992–1005.

66. Zeisler H, Llurba E, Chantraine F, et al. Predictive value of the sFlt-1:PlGF ratio in women with suspected preeclampsia. N Engl J Med 2016;374(1):13–22.

67. National Institute for Health and Care Excellence (NICE). Diagnostics guidance DG49. 2022. Available at: https://www.nice.org.uk/guidance/dg49.

68. Verlohren S, Herraiz I, Lapaire O, et al. New gestational phase-specific cutoff values for the use of the soluble fms-like tyrosine kinase-1/placental growth factor ratio as a diagnostic test for preeclampsia. Hypertension 2014;63(2):346–52.

69. Beernink RHJ, Zwertbroek EF, Schuitemaker JHN, et al. First trimester serum biomarker discovery study for early onset, preterm onset and preeclampsia at term. Placenta 2022;128:39–48.

70. Chen H, Aneman I, Nikolic V, et al. Maternal plasma proteome profiling of biomarkers and pathogenic mechanisms of early-onset and late-onset preeclampsia. Sci Rep 2022;12(1):19099.

71. Ouyang Y, Chen H, Chen H. Reduced plasma adiponectin and elevated leptin in pre-eclampsia. Int J Gynaecol Obstet 2007;98(2):110–4.

72. Taylor BD, Ness RB, Olsen J, et al. Serum leptin measured in early pregnancy is higher in women with preeclampsia compared with normotensive pregnant women. Hypertension 2015;65(3):594–9.

73. Luewan S, Teja-Intr M, Sirichotiyakul S, et al. Low maternal serum pregnancy-associated plasma protein-A as a risk factor of preeclampsia. Singapore Med J 2018;59(1):55–9.

74. Poon LC, Nicolaides KH. Early prediction of preeclampsia. Obstet Gynecol Int 2014;2014:297397.

75. Wright D, Tan MY, O'Gorman N, et al. Predictive performance of the competing risk model in screening for preeclampsia. Am J Obstet Gynecol 2019;220(2):199 e1–e13.

76. Lunke S, Bouffler SE, Patel CV, et al. Integrated multi-omics for rapid rare disease diagnosis on a national scale. Nat Med 2023;29(7):1681–91.

77. Baltrusaitis T, Ahuja C, Morency LP. Multimodal machine learning: a survey and taxonomy. IEEE Trans Pattern Anal Mach Intell 2019;41(2):423–43.

78. Breiman L. Stacked regressions. Mach Learn 1996;24:49–64.

79. Cnattingius S, Villamor E, Johansson S, et al. Maternal obesity and risk of preterm delivery. JAMA 2013;309(22):2362–70.

80. Koire A, Chu DM, Aagaard K. Family history is a predictor of current preterm birth. Am J Obstet Gynecol MFM 2021;3(1):100277.

81. Schummers L, Hutcheon JA, Hernandez-Diaz S, et al. Association of short interpregnancy interval with pregnancy outcomes according to maternal age. JAMA Intern Med 2018;178(12):1661–70.

82. American College of Obstetrics and Gynecology. Low-dose aspirin use for the prevention of preeclampsia and related morbidity and mortality. Practice Advisory 2021;1–6.
83. Marić I, Tsur A, Aghaeepour N, et al. Early prediction of preeclampsia via machine learning. Am J Obstet Gynecol MFM 2020;2(2):100100.
84. Higdon R, Earl RK, Stanberry L, et al. The promise of multi-omics and clinical data integration to identify and target personalized healthcare approaches in autism spectrum disorders. OMICS 2015;19(4):197–208.

Estimating Gestational Age and Prediction of Preterm Birth Using Metabolomics Biomarkers

Victoria C. Ward, MD[a,1], Steven Hawken, PhD[b,c,1,*],
Pranesh Chakraborty, MD[d,e], Gary L. Darmstadt, MD, MS[f,2],
Kumanan Wilson, MD, MSc[b,g,h,2]

KEYWORDS

- Metabolomics • Preterm birth • Gestational age • Newborn screening
- Maternal newborn health • Perinatal epidemiology • Machine learning
- Prediction modeling

KEY POINTS

- Preterm birth (PTB) is a leading cause of morbidity and mortality globally in children aged under 5 years, particularly in low-resource settings.
- Accurate measurement of gestational age (GA) and PTB status in newborns are often a challenge in low-resource settings where access to prenatal care and ultrasound GA dating may be limited.
- Algorithms utilizing metabolomic biomarkers could allow accurate prediction of high-risk pregnancies for PTB and accurate GA dating.

Continued

[a] Department of Pediatrics, Stanford University School of Medicine, 291 Campus Drive Li Ka Shing Building, Stanford, CA 94305, USA; [b] Clinical Epidemiology Program, Ottawa Hospital Research Institute, Centre for Practice Changing Research, 501 Smyth Road, Box 201-B, Ottawa, Ontario, Canada K1H 8L6; [c] School of Epidemiology and Public Health, University of Ottawa, 600 Peter Morand Crescent, Ottawa, Ontario, Canada K1G 5Z3; [d] Newborn Screening Ontario, Children's Hospital of Eastern Ontario, 415 Smyth Road, Ottawa, Ontario K1H 8M8, Canada; [e] Department of Pediatrics, University of Ottawa, Roger Guindon Hall, 451 Smyth Rd, Ottawa Ontario, Canada K1H 8M5; [f] Prematurity Research Center, Department of Pediatrics, Stanford University School of Medicine, 453 Quarry Road, Palo Alto, CA 94304, USA; [g] Department of Medicine, University of Ottawa, Roger Guindon Hall, 451 Smyth Road, Ottawa, Ontario, Canada K1H 8M5; [h] Bruyère Research Institute, 85 Primrose Avenue, Ottawa, Ontario, Canada K2A2E5
[1] Equally contributing first authors.
[2] Equally contributing senior authors.
* Corresponding author. Centre for Practice Changing Research, 451 Smyth Road, L1294 Box 201-B, Ottawa, Ontario, Canada K1H 8L6.
E-mail address: shawken@ohri.ca

Clin Perinatol 51 (2024) 411–424
https://doi.org/10.1016/j.clp.2024.02.012
0095-5108/24/© 2024 Elsevier Inc. All rights reserved.
perinatology.theclinics.com

Continued

- Accurate metabolomic prediction algorithms would provide the opportunity for more appropriate newborn care, and improved surveillance of the burden of PTB, especially in low-resource countries with limited access to ultrasound and prenatal care.
- Postnatal metabolomics algorithms for GA estimation and PTB status have been developed and extensively externally validated that can estimate GA within less than 1 week of ultrasound GA.

INTRODUCTION

Complications from preterm birth (PTB), defined as birth occurring before 37 weeks' gestation, are the leading cause of death in children aged under 5 years, accounting for over a third of neonatal deaths globally.[1,2] Despite the importance and impact of PTB, it remains a global challenge to accurately measure the true burden, especially in low-resource settings. The reference standard for an accurate gestational age (GA) dating is first trimester ultrasound coupled with standardized training and use of appropriate growth metrics.[3,4] Yet in many places, there is limited availability of accurate measures of GA such as first trimester ultrasound, as well as the implementation of standardized training and tools. In the absence of this gold standard, other methods are available to estimate GA postnatally, including tools such as the Ballard and Dubowitz scores based on a combination of physical, neurologic, and developmental measures.[5] These tools are less accurate than ultrasound and require training and standardized methodologies to be consistently applied in different settings. Furthermore, there is often inadequate access to high-quality prenatal care and thus incomplete or inaccurate documentation of date of last menstrual period, making the estimation of GA, and hence of PTB, challenging at both individual and population levels. In recent years, a number of alternative approaches to prenatal and postnatal GA assessments have leveraged laboratory-based assessments of multiomics to explore their feasibility and reliability for accurate GA dating. Genomics, proteomics, transcriptomics, lipidomics, and metabolomic markers have been investigated for predictive utility in characterizing both GA and the risk of PTB. Metabolomics—or the field of study involving metabolites or small molecules ($\leq$1.5 kDa) involved in the biochemical processes and pathways that comprise the metabolism of an organism—have been thought to be particularly promising in this regard. Metabolomics is a field undergoing rapid growth, particularly in research studies of disease risk and health prognoses.[6,7] Metabolomics markers are of particular interest among multiomics in studying health-related states because they most closely reflect phenotype, physiology and response to environmental exposures, infection, drugs, diet, and health-related behaviors.[8,9] While targeted metabolomics analyses measure a limited number of labeled analytes with known molecular weight, untargeted metabolomics is primarily a hypothesis generating process whereby all measurable analytes in a sample are characterized. This often leads to the detection of hundreds, potentially thousands of analytes, both known and unknown.[10–12]

To date, there is no universal approach for the detection and analysis of metabolites. However, laboratory technologies such as liquid chromatography and mass spectrometry (MS) are used in many settings for the detection and measurement of metabolite concentrations in biofluids. Multiple biofluids and tissues have been identified for their potential in characterizing GA and risk of PTB. These include maternal sources such as blood, urine, or cervicovaginal fluid or amniotic fluid (AF) collected during pregnancy, as well as postpartum maternal and neonatal sources including placenta, umbilical cord blood, or newborn blood or urine.[13,14] In addition, the metabolomics of breast milk composition has been studied in order to characterize the trajectory of nutritional characteristics, specifically to capture when full-term nutritional status is achieved.[13,15] Metabolomics biomarkers derived from noninvasive sources, especially maternal urine or blood, or neonatal samples such as heel-prick-derived blood or cord blood, are of particular value in clinical prediction and care management, given the feasibility and acceptability of their collection.

There are distinct differences in the goals of metabolomics biomarker discovery and prediction algorithms. A number of studies have focused on identifying metabolomic biomarkers early in pregnancy from maternal blood, urine, or cervicovaginal fluid or AF to prospectively identify those at high risk of PTB with the aim of early intervention and management of complications.[16–23] Conversely, several studies focused on postnatal metabolites derived from newborn dried blood spots (DBS) with the aim of estimating GA and preterm-status at birth in low-resource settings, both for surveillance and potentially care management where prenatal care and GA dating tools such as first trimester ultrasound have limited availability.[24–31] In this review, we aim to examine the current state of the evidence for the use of metabolomic biomarkers to predict the risk of PTB prospectively, and for postnatal estimation of GA and PTB status.

MATERNAL METABOLOMIC FACTORS

Biorepositories of maternal samples are being applied to identify maternal metabolites predictive of PTB and GA at birth. Multiple studies have investigated the predictive utility of maternal plasma metabolites for PTB.[17,18] Other studies have pursued multiomics approaches involving multiple biofluids. For instance, Jehan and colleagues[16] utilized a multiomics strategy to characterize maternal biological factors associated with PTB. Blood and urine specimens were collected in 81 women early in pregnancy, and targeted proteomics and untargeted transcriptomics assays were conducted on plasma and metabolomics analyses were conducted on urine. A machine-learning algorithm was applied to each individual omics dataset, and then an integrated machine-learning approach was used to develop a combined prediction algorithm. The primary biological features associated with prematurity were plasma inflammatory biomarkers and urine metabolomics biomarkers involved in the glutamine and glutamate metabolism, as well as amino acid biosynthesis pathways for valine, leucine, and isoleucine.

AMNIOTIC AND CERVICOVAGINAL FLUIDS

AF collection is an invasive specialized procedure whereby fluid is collected early in pregnancy from the amniotic sac surrounding the developing fetus. This procedure carries the risk of complications including miscarriage, infection, preterm labor, and bleeding. Romero and colleagues[18–20,22,23] reported differences in amino acid and carbohydrate profiles in AF samples from women with preterm labor with and without intra-amniotic inflammation or infection. Menon and colleagues[22] collected AF samples during labor in 25 women with PTB prior to 34 weeks (excluding preterm premature rupture of membranes) and 25 with full-term deliveries. They identified 350 metabolites via MS and further identified differences in metabolites in biochemical pathways related to histidine, steroids, xanthine, bile acids, and fatty acids as well as metabolism of drugs and detoxification of xenobiotics. Although promising predictive performance in discriminating between preterm and full-term births was reported in these and other metabolomic studies of AF, the invasiveness and risk of complications makes it unlikely that the use of AF would become commonplace except in cases where amniocentesis was medically indicated.

POSTNATAL METABOLOMIC ANALYSIS OF NEWBORN PERIPHERAL BLOOD AND UMBILICAL CORD BLOOD SAMPLES

In settings where prenatal assessments of GA are limited, postnatal assessments can potentially be conducted. Postnatal assessments can be particularly valuable when an infant is born small to help determine whether the child is small due to prematurity or whether they experienced restricted intrauterine growth resulting in small-for-gestational age. At a population level, these assessments can provide estimates of the prevalence of PTB. At an individual level, personalized GA estimates would facilitate the provision of appropriate clinical interventions employed to support the infant and thus improve their likelihood of survival and long-term health and development.

A number of studies have been conducted by our research group and others to develop and validate metabolomics models to estimate GA at birth and PTB status.[24–26,30,31] These studies have used large retrospective cohorts with metabolomics markers measured from newborn heel-prick-derived DBS samples for purposes of newborn screening for rare inborn errors of metabolism and other serious conditions. Many countries have implemented newborn screening programs, which routinely collect and analyze neonatal biosamples for concentrations of targeted metabolites, among other markers (such as genomic and immunologic factors), to identify newborns at high risk of inborn errors of metabolism and other rare and serious conditions.[32,33] The clear advantage of investigating the utility of these markers in characterizing GA and PTB is that the infrastructure and laboratory processes for these biomarkers are already in place in some settings. Although the screening analytes available in newborn screening panels are tailored to the detection of specific disorders, these analytes are also reflective of the newborn's physiologic and developmental state, and hence they have utility in assessing general health and developmental status.

In traditional newborn screening, DBS are collected from newborn heel-prick blood samples within 72 hours of birth, and metabolites are analyzed to assess for various genetic and metabolic diseases such as cystic fibrosis, sickle cell disease, and amino acid metabolism diseases. Similar sets of these analytes were investigated for their associations with levels of prematurity using algorithms developed in North American cohorts of newborns to estimate an infant's GA postnatally.[24–26,30,31] We will discuss in more detail algorithms for which prospective external validation has been undertaken.

MODEL DEVELOPMENT

A number of algorithms have been developed by our research group and others utilizing a variety of statistical modeling and machine-learning approaches, including multivariable linear and logistic regression analyses. A number of postnatal GA dating algorithms have been developed in large North American cohorts of newborns with clinical data linked to newborn screening results from heel-prick DBS samples. These models incorporated large numbers of candidate predictors, including clinical covariates (sex, birthweight, and multiple gestation) and screening analyte levels (**Table 1**), pairwise interactions among covariates, and nonlinear relationships between covariates and outcomes. GA in weeks has been modeled as a continuous outcome, as well as PTB status as a dichotomous outcome. The incorporation of nonlinear relationships and interaction effects among predictors quickly results in large numbers of predictors relative to sample size. Because of the large number of predictors used in model development, regularization algorithms have been applied during model training for models developed by our team.[25] Specifically, we applied elastic net regularization, which uses a 2 fold penalization approach that blends lasso and ridge regression which penalizes model complexity by shrinking regression coefficients toward 0. The elastic net algorithm allows model fitting that can accommodate large numbers of predictors, including the scenario where there are potentially more candidate predictors than observations in the dataset (p >> n).[34,35] These regularization methods were developed in response to the challenges of large omics datasets where hundreds or even thousands of features may be measured for each participant (genomic or gene expression arrays, for example). Standard statistical modeling approaches start to fail when p is large in relation to n. Variable screening and automatic selection procedures are not necessarily helpful in these situations because biases can be introduced through bivariate screening of individual predictors. Regularization approaches can either eliminate the need for variable selection or in the case of the lasso/elastic net approaches can act as a form of automatic variable selection by shrinking some model coefficients to 0 or near 0, without the inherent biases that can be introduced by other variable selection methods (such as stepwise/stepdown algorithms and bivariate prescreening of candidate predictors).

DATA PREPARATION

There are multiple sources of bias and heterogeneity that can impact metabolite levels such as differences in assays, seasonality, laboratory, and equipment effects.[36] If samples are analyzed in the same central laboratory using the same equipment and assays, then the problem will be less severe. However, when applying algorithms developed in one population to samples collected in another population and setting with different ethnic, sociodemographic, and environmental conditions, these factors can impact model generalizability. A rigorous data-preprocessing strategy can potentially mitigate some of these effects.

Normalization

Data normalization is a process that may include centering and scaling of covariate values. Centering is carried out by subtracting the grand mean of analyte levels from each individual value such that the mean for all analytes is 0. Scaling can be

Table 1	
Newborn screening analytes used in postnatal gestational age-dating models	
Hemoglobins	Adult: HbA(A) Fetal: HbF (F), Acetylated HbF (F1)
Endocrine markers	17-hydroxyprogesterone, thyroid-stimulating hormone
Amino acids	Arginine; phenylalanine; alanine; leucine; ornithine; citruline; tyrosine; glycine; methionine; valine
Acylcarnitines	C0; C2; C3; C4; C5; C5:1; C6; C8; C8:1; C10; C10:1; C12; C12:1; C14; C14:1; C14:2; C16; C18; C18:1; C18:2; C10:1; C12:1; C14:1; C14:2; C4OH; C5:1; C5DC; C5OH; C6DC; C16:OH; C16:1OH; C18OH; C18:1OH; C3DC; C4DC
Enzyme markers	Biotinidase; immunotripsinogen; galactose-1-phosphate uridylyltransferase
T-cell function	T-cell receptor excision circles

conducted by dividing individual analyte values by the overall standard deviation of each analyte. Both centering and scaling results in each analyte having an overall mean of 0 and standard deviation of 1. This has the advantage of bringing all analytes onto a level playing field such that a 1 unit change in any individual analyte represents a 1 SD change. Other variations on normalization are also commonly applied, such as Pareto scaling in which the grand mean is subtracted from each analyte value, but scaling is by the square root of the standard deviation. This has the general impact of preserving more natural biological variation in a given analyte and is often used in normalizing biomarker data.[37,38] Normalization can help prepare analyte covariates for model development and is often recommended as a crucial preprocessing step in many statistical and machine-learning models.

Normalization can reduce the impact of many sources of nonbiological bias; however, it may not address issues in the distribution of analyte values. Many analytes will be highly right skewed, with some values potentially orders of magnitude larger than the bulk of values. These may be characterized as extreme outliers, but they reflect true biological variation and thus must be carefully addressed.

Transformations

Power transformations can often overcome the impact of highly right-skewed distributions and stabilize variance, but for some analytes where there may be very extreme outliers, there may still be highly influential observations that lie far to the right of the bulk of values. In these cases, if the number of extreme outliers is small and they do not disproportionately occur in preterm infants, it may be reasonable to exclude these values. However, in our experience, these values are not rare enough to ignore and do occur more often in preterm or other important subgroups. Hence, we have used the approach of Winsorizing extreme values that are either at least 3 interquartile ranges (IQRs) above the third quartile value or at least 3 IQRs below the first quartile value. Values beyond these boundaries are assigned the value of the boundary. This has the effect of preserving most of the "extremeness" of outlying values while reducing their potential deleterious effect on model fitting.

Nonlinear Associations

In order to allow for nonlinear effects of covariates on the continuous outcome, in developing algorithms for GA dating of North American cohorts, we applied an approach whereby we identified the covariates with the strongest general correlations with GA using partial Spearman correlations.[39] We identified a subset of clinical and analyte predictors with markedly stronger correlations with GA, adjusting for all other predictors. We allocated additional degrees of freedom to these predictors and used restricted cubic splines to model this subset of predictors rather than simple linear terms.

Internal Validation, Overfitting Optimism Correction

Model development must include strategies to avoid overfitting, which occurs when model performance is evaluated simultaneously in the same data in which the model is generated. If a relatively large number of covariates are included relative to the training data, the model's apparent accuracy will be deceptively high compared to future performance in new data. Therefore, the study data are often randomly split into training and testing/validation subsets. The model is fit in one subset, but then evaluated in a separate subset, thereby mimicking performance in an "unseen" population. An alternate approach is to use cross-validation or bootstrap optimism correction, which uses resampling to iteratively train models in one subset of the data and evaluate performance in a separate subset of the data.[39–41] In model development by our group, we employed data splitting, given our large cohorts. We utilized 50% of data for model training, 25% for internal validation/hyperparameter tuning, and 25% to evaluate model performance. For models aimed at estimating GA as a continuous variable, validation metrics for model accuracy include root mean square error (RMSE), which is the square root of the residual variance or mean squared error (MSE) from the model, and mean absolute error (MAE), which is the average deviation between model estimates and true GA. MAE uses absolute value of model errors, compared to MSE, which is the average squared error. Because MSE is based on squared differences, it tends to inflate larger residuals and overpenalizes the average squared error. Hence, MAE arguably provides a more balanced metric reflecting average model accuracy and is increasingly applied as a performance metric for models estimating continuous outcomes.

The final models derived by our research team included birthweight, sex, and multiple gestation, as well as newborn screening analyte values, with birthweight and several highly predictive analytes modeled using restricted cubic splines with 5 knots (optimized using cross-validation) to allow for nonlinearity. The model included pairwise interactions among the clinical and analyte predictors and utilized elastic net regularization to minimize overfitting and accommodate the large number of predictors. This final model was able to accurately predict GA within an average of ±5 days of gold standard ultrasound values (MAE: 0.71; 95% confidence interval [CI]: 0.95, 0.97 weeks), RMSE of 1.04 and AUROC of 0.991 for PTB classification in the internal validation test cohort from Ontario, Canada (**Table 2**).[26] By comparison, internal validation of a model derived independently in Iowa newborns had an internal validation RMSE of 1.5 and area under the receiver-operator curve (AUROC) of 0.938 (see **Table 2**).

EXTERNAL VALIDATION OF NORTH-AMERICAN MODELS

Following the development and internal validation of models in North American heel-prick blood samples, focus shifted to external validation of these models in low-resource settings, given that the majority of prematurity-associated morbidity and mortality occurs in Sub-Saharan Africa and Southeast Asia.[1,2] Validation results are summarized in **Table 2**. We first conducted a validation using data for recent immigrants to Canada according to ethnicity/country of origin and reported very similar accuracy of approximately ±1 week compared with ultrasounds results for nonimmigrant Ontario residents in relation to recent immigrants from India, China, Pakistan, the Philippines, and several other countries of origin.[42] We then conducted external validation studies in existing newborn screening programs and data repositories with collaborators in The Philippines and China and reported lower accuracy compared to the Ontario results, but still within about ±1 week of reference GA determined by ultrasound.[27] Next, we conducted external validation studies in prospective birth cohorts in Bangladesh and Zambia, where we also collected cord blood samples and evaluated the performance of our models compared with those developed in Ontario heel-prick samples. Although model estimates using cord blood were less accurate than those in heel-prick samples, cord blood samples still provided moderate accuracy.[26,28] Finally, we conducted additional external validation studies in prospective birth cohorts in Kenya, Zimbabwe, Zambia, and Bangladesh to further explore accuracy of GA dating algorithms in heel-prick and cord blood, as well as feasibility of implementation in low-income settings. Our findings highlighted the importance of proper timing of reference first trimester GA-dating ultrasounds; the apparent accuracy of model estimates in

Table 2
Internal and external model validation results

Validation Cohort	Study Type	Sample Type	n total/n Preterm	External Validation Accuracy MAE or RMSE (Weeks) for GA Estimation, AUROC for Prediction of Preterm Status 95% CI Included When Reported
Ontario[26]	Retrospective internal validation	Heel-prick	39,666/2226	MAE: 0.71 (95% CI: 0.71, 0.72) RMSE: 1.04 AUROC: 0.991
Iowa[31,45]	Retrospective internal validation	Heel-prick Cord	76,671/6812 933/460	AUROC: 0.938 (95% CI: 0.934, 0.941) RMSE: 1.5 AUROC: 0.982 (95% CI: 0.974, 0.989) RMSE: 1.55
Tanzania (Iowa model)[44]	Prospective external validation	Heel-prick	736/67	RMSE: 1.53 AUROC: 0.83 (95% CI: 0.80, 0.85)
Pakistan and Bangladesh (Iowa model)[44]	Prospective external validation	Heel-prick	575/83	RMSE: 1.52 AUROC: 0.90 (95% CI: 0.88, 0.93)
Uganda (Iowa model)[43,45]	Prospective external validation	Heel-prick Cord (Iowa cord blood model)	666/39 150/11	45.8% within ±1 wk of true GA AUROC: 0.851
Ontario Ethnic Subgroups (Ontario model)[42]	Retrospective internal validation	Heel-prick Nonimmigrants India China Pakistan Philippines Vietnam Bangladesh Somalia Nigeria	230,034/17,045 10,038/681 7468/362 5824/377 5441/451 1408/86 1182/85 833/58 800/56	RMSE: 1.05 RMSE: 1.04 RMSE: 0.98 RMSE: 1.05 RMSE: 1.05 RMSE: 1.00 RMSE:1.14 RMSE: 1.15 RMSE: 1.08

Study (model)	Validation	Sample type	N	MAE
Ontario Assisted Reproduction Conceptions (Ontario model)[46]	Retrospective internal validation	Heel-prick Spontaneous conception Assisted Reproductive Technology conception	50,735/3543 1924/260	MAE(US): 0.70 (95% CI: 0.69, 0.70) MAE (US): 0.70 (95% CI: 0.68, 0.73) MAE(DET): 0.68 (95% CI: 0.66, 0.71)
Philippines (Ontario model)[27]	Retrospective external validation	Heel-prick	82,909/3828	MAE: 0.90 (95% CI: 0.90, 0.91)
China (Ontario model)[27]	Retrospective external validation	Heel-prick	4448/215	MAE: 0.89 (95% CI: 0.86, 0.91)
Bangladesh (Ontario model)[26,28]	Prospective external validation	Heel-prick Cord	520/35 1139/108	MAE: 0.81 (95% CI: 0.75, 0.86) MAE: 0.95 (95% CI: 0.90, 0.99)
Zambia (Ontario model)[26]	Prospective external validation	Heel-prick Cord	142/11 265/22	MAE: 0.79 (95% CI: 0.69, 0.90) MAE: 1.02 (95% CI: 0.90, 1.15)
Kenya (Ontario model)[29]	Prospective external validation	Heel-prick Heel-prick (US at 9–13 wk) Cord Cord (US at 9–13 wk)	1039/93 120/10 1012/91 121/10	MAE: 1.35 (95% CI: 1.27, 1.43) MAE: 1.04 (95% CI: 0.87, 1.22) MAE: 1.44 (95% CI: 1.36, 1.53) MAE: 1.08 (95% CI: 0.90, 1.27)
Zimbabwe (Ontario model) (in preparation)	Prospective external validation	Heel-prick Cord	583/82 562/75	MAE: 1.23 (95% CI: 1.14,1.33) MAE: 1.36 (95% CI: 1.26,1.47)
Zambia (Ontario model) (in preparation)	Prospective external validation	Heel-prick Cord	305/18 528/40	MAE: 0.93 (95% CI: 0.83,1.05) MAE: 1.15 (95% CI: 1.06,1.25)

Kenya was markedly lower than in other cohorts, but when we looked only at newborn samples where the reference GA was estimated between 9 and 13 weeks, model accuracy increased sharply and compared more favorably to other cohorts.[29] Another North-American model derived from an Iowa, United States cohort was externally validated in prospective birth cohorts in Sub-Saharan Africa (Tanzania, Uganda), and South Asia (Pakistan and Bangladesh),[31,43–45] and found similar results to those from Ontario, Canada. **Table 2** lists postnatal GA algorithms developed by our team and other North-American teams and details of model performance metrics for internal and external validation investigations of these algorithms.

DISCUSSION

PTB is the leading cause of morbidity and mortality in children aged under 5 years globally, yet diagnostic assessment tools have continued to be lacking. In the past 10 years, multiomics approaches have advanced as a promising area of research for leveraging multiple types of body fluids to analyze physiologic and pathophysiologic biomarkers for estimating GA and predicting PTB. Studies have explored proteomics, transcriptomics, lipidomics, metabolomics, genomics, immunomics, and others. Lipidomics have demonstrated significant promise, particularly related to the pathways associated with PTB.[47,48] Metabolomics have also been shown to be particularly useful in that metabolites reflect cellular physiology both from underlying genetic material and from the body's response to environmental stressors such as infection and malnutrition leading to characterization of specific disease states. To date, metabolomics have been studied in multiple biosamples including AF, cervicovaginal fluid, urine, or feces in addition to blood from maternal, cord, and neonatal samples.

Given the immense burden of disease associated with PTB, biomarker discovery for the prediction of PTB has been an active area of research in hopes of identifying diagnostic or therapeutic assays to inform development and selection of prenatal and postnatal interventions to avert morbidity and mortality. Metabolite analysis in combination with advanced bioinformatics has led to identification of potential biomarkers and biochemical pathways associated with adverse physiologic states that may lead to PTB or risk of various complications of pregnancy and prematurity. The models we have described demonstrate that metabolomics models can estimate GA to within a week or less of GA via dating ultrasound. Similarly, models for classifying preterm status have achieved a high level of accuracy in classifying preterm infants. There have been promising results in studies aimed at predicting the risk of preterm delivery at various stages of pregnancy from markers and models derived from maternal biofluids; however, none of these markers and models have achieved a level of accuracy that would be useful for clinical intervention and management. Additional research coupled with extensive replication and validation work would be important to advance this area of PTB risk modeling.

While multiple studies have been undertaken to estimate GA and risk of PTB, limitations in sample size and generalizability have hampered success in this endeavor. Metabolomics analysis requires MS or nuclear magnetic resonance spectroscopy and thus is an expensive science,[49] frequently limited to high-income countries or regional laboratories. Furthermore, concordance studies between laboratories for metabolomics measurement in biosamples have rarely been successfully undertaken to ensure generalizability across assays where results from a single study/site show promise. In many instances, biomarker discovery, especially in untargeted metabolomics analyses, is hypotheses generating rather than providing immediately useful tools for diagnoses. Another critique encompasses the findings that in some instances, the assessment of observable clinical factors with or without combination of simple blood tests, such as 17-OHP, TSH, or fetal hemoglobin, for instance in the assessment of preeclampsia[50,51] or even in GA dating,[25] could potentially obviate expensive metabolomics. However, these approaches have not yet proven sufficiently reliable in their accuracy for prediction. And yet, given that over 90% of the burden of mortality and morbidity of premature birth occurs in low-income and middle-income countries where access to ultrasound as well as early intervention and life-saving treatments may be limited, further studies are needed to validate cost-effective dating and risk analysis tools for the identification of fetal and perinatal risks. Therefore, while validation of metabolomics analyses is compelling, metabolomics perhaps best serves as an intermediary step to identify those metabolites that could be leveraged in the future by a simple, cost-effective, and noninvasive point-of-care test such as enzyme-linked immunosorbent assay that not only enables identification of PTB but also provides risk prediction early enough to enable preventive interventions. Only then can we hope to reduce the massive burden of PTB and its associated complications in the expansive burden of morbidity and mortality it causes the world's infants.

DISCLOSURE

The authors have no disclosures to report.

FUNDING

We would like to acknowledge funding from the Bill and Melinda Gates Foundation: Ottawa Hospital Research Institute: OPP1184574; Stanford: OPP1182996.

REFERENCES

1. Ohuma EO, Moller AB, Bradley E, et al. National, regional, and global estimates of preterm birth in 2020, with trends from 2010: a systematic analysis. Lancet 2023;402(10409):1261–71.
2. Ashorn P, Ashorn U, Muthiani Y, et al. Small vulnerable newborns – big potential for impact. Lancet 2023;401(10389):1692–706.
3. Butt K, Lim KI. Guideline No. 388-Determination of gestational age by ultrasound. J Obstet Gynaecol Can 2019;41(10):1497–507.
4. Committee Opinion No 700. Obstet Gynecol 2017;129(5):e150–4.
5. Locham KK, Garg R, Sodhi M, et al. Comparison of assessment of gestational age by Dubowitz scoring system and New Ballard scoring system. J Neonatol 2003;17(2):58–64.
6. Joshi AD, Rahnavard A, Kachroo P, et al. An epidemiological introduction to human metabolomic investigations. Trends Endocrinol Metab 2023;34(9):505–25.
7. Tolstikov V, Moser AJ, Sarangarajan R, et al. Current status of metabolomic biomarker discovery: impact of study design and demographic characteristics. Metabolites 2020;10(6):224.
8. Lasky-Su J, Kelly RS, Wheelock CE, et al. A strategy for advancing for population-based scientific discovery using the metabolome: the establishment of the Metabolomics Society Metabolomic Epidemiology Task Group. Metabolomics 2021;17(5):45.
9. Roekel EH van, Loftfield E, Kelly RS, et al. Metabolomics in epidemiologic research: challenges and opportunities for early-career epidemiologists. Metabolomics 2019;15(1):9.

10. Parfieniuk E, Zbucka-Kretowska M, Ciborowski M, et al. Untargeted metabolomics: an overview of its usefulness and future potential in prenatal diagnosis. Expert Rev Proteomics 2018;15(10):809–16.
11. Zhuang YJ, Mangwiro Y, Wake M, et al. Multi-omics analysis from archival neonatal dried blood spots: limitations and opportunities. Clin Chem Lab Med CCLM 2022;60(9):1318–41.
12. Trifonova OP, Maslov DL, Balashova EE, et al. Evaluation of dried blood spot sampling for clinical metabolomics: effects of different papers and sample storage stability. Metabolites 2019;9(11):277.
13. Pintus R, Dessì A, Mussap M, et al. Metabolomics can provide new insights into perinatal nutrition. Acta Paediatr 2023;112(2):233–41.
14. Monni G, Atzori L, Corda V, et al. Metabolomics in prenatal medicine: a review. Front Med 2021;8:645118.
15. Dessì A, Briana D, Corbu S, et al. Metabolomics of breast milk: the importance of phenotypes. Metabolites 2018;8(4):79.
16. Jehan F, Sazawal S, Baqui AH, et al. Multiomics characterization of preterm birth in low- and middle-income countries. JAMA Netw Open 2020;3(12):e2029655.
17. Espinosa CA, Khan W, Khanam R, et al. Multiomic signals associated with maternal epidemiological factors contributing to preterm birth in low- and middle-income countries. Sci Adv 2023;9(21):eade7692.
18. Baraldi E, Giordano G, Stocchero M, et al. Untargeted metabolomic analysis of amniotic fluid in the prediction of preterm delivery and bronchopulmonary dysplasia. PLoS One 2016;11(10):e0164211.
19. Romero R, Mazaki-Tovi S, Vaisbuch E, et al. Metabolomics in premature labor: a novel approach to identify patients at risk for preterm delivery. J Matern Fetal Neonatal Med 2010;23(12):1344–59.
20. Ghartey J, Anglim L, Romero J, et al. Women with symptomatic preterm birth have a distinct cervicovaginal metabolome. Am J Perinatol 2017;34(11):1078–83.
21. Jelliffe-Pawlowski LL, Shaw GM, Currier RJ, et al. Association of early-preterm birth with abnormal levels of routinely collected first- and second-trimester biomarkers. Am J Obstet Gynecol 2013;208(6):492.e1–11.
22. Menon R, Jones J, Gunst PR, et al. Amniotic fluid metabolomic analysis in spontaneous preterm birth. Reprod Sci 2014;21(6):791–803.
23. Romero R, Espinoza J, Gotsch F, et al. The use of high-dimensional biology (genomics, transcriptomics, proteomics, and metabolomics) to understand the preterm parturition syndrome. BJOG 2006;113(Suppl 3):118–35.
24. Wilson K, Hawken S, Potter B, et al. Accurate prediction of gestational age using newborn screening analyte data. Am J Obstet Gynecol 2016;214(4):513.e1–9.
25. Wilson K, Hawken S, Murphy MSQ, et al. Postnatal prediction of gestational age using newborn fetal hemoglobin levels. EBioMedicine 2017;15:203–9.
26. Hawken S, Ducharme R, Murphy MSQ, et al. Development and external validation of machine learning algorithms for postnatal gestational age estimation using clinical data and metabolomic markers. PLoS One 2023;18(3):e0281074.
27. Hawken S, Murphy MSQ, Ducharme R, et al. External validation of machine learning models including newborn metabolomic markers for postnatal gestational age estimation in East and South-East Asian infants. Gates Open Res 2021;4:164.
28. Murphy MS, Hawken S, Cheng W, et al. External validation of postnatal gestational age estimation using newborn metabolic profiles in Matlab, Bangladesh. Elife 2019;8:e42627.

29. Hawken S, Ward V, Bota AB, et al. Real world external validation of metabolic gestational age assessment in Kenya. PLoS Glob Public Health 2022;2(11): e0000652.

30. Jelliffe-Pawlowski LL, Norton ME, Baer RJ, et al. Gestational dating by metabolic profile at birth: a California cohort study. Am J Obstet Gynecol 2016;214(4): 511.e1–13.

31. Ryckman KK, Berberich SL, Dagle JM. Predicting gestational age using neonatal metabolic markers. Am J Obstet Gynecol 2016;214(4):515.e1–13.

32. Therrell BL, Padilla CD, Loeber JG, et al. Current status of newborn screening worldwide: 2015. Semin Perinatol 2015;39(3):171–87.

33. Fabie NAV, Pappas KB, Feldman GL. The current state of newborn screening in the United States. Pediatr Clin North Am 2019;66(2):369–86.

34. James G, Witten D, Hastie T, et al. An introduction to statistical learning: with applications in R. 2nd edition. New York: Springer; 2021. p. 607.

35. Zou H, Hastie T. Regularization and variable selection via the elastic net. J R Stat Soc Ser B Stat Methodol 2005;67(2):301–20.

36. Sun J, Xia Y. Pretreating and normalizing metabolomics data for statistical analysis. Genes Dis 2024;11(3):100979.

37. Vu T, Riekeberg E, Qiu Y, et al. Comparing normalization methods and the impact of noise. Metabolomics 2018;14(8):108.

38. Karaman I. Metabolomics: from fundamentals to clinical applications. Adv Exp Med Biol 2017;965:145–61.

39. Harrell FE. Regression modeling strategies: with applications to linear models, logistic and ordinal regression, and survival analysis. 2nd edition. Cham Heidelberg New York: Springer; 2015. p. 582.

40. Steyerberg EW. Clinical prediction models: a practical approach to development, validation, and updating. 2nd edition. Cham (Switzerland): Springer; 2019. p. 558.

41. Steyerberg EW, Harrell FE. Prediction models need appropriate internal, internal-external, and external validation. J Clin Epidemiol 2016;69:245–7.

42. Hawken S, Ducharme R, Murphy MSQ, et al. Performance of a postnatal metabolic gestational age algorithm: a retrospective validation study among ethnic subgroups in Canada. BMJ Open 2017;7(9):e015615.

43. Oltman SP, Jasper EA, Kajubi R, et al. Gestational age dating using newborn metabolic screening: a validation study in Busia, Uganda. J Glob Health 2021; 11:04012.

44. Sazawal S, Ryckman KK, Mittal H, et al. Using AMANHI-ACT cohorts for external validation of Iowa new-born metabolic profiles based models for postnatal gestational age estimation. J Glob Health 2021;11:04044.

45. Jasper EA, Oltman SP, Rogers EE, et al. Targeted newborn metabolomics: prediction of gestational age from cord blood. J Perinatol 2022;42(2):181–6.

46. Hawken S, Olibris B, Ducharme R, et al. Validation of gestational age determination from ultrasound or a metabolic gestational age algorithm using exact date of conception in a cohort of newborns conceived using assisted reproduction technologies. AJOG Glob Rep 2022;2(4):100091.

47. Hong SH, Lee JY, Seo S, et al. Lipidomic analysis of cervicovaginal fluid for elucidating prognostic biomarkers and relevant phospholipid and sphingolipid pathways in preterm birth. Metabolites 2023;13(2):177.

48. Chen Y, He B, Liu Y, et al. Maternal plasma lipids are involved in the pathogenesis of preterm birth. GigaScience 2022;11:giac004.

49. Coyle K, Quan AML, Wilson LA, et al. Cost-effectiveness of a gestational age metabolic algorithm for preterm and small-for-gestational-age classification. Am J Obstet Gynecol MFM 2021;3(1):100279.

50. Marić I, Contrepois K, Moufarrej MN, et al. Early prediction and longitudinal modeling of preeclampsia from multiomics. Patterns (NY) 2022;3(12):100655.

51. Fox R, Kitt J, Leeson P, et al. Preeclampsia: risk factors, diagnosis, management, and the cardiovascular impact on the offspring. J Clin Med 2019;8(10):1625.

Untangling Associations of Microbiomes of Pregnancy and Preterm Birth

Anna Maya Powell, MD, MSCR[a,1],
Fouzia Zahid Ali Khan, MBBS, MSPH[a,1], Jacques Ravel, PhD[b],
Michal A. Elovitz, MD[c],*

KEYWORDS

- Microbiomes • Community state types • Preterm birth • Metabolomics
- Metagenomics • Meta transcriptomics

KEY POINTS

- There are strong associative data between *Lactobacillus*-deficient vaginal microbiomes and spontaneous preterm birth (sPTB), preliminary or inconclusive associative data linking oral and gut dysbiosis to sPTB and no inherent placental microbiome.
- Pregnancy microbiome studies lack mechanistic data to explain an increased risk of sPTB in the setting of "dysbiosis" or *Lactobacillus*-deficient, anaerobe-rich vaginal microbial communities.
- PTB phenotyping and standardized reporting of microbiome parameters will allow for easier and more accurate comparisons of results between studies.

INTRODUCTION

Preterm birth (PTB), a live birth prior to 37 weeks, is a leading cause of neonatal morbidity and mortality globally, with rates ranging from 8.7% to 41.4%, with few measurable changes in the PTB rate over the last decade on a global scale.[1,2]

Funding: A.M. Powell is funded by NIH, Unites States/NIAID grant K23-AI155296 and receives royalty payments from UpToDate for authorship. M.A. Elovitz is funded by National Institutes of Health (NIH) (National Institute of Allergy and Infectious Diseases [NIAID]; National Institute of Child Health and Human Development [NICHD]; National Institute of Nursing Research [NINR]). M.A. Elovitz is a consultant with equity in Mirvie.
^a Department of Gynecology and Obstetrics, Johns Hopkins University School of Medicine, 600 North Wolfe Street, Phipps 249, Baltimore, MD 21287, USA; ^b Department of Microbiology and Immunology, Institute for Genome Sciences, 670 West Baltimore Street, 3rd Floor, Room 3173, Baltimore, MD 21201, USA; ^c Department of Obstetrics and Gynecology, Women's Health Research, Icahn School of Medicine at Mount Sinai, Women's Biomedical Research Institute, 1468 Madison Avenue, New York, NY 10029, USA
¹ Authors contributed equally.
* Corresponding author.
E-mail address: michal.elovitz@mssm.edu

Clin Perinatol 51 (2024) 425–439
https://doi.org/10.1016/j.clp.2024.02.009
0095-5108/24/© 2024 Elsevier Inc. All rights reserved.

Approximately a third of PTBs is medically indicated due to maternal health conditions such as pre-eclampsia or fetal conditions such as severe growth restriction. The remaining two-thirds of PTBs are considered "spontaneous" (sPTB). The concept of sPTB implies that the process is similar to a term parturition but just occurring at an early time point. However, several studies suggest that this idea is in error, with research suggesting divergent molecular pathways involved in a preterm compared to a term parturition.[3,4] While etiology of sPTB is likely diverse, there is an overwhelming amount of evidence that demonstrates a role for infection and inflammation.[5,6] Recently, attention has been focused on a role of eubiotic and dysbiotic maternal microbiomes in the etiology of sPTB, including oral, gastrointestinal, and vaginal as drivers of infection and inflammation in the reproductive tract and maternal–fetal interface. Deep sequencing explorations of the maternal microbiomes have expanded knowledge of host–microbiome interactions and has allowed for more comprehensive classifications of the presence or absence of these microbiomes during pregnancy. While several studies have now demonstrated an association between these microbiomes and PTB, these studies were unable to inform whether the microbiomes—or their components—are mechanistically and critically involved in the pathogenesis of sPTB. In this review, we described the current knowledge landscape within each maternal microbiome (oral, gastrointestinal, and vaginal), discussed emerging areas of research, incorporating more holistic metadata for microbiome studies, and finally reviewed future directions.

OVERVIEW OF PREGNANCY MICROBIOMES
The Oral Microbiome

The oral cavity is colonized with over 700 commensals that have been identified from the Human Oral Microbiome Database.[7] The total number of cultivable microorganisms appears to be higher among pregnant versus nonpregnant women.[8,9] Streptococcus mutans carriage increases over the course of pregnancy with significant differences seen between the first trimester versus nonpregnant states.[8,10,11] Several studies revealed that the oral microbiome remains stable throughout pregnancy in terms of richness, diversity, and composition,[8] though composition can vary significantly in the postpartum period with reduced total bacterial counts and altered levels of particular bacterial and pathogenic species.[8,12]

The relationship between maternal periodontal disease and the delivery of a preterm infant was first reported in 1996 by Offenbacher and colleagues.[13] Recent epidemiologic studies have consistently reported that maternal periodontal disease is associated with PTB[14] and emphasized the need for integrated health care approaches that include oral health as a key component of prenatal care. Some studies have demonstrated a higher risk of delivering preterm, low birthweight (LBW) infants, and pre-eclampsia among women with periodontal diseases.[15] The reported associations of periodontal disease and increased risk for adverse pregnancy outcomes, including PTB (relative risk: 1.6; 95% confidence interval [CI]: 1.3, 2.0; 17 studies, 6741 participants) with estimated population-attributable fractions for periodontal disease are 5% to 38% for PTB, 6% to 1% for LBW, and 10% to 55% for pre-eclampsia.[8,15] The most commonly found oral pathogen among women with preterm deliveries is Porphyromonas gingivalis,[8] the major etiologic microorganism that contributes to chronic periodontal disease. The prevalence of this microorganism is statistically significant in women experiencing threatened preterm labor leading to preterm birth, as compared with those with threatened preterm labor resulting in term birth.[16–18] Research to date has not explicitly examined the correlation between P gingivalis and sPTB or iatrogenic PTB.

While the OMB remains stable in composition throughout pregnancy,[8] there are distinct changes in the composition and abundance of oral microorganisms compared with the postpartum or nonpregnant states. Notably, colony-forming unit counts of red and orange complex pathogens, including P gingivalis, were found to be more abundant in subgingival plaque of women with PTBs in contrast to term births ($P < .01$).[14] The levels of Fusobacterium nucleatum, Treponema forsythia, Treponema denticola, and Aggregatibacter actinomycetemcomitans were also closely linked to PTB.[8] These findings suggest that while there is a correlation among OMB, periodontal diseases, and PTB, the relationship is complex and may depend on various factors, including the specific types of bacteria involved and individual host responses. In contrast to this body of study, other studies negate the correlation. For instance, Costa and colleagues[19] reported that the risk of PTB is not directly correlated to an increased amount of periodonto-pathogenic bacteria.

The debate continues regarding the impact of dental treatment during pregnancy on the risk of PTB. Studies indicate a potential reduction in PTB prevalence among pregnant individuals who received dental cleanings.[20] Additionally, evidence suggests that administering periodontal treatment to pregnant patients with mild-to-moderate periodontal disease before 21 weeks of gestation could potentially decrease the risk of PTB by 6%.[20,21] However, other studies have failed to find any associations between periodontal disease and PTB.[22,23]

Whereas optimizing dental health is desired for overall maternal health, there is currently insufficient evidence that targeting the OMB will impact sPTB risk. Research suggests a decrease in the prevalence of S mutans subsequent to the implementation of oral health care intervention, but the outcomes derived from a recent meta-analysis failed to demonstrate statistically significant alterations in S mutans levels after prenatal dental treatment and its effect on PTB.[5] A role for the host–microbiome interaction in the oral cavity to drive inflammation as a contributor to adverse pregnancy outcome is an intriguing and biologically plausible hypothesis, but as of yet, has not been conclusively demonstrated.

The Gut Microbiome

Advances in molecular diagnostic methods have shed light on the role of gut microbiome (GMB) on the risk of PTB. Notably, a study by Shiozaki and colleagues[24] found differences in the GMB of all women who had PTB compared with those with term pregnancies, with a decrease in Clostridium subcluster XVIII, Clostridium cluster IV, Clostridium subcluster XIVa, and Bacteroides observed in the former group. While it was not specified if PTBs were spontaneous or iatrogenic, it was found that concentrations of Clostridium subclusters XVIII and XIVa were observed to be significantly diminished in the PTB cohort compared with the threatened preterm labor without delivery cohort. Furthermore, these concentrations in the threatened preterm labor without delivery cohort were notably reduced in comparison to the PTB group.

Even though the changes in the maternal vaginal microbiome (VMB) and the development of the infant microbiome across different body sites have been well studied, the relationship between the maternal GMB and PTB has not been widely reported. A highly diverse and compositionally stable GMB is considered ideal in supporting intestinal barrier function and metabolite production to maintain an anti-inflammatory environment, particularly from short chain fatty acid (SCFA) production.[25–27] Changes in the GMB over the course of pregnancy include a convergence on a less diverse profile in terms of bacterial richness/abundance, as well as one that metabolically more closely resembles a microbiome associated with metabolic syndrome.[28] Between the first and third trimesters of pregnancy, the alpha diversity (within-subject bacterial diversity) of the gastrointestinal tract decreases while the beta diversity (between subjects bacterial diversity) increases, suggesting a physiologic adaptation to pregnancy.[28] Further aberrations because of poor diet or other underlying conditions, for example, obesity, may be associated with adverse pregnancy outcomes, including pre-eclampsia, PTB, and gestational diabetes.[29–32] In particular, sPTB has been associated with reduced maternal GMB alpha diversity and altered beta diversity. Poor diet (eg, high saturated fat intake) is also noted to be greater among sPTB cases compared with controls.[31,33] Increased maternal GMB alpha-diversity was associated with a 48% lower odds of sPTB (95% CI: 4.2%, 72%) following adjustment for maternal age, marital status, ethnicity, parity, body mass index (BMI), education, antibiotic use, household pets, income, and smoking.[34] Gastrointestinal metabolites, primarily SCFA, are thought to play a critical role in inflammation modulation, and maintenance of intestinal barrier function.[35,36] Microbial dysbiosis may decrease SCFA production which in turn worsens dysbiosis with promotion of more proinflammatory properties. In a case–control study comparing the fecal microbiome of pregnant women with pre-eclampsia (n = 67) to normotensive pregnant individuals by 16S rRNA gene amplicons sequencing, Chen and colleagues investigated microbiome differences by hypertensive disorder status.[30] Fecal material transplants (FMTs) from pregnant participants were then administered to mice, which then demonstrated similar pre-eclampsia phenotypes (increased proteinuria, embryonic resorption, elevated blood pressures, and lower fetal and placental weights). These authors identified impaired intestinal barrier function in the mice with reduced expression of zonulin-1, claudin-4, and occludin tight junction proteins in those receiving FMTs from participants with pre-eclampsia.

Overall, there are preliminary and associative, but not conclusive, data that shift in GMB composition and structure during pregnancy, which are critically involved in the pathogenesis of sPTB and other adverse pregnancy outcomes. It is also noted that there are very preliminary data on the role components of the GMB (eg, microbial metabolites) might contribute to sPTB. Similarly, research on how the GMB might drive inflammatory processes systemically or in the reproductive track is limited.

The Absence of a Placental Microbiome

While the placenta has long been considered to be sterile in normal gestation, about a decade ago, a highly discussed report suggested that the placenta has its own microbiome.[11] In 2014, Aagaard and colleagues[37] found bacterial DNA sequences in a population-based cohort of placental tissues, which raised significant interest in the idea that the placenta might harbor a microbiome. A distinct placental microbiome niche was reported, made up of nonpathogenic commensal microbiota from the phyla Firmicutes, Tenericutes, Proteobacteria, Bacteroidetes, and Fusobacteria, using metagenomic analysis.[37] Though the bacteria were few in absolute number, these various bacteria were thought to represent a metabolically diverse endogenous microbial community in the placenta.

Upon further evaluation, it was found that the isolation of bacteria from placenta had been confounded in prior studies by a variety of factors, including methodology with insufficient infection control, lack of negative controls, and poor descriptions of healthy cases.[38–41] In addition, both the environment of placental collection and mode of delivery can significantly influence bacterial DNA signals from term-delivered placentas.[41] A re-analysis of 15 microbiota studies by Panzer and colleagues[41] found that the high prevalence of *Lactobacillus* amplicon sequence variants was most likely due to contamination, likely from the birth canal during delivery and background DNA contamination. Similarly, another study conducted in Sweden on 76 pregnancies, with 50 women with cesarean deliveries and 26 with vaginal deliveries, did not find placental microbiomes by polymerase chain reaction analysis, sequencing approaches, or bacterial culture experiments.[40] Indeed, many studies have concluded that the placenta, while able to be pathogenically colonized with bacteria, does not have an inherent microbiome.[39,42,43]

The missteps with the research on a nonexisting placental microbiome created calls on the best protocols and processes when investigating low-biomass (or absent) microbiomes.[44,45] Lessons learned should be heeded as we proceed to understand how microbiomes do or do not contribute to sPTB and all aspects of maternal–fetal health.

The Vaginal Microbiome

Low diversity *Lactobacillus*-dominated microbiomes are considered favorable within the vaginal environment, and the pregnancy VMB converges upon one characterized by *Lactobacillus*-predominance.[33] Bacterial vaginosis (BV) is a condition characterized by strict and facultative anaerobic bacterial overgrowth, absence of protective lactobacilli, abnormal vaginal discharge and odor.[34] Almost a third of women of reproductive age will be affected within their lifetimes, with Black/Hispanic women are disproportionately affected.[46,47] Women with a baseline VMB in early pregnancy that is predominantly anaerobe-dominant or non-*Lactobacillus crispatus*-dominant appear to be at higher risk for sPTB.[48–50] In a systematic review and network meta-analysis of 17 studies conducted between 2014 and 2021 (38–539 pregnancies, 8–107 PTB) demonstrated that women presenting with "low-lactobacilli" VMB were at an increased risk (odds ratio [OR]: 1.69; 95% CI: 1.15, 2.49) for PTB compared to women with *L crispatus*-dominant VMB.[51] Limitations of these studies were their inability to dissect the contributions of the VMB to sPTB compared with all PTBs.

The foundational discovery of *Lactobacillus* dominance among vaginal bacteria in 1891[52] was further expanded upon in 2011 by Ravel and colleagues,[53] utilizing advanced 16S rRNA gene amplicon sequencing techniques to characterize the VMB bacterial composition of 396 healthy North American reproductive age women. They categorized the VMB into 5 distinct community state types (CSTs). Notably, 4 of these CSTs were predominantly characterized by *Lactobacillus* species: CST-I by *L crispatus*, CST-II by *Lactobacillus gasseri*, CST-III by *Lactobacillus iners*, and CST-V by *Lactobacillus jensenii*. In contrast, CST-IV was marked by a more diverse composition of non-*Lactobacillus* bacterial groups including *Prevotella*, *Dialister*, *Fannyhessae*, *Gardnerella*, *Megasphaera*, *Peptoniphilus*, *Sneathia*, *Eggerthella*, *Aerococcus*, *Finegoldia*, and *Mobiluncus*.[53]

Fettweis and colleagues[50] used samples from the Multi-Omics Microbiome Study-Pregnancy Initiative to perform longitudinal analysis of the VMB using 16S rRNA gene amplicon sequencing, metagenomics, metratranscriptomics, and cytokine profiles from 45 PTB and 90 term births. Primary findings included that *L crispatus* was greatly reduced in PTB samples, which had higher abundance of *Prevotella* cluster 2 and *Sneathia amnii*. Modeling of relative abundances of vaginal bacterial taxa incorporated BMI, vaginal pH, pregnancy outcome (PTB or TB), gestational age, and random subject effect. When plotted over the duration of gestational age, differential relative abundances can be demonstrated by race and by pregnancy outcomes.[50] This finding suggested that early pregnancy VMB may be helpful in firming up associations with PTB and potential timing for interventions. Additional findings from the study included that bacterial taxa associated with dysbiosis were associated with proinflammatory cytokine elaboration and that PTB risk may differ by carriage of different *Gardnerella vaginalis* clades and transcriptional activities, though the strength of the conclusions is limited by the small number of sPTB cases within the cohort.

Elovitz and colleagues[49] performed a nested case–control study of 107 sPTB cases and 432 term birth controls from a cohort of 2000 pregnant individuals with singleton pregnancies from the motherhood and microbiome study. Key findings included that Black women are more likely to have baseline VMBs classified as CST IV-A or IV-B (more diverse VMB compositions). Additionally, Black participants were more likely to have higher abundance of anaerobic bacteria associated with sPTB (eg, *Mobiluncus curtsii*).[49] The risk profile for sPTB was modulated by a relative mean abundance of *Lactobacillus* spp and vaginal antimicrobial peptide β-defensin-2. In participants with a high relative abundance of *M curtsii*/*Mobiluncus mulieris*, those with high *Lactobacillus* spp abundance had significantly lower sPTB risk compared with those with low *Lactobacillus* spp abundance. Additionally, highest quartiles of β-defensin-2 offered protection against sPTB even in the face of high abundance of bacteria associated with sPTB, for example, genus *Fannyhessea*.[49] Thus, a more nuanced approach is needed to examine the interplay between bacterial presence, relative bacterial abundance, and protective factors that ultimately may modulate sPTB risk.

INTERPLAY BETWEEN SOCIAL HEALTH DETERMINANTS, MICROBIOME, AND PRETERM BIRTH

VMBs are sensitive to environmental chemical exposures that may also be associated with adverse pregnancy outcomes.[47,54] Minority populations may be disproportionately exposed to various environmental chemicals or endocrine disrupting chemicals from food, clothing, and personal care products targeting particular hair textures and skin tones.[55] Environmental exposures and unequal access to green spaces or healthy food may be related to historic practices such as blockbusting and redlining.[56,57] *Lactobacillus*-deficient VMBs have been previously shown to be associated with sPTB and to be more common among Black pregnant people, though the extent to which racial differences in neighborhood conditions may contribute to the disparity in *Lactobacillus*-deficient cervicovaginal microbiomes is unknown. In a Philadelphia-based study, census tract neighborhood deprivation was associated with a *Lactobacillus*-deficient cervicovaginal microbiome in a secondary analysis of the motherhood and microbiome study.[58] Several studies similarly tied in socioeconomic factors and *Lactobacillus* predominance, particularly among Black pregnant women.[48,59–61] *Lactobacillus* dominance has also been associated with avoiding marijuana use,[60] cohabitating with a sexual partner,[60] education level,[59,61] private (vs public) insurance,[59] and private (vs public) hospital use.[59]

In a study of 232 second trimester pregnancy vaginal samples (with 80 PTB), untargeted metabolomics revealed that subjects experiencing sPTB had higher levels of diethanolamine, a chemical commonly used in cosmetics, shampoos, and moisturizers, which is classified as a xenobiotic to the VMB and is thought to disrupt choline and betaine production, processes thought to support term birth.[62] Another highly prevalent metabolite associated with PTB in this cohort, ethyl glucoside, is found in alcohol-containing products, hygienic, and cosmetic products.[63–65]

Cigarette smoking is associated with an independent risk for BV acquisition[66] and lower proportion of vaginal *Lactobacillus* spp[67,68] and may be mediated through the antiestrogenic effects of smoking and small amounts of benzo[a]pyrene diol epoxide.[67] Metabolomics profiles in smokers also differ from nonsmokers, with increased concentrations of biogenic amines such as agmatine, cadaverine, putrescine, tryptamine, and tyramine, known to contribute the malodor associated with BV.[68]

Additionally, social health determinants such as exposure to chronic psychosocial stress may impact vaginal health. Psychosocial stressors including relationships, occupational or housing or food insecurity, and domestic violence can stimulate the hypothalamic–pituitary axis which, in turn, leads to elevated cortisol levels.[69] Both elevated cortisol and norepinephrine levels are associated with vaginal dysbiosis, potentially due to a dysregulated immune response or cortisol-induced inhibition of vaginal glycogen deposition,[70] a key host-produced nutrient supporting the growth and acidification of the vagina by *Lactobacillus* spp in the vagina.

There is emerging evidence that features of the maternal GMB are associated with adverse pregnancy outcomes and that these features may be influenced by diet. Poor diet may act as a risk factor to push physiologic maternal GMB changes to pathogenic alterations. Additionally, poor diet may be a function of access to healthy food which, in turn, may be affected by historic practices such as redlining and blockbusting that are credited with food desert creation.[47] Residence in a food desert is associated with pregnancy morbidity. The rate of having at least one pregnancy morbidity (hypertensive disorder of pregnancy, gestational diabetes, intrauterine growth restriction, preterm premature rupture of membranes, or preterm labor) was higher among women living in food deserts (adjusted OR: 1.64; 95% CI: 1.18, 2.29).[71] Previous study by Salow and colleagues[72] showed that residents in neighborhoods with higher levels of racial residential segregation were at higher risk for PTB. Proinflammatory changes in maternal microbiota are associated with levels of fat-soluble vitamins, higher saturated and mono-unsaturated fats, and higher cholesterol intake in pregnancy.[73] Key differences in the GMB between vegetarian and omnivorous diets have been detected during pregnancy, with vegetarian diets enriched with increased SCFA-producing gut bacteria, which are involved in immune modulation.[74] Other studies have established associations between diet, alterations in the GMB, and development of gestational diabetes.[75–79] Ferrocino and colleagues[78,79] examined fecal microbiota (by 16S rRNA gene amplicons sequencing) of pregnant individuals with gestational diabetes at 24 to 28 weeks and again at 38 weeks of gestation after receiving dietary counseling. Participants who adhered to dietary recommendations as evaluated by a food diary had less *Bacteroides*, bacteria implicated in risk of type 2 diabetes.

LIMITATIONS OF MICROBIOME STUDIES AND ADVERSE PREGNANCY OUTCOMES

Over the last decade, there has been a surge in studies focused on the role of microbiomes at different biological niches and adverse pregnancy outcomes specifically sPTB. To date, the studies support the association of a non-*Lactobacillus*-dominated VMBs with PTB. The association of microbiomes (oral, gut) and sPTB remain unconfirmed. While there are clear associations between the VMB and PTB, progress has been hampered by a reliance on observational studies and 16S rRNA gene amplicons sequencing-based compositional survey data, limiting a mechanistic understanding of these microbiomes and their impact on host physiology.[80] One potential challenge is the lack of in vitro model systems to accurately recapitulate the lower reproductive tract with the presence of epithelial, immune, and stromal cells in varying compositions and known responsiveness to sex-steroids. Additionally, we need to recognize the deep complexity of the vaginal ecosystem, noting that microbial composition alone cannot explain the functional capacity of microbiomes. As such, integrated multiomics (metagenomics, metatranscriptomics, and metabolomics) approaches are required to better understand the host–microbiome relationship. While multiomics studies are needed, for these studies to be clinically impactful, they must not be limited to small samples sizes and/or fail to adequately phenotype the condition of interest. Phenotyping PTB is of critical importance, as broad classifications (eg, by gestational age at delivery or general clinical presentation) are not sufficiently precise to define underlying etiologies.[81] At a simple level, "grouping" of medically indicated PTB and sPTB must not occur. Additionally, sufficient metadata and biological information must be obtained to better delineate the different etiologies of sPTB and allow for more targeted interventions in the future. Low biomass microbiomes may also be more difficult to describe and require special techniques (eg, maternal breastmilk). Maternal microbiomes should also not be regarded in isolation; as more information about associations between dysbiosis in different compartments with sPTB emerges, we need to be thoughtful about investigating cross-talk between microbiomes (**Fig. 1**).

EMERGING AREAS OF RESEARCH

Advancements in culture-independent profiling, particularly through 16S rRNA gene amplicons sequencing and metagenomics, have significantly impacted biology and medicine, leading to initiatives like the NIH's Human Microbiome Project, Europe's MetaHit Project, and the International Human Microbiome Consortium. A shift from culture-based methods to these sequencing-based approaches has advanced our understanding of the composition, structure, and function of microbiomes. However, a lack of consensus protocol may limit comparisons among studies.[82]

While the first decade of microbiome research was characterized by the usage of DNA sequencing-based 16S rRNA gene amplicon and shotgun metagenomics sequencing to describe microbial composition, structure, and functions, genomic technological advances provide the ability to report host and microbial gene activity and expression in complex samples via metatranscriptomics.[83] This technique can elucidate the functioning of microbiomes and make inferences about how environmental factors impact their gene expression, hence the microbiome functions.[83,84] Similarly, metabolomics further our understanding of the mechanism by which the microbiomes exert its effect on the host, by elucidating the effector metabolites. Studies that investigate these crossroads will provide richer data to further explore mechanisms by which the microbiome contribute to healthy and disease states.

Microbiomes that May Impact Preterm Birth

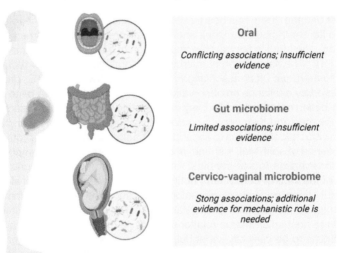

Oral

Conflicting associations; insufficient evidence

Gut microbiome

Limited associations; insufficient evidence

Cervico-vaginal microbiome

Stong associations; additional evidence for mechanistic role is needed

Fig. 1. Summary of microbiomes that may impact preterm birth. (Created with BioRender. com.).

Maternal microbiomes do not exist in a vacuum. As one example, the GMB and VMB both represent complex biological ecosystems that are in communication with each other,[25] and this cross-talk impacts host physiologic, immunologic, and metabolic homeostasis. In mice, *G vaginalis*-induced BV was alleviated by oral gavage of *Lactobacillus plantarum* NK3 and *Bifidobacterium longum* NK49 by inhibiting nuclear factor-κB activation and tumor necrosis factor alpha expression in the vagina, uterus, and colon.[85] In humans, oral probiotics have historically yielded mixed results in treating BV.[86–92] Recently, the live vaginal biotherapeutic *L crispatus* CTV-05 (LACTIN-V) was administered to those at high risk for PTB during an observational clinical study of pregnant individuals and was found to be well tolerated and easy to use.[93] Compared with a historic control cohort, the PTB rate from the study participants was lower (3.3% vs 7%).[93] In nonpregnant individuals, LACTIN-V was found to be very effective in reducing the risk of recurrent BV following vaginal metronidazole treatment in a randomized, double-blind, placebo-controlled phase 2b trial.[94] Further studies are needed to better assess colonization of *L crispatus* CTV-05, but vaginal probiotic use may certainly play a strong role in future PTB interventions. However, it must be noted that, revealing how (and if) these probiotics mechanistically prevent PTB will be essential for the optimization of their use or other therapeutics to impact this condition.

Microbiome transplant therapy is an emerging technology that has proven successful in the restoration of eubiotic GMB following *Clostridioides difficile* infection,[95,96] with some evidence it may be an intervention to treat BV as well.[97] Current investigations are underway to explore vaginal microbiota transplant as a treatment for recurrent BV and other indications but may be difficult to scale up as small amount of sample is collected and the procedure requires extensive vaginal pathogen testing (sexually transmitted infections and viruses such as human papilloma virus and herpes simplex virus) of the samples prior to transplant.[80]

DISCUSSION

In order to continue moving the field forward, it may be time to consider standardization of microbiome reporting in pregnancy studies, mandated phenotyping of PTB, as well as incorporating next-generation sequencing techniques to provide a more complete picture of the maternal and in particular, the VMB.

DISCLOSURE

None.

Best Practices

What is the current practice for microbiome reporting in pregnancy and PTB?

PTB is a complex syndrome and characterized by the heterogeneity of its etiologic origins, rendering the establishment of standardized protocols for prevention and diagnosis a challenging endeavor. While various clinical and biological biomarkers like short cervical length, and fetal fibronectin are used to predict PTB, the sequencing of the vaginal microbiome in pregnancy as a predictive tool is still in its embryologic stage and yet to be fully established in the current clinical practices.

What changes in current practice are likely to improve outcomes?

The complexity of etiologic factors in PTB underscores the challenges in developing universally effective protocols for its prevention, diagnosis, and treatment. Emphasizing universal phenotyping of PTB, leveraging advanced gene sequencing techniques, and viewing maternal microbiomes holistically (understanding complex ecosystems complete with metabolomics and host immunity) may enhance our capability to mitigate the risk of adverse pregnancy outcomes.

Major recommendations:

- Advocate the need for uniformity in microbiome reporting across pregnancy studies to foster comparability and reliability of data.
- Integrate PTB phenotyping and predictive models for PTB.
- Integrate next-generation multiomics sequencing not only in research but also in clinical practice to enrich the depth of analysis and understanding role of the maternal microbiomes in pregnancy.

REFERENCES

1. Ohuma EO, Moller AB, Bradley E, et al. National, regional, and global estimates of preterm birth in 2020, with trends from 2010: a systematic analysis. Lancet 2023;402(10409):1261–71.
2. Chawanpaiboon S, Vogel JP, Moller AB, et al. Global, regional, and national estimates of levels of preterm birth in 2014: a systematic review and modelling analysis. Lancet Glob Health 2019;7(1):e37–46.
3. Gonzalez JM, Xu H, Chai J, et al. Preterm and term cervical ripening in CD1 Mice (Mus musculus): similar or divergent molecular mechanisms? Biol Reprod Dec 2009;81(6):1226–32.
4. Timmons BC, Reese J, Socrate S, et al. Prostaglandins are essential for cervical ripening in LPS-mediated preterm birth but not term or antiprogestin-driven preterm ripening. Endocrinology 2014;155(1):287–98.
5. Areia AL, Mota-Pinto A. Inflammation and preterm birth: a systematic review. Reprod Med 2022;3(2):101–11.
6. Goldenberg RL, Hauth JC, Andrews WW. Intrauterine infection and preterm delivery. N Engl J Med 2000;342(20):1500–7.
7. Escapa IF, Chen T, Huang Y, et al. New Insights into human nostril microbiome from the expanded human oral microbiome database (eHOMD): a resource for the microbiome of the human aerodigestive tract. mSystems 2018;3(6). 001877-18.
8. Jang H, Patoine A, Wu TT, et al. Oral microflora and pregnancy: a systematic review and meta-analysis. Sci Rep 2021;11(1):16870.
9. Fujiwara N, Tsuruda K, Iwamoto Y, et al. Significant increase of oral bacteria in the early pregnancy period in Japanese women. J Investig Clin Dent 2017;8(1).
10. Xiao J, Fogarty C, Wu TT, et al. Oral health and Candida carriage in socioeconomically disadvantaged US pregnant women. BMC Pregnancy Childbirth 2019; 19(1):480.
11. Kamate WI, Vibhute NA, Baad RK. Estimation of DMFT, Salivary streptococcus mutans count, flow rate, ph, and salivary total calcium content in pregnant and non-pregnant women: a prospective study. J Clin Diagn Res 2017;11(4): Zc147–51.
12. Balan P, Chong YS, Umashankar S, et al. Keystone species in pregnancy gingivitis: a snapshot of oral microbiome during pregnancy and postpartum period. Front Microbiol 2018;9:2360.
13. Offenbacher S, Katz V, Fertik G, et al. Periodontal infection as a possible risk factor for preterm low birth weight. J Periodontol 1996;67(10 Suppl):1103–13.

14. Saadaoui M, Singh P, Al Khodor S. Oral microbiome and pregnancy: a bidirectional relationship. J Reprod Immunol 2021;145:103293.

15. Koerner R, Prescott S, Alman A, et al. The oral microbiome throughout pregnancy: a scoping review. MCN Am J Matern Child Nurs 2023;48(4):200–8.

16. Ye C, Katagiri S, Miyasaka N, et al. The anti-phospholipid antibody-dependent and independent effects of periodontopathic bacteria on threatened preterm labor and preterm birth. Arch Gynecol Obstet 2013;288(1):65–72.

17. Ye C, Katagiri S, Miyasaka N, et al. The periodontopathic bacteria in placenta, saliva and subgingival plaque of threatened preterm labor and preterm low birth weight cases: a longitudinal study in Japanese pregnant women. Clin Oral Investig 2020;24(12):4261–70, d.

18. Ye C, Kobayashi H, Katagiri S, et al. The relationship between the anti-Porphyromonas gingivalis immunoglobulin G subclass antibody and small for gestational age delivery: a longitudinal study in pregnant Japanese women. Int Dent 2020;70(4):296–302.

19. Cobb CM, Kelly PJ, Williams KB, et al. The oral microbiome and adverse pregnancy outcomes. Int J Womens Health 2017;9:551–9.

20. Zhang X, Lu E, Stone SL, et al. Dental cleaning, community water fluoridation and preterm birth, Massachusetts: 2009-2016. Matern Child Health J 2019;23(4):451–8.

21. Daalderop LA, Wieland BV, Tomsin K, et al. Periodontal disease and pregnancy outcomes: overview of systematic reviews. JDR Clin Trans Res 2018;3(1):10–27.

22. Srinivas SK, Sammel MD, Stamilio DM, et al. Periodontal disease and adverse pregnancy outcomes: is there an association? Am J Obstet Gynecol 2009;200(5):497.e1–8.

23. Costa EM, de Araujo Figueiredo CS, Martins RFM, et al. Periodontopathogenic microbiota, infectious mechanisms and preterm birth: analysis with structural equations (cohort-BRISA). Arch Gynecol Obstet 2019;300(6):1521–30.

24. Shiozaki A, Yoneda S, Yoneda N, et al. Intestinal microbiota is different in women with preterm birth: results from terminal restriction fragment length polymorphism analysis. PLoS One 2014;9(11):e111374.

25. Amabebe E, Anumba DOC. Female gut and genital tract microbiota-induced crosstalk and differential effects of short-chain fatty acids on immune sequelae. Front Immunol 2020;11:2184.

26. Bilotta AJ, Cong Y. Gut microbiota metabolite regulation of host defenses at mucosal surfaces: implication in precision medicine. Precis Clin Med 2019;2(2):110–9.

27. Parada Venegas D, De la Fuente MK, Landskron G, et al. Short chain fatty acids (SCFAs)-mediated gut epithelial and immune regulation and its relevance for inflammatory bowel diseases. Front Immunol 2019;10:277.

28. Koren O, Goodrich JK, Cullender TC, et al. Host remodeling of the gut microbiome and metabolic changes during pregnancy. Cell 2012;150(3):470–80.

29. Boakye E, Kwapong YA, Obisesan O, et al. Nativity-related disparities in preeclampsia and cardiovascular disease risk among a racially diverse cohort of US women. JAMA Netw Open 2021;4(12):e2139564.

30. Chen X, Li P, Liu M, et al. Gut dysbiosis induces the development of preeclampsia through bacterial translocation. Gut. Mar 2020;69(3):513–22.

31. Gershuni V, Li Y, Elovitz M, et al. Maternal gut microbiota reflecting poor diet quality is associated with spontaneous preterm birth in a prospective cohort study. Am J Clin Nutr 2021;113(3):602–11.

32. Hasain Z, Mokhtar NM, Kamaruddin NA, et al. Gut microbiota and gestational diabetes mellitus: a review of host-gut microbiota interactions and their therapeutic potential. Front Cell Infect Microbiol 2020;10:188.

33. Li M, Grewal J, Hinkle SN, et al. Healthy dietary patterns and common pregnancy complications: a prospective and longitudinal study. Am J Clin Nutr 2021;114(3): 1229–37.

34. Dahl C, Stanislawski M, Iszatt N, et al. Gut microbiome of mothers delivering prematurely shows reduced diversity and lower relative abundance of Bifidobacterium and Streptococcus. PLoS One 2017;12(10):e0184336.

35. Fuhler GM. The immune system and microbiome in pregnancy. Best Pract Res Clin Gastroenterol 2020;44-45:101671.

36. Dalile B, Van Oudenhove L, Vervliet B, et al. The role of short-chain fatty acids in microbiota-gut-brain communication. Nat Rev Gastroenterol Hepatol 2019;16(8): 461–78.

37. Aagaard K, Ma J, Antony KM, et al. The placenta harbors a unique microbiome. Sci Transl Med 2014;6(237):237ra65.

38. Zakis DR, Paulissen E, Kornete L, et al. The evidence for placental microbiome and its composition in healthy pregnancies: a systematic review. J Reprod Immunol 2022;149:103455.

39. Theis KR, Romero R, Winters AD, et al. Does the human placenta delivered at term have a microbiota? Results of cultivation, quantitative real-time PCR, 16S rRNA gene sequencing, and metagenomics. Am J Obstet Gynecol 2019; 220(3):267.e1–39.

40. Sterpu I, Fransson E, Hugerth LW, et al. No evidence for a placental microbiome in human pregnancies at term. Am J Obstet Gynecol 2021;224(3):296.e1–23.

41. Panzer JJ, Romero R, Greenberg JM, et al. Is there a placental microbiota? A critical review and re-analysis of published placental microbiota datasets. BMC Microbiol 2023;23(1):76.

42. Leiby JS, McCormick K, Sherrill-Mix S, et al. Lack of detection of a human placenta microbiome in samples from preterm and term deliveries. Microbiome 2018;6(1):196.

43. Lauder AP, Roche AM, Sherrill-Mix S, et al. Comparison of placenta samples with contamination controls does not provide evidence for a distinct placenta microbiota. Microbiome 2016;4(1):29.

44. Kennedy KM, de Goffau MC, Perez-Muñoz ME, et al. Questioning the fetal microbiome illustrates pitfalls of low-biomass microbial studies. Nature 2023;613(7945): 639–49.

45. Blaser MJ, Devkota S, McCoy KD, et al. Lessons learned from the prenatal microbiome controversy. Microbiome 2021;9(1):8. https://doi.org/10.1186/s40168-020-00946-2.

46. Culhane JF, Rauh V, McCollum KF, et al. Exposure to chronic stress and ethnic differences in rates of bacterial vaginosis among pregnant women. Am J Obstet Gynecol 2002;187(5):1272–6.

47. Hadley M, Oppong AY, Coleman J, et al. Structural racism and adverse pregnancy outcomes through the lens of the maternal microbiome. Obstet Gynecol 2023;142(4):911–9.

48. Dunlop AL, Satten GA, Hu YJ, et al. Vaginal microbiome composition in early pregnancy and risk of spontaneous preterm and early term birth among African American women. Front Cell Infect Microbiol 2021;11:641005.

49. Elovitz MA, Gajer P, Riis V, et al. Cervicovaginal microbiota and local immune response modulate the risk of spontaneous preterm delivery. Nat Commun 2019;10(1):1305.
50. Fettweis JM, Serrano MG, Brooks JP, et al. The vaginal microbiome and preterm birth. Nat Med 2019;25(6):1012–21.
51. Gudnadottir U, Debelius JW, Du J, et al. The vaginal microbiome and the risk of preterm birth: a systematic review and network meta-analysis. Sci Rep 2022; 12(1):7926.
52. Cruickshank R. Döderlein's Vaginal bacillus: a contribution to the study of the lacto-bacilli. J Hyg 1931;31(3):375–81.
53. Ravel J, Gajer P, Abdo Z, et al. Vaginal microbiome of reproductive-age women. Proc Natl Acad Sci USA 2011;108(Suppl 1):4680–7.
54. Padula AM, Monk C, Brennan PA, et al. A review of maternal prenatal exposures to environmental chemicals and psychosocial stressors-implications for research on perinatal outcomes in the ECHO program. J Perinatol 2020;40(1):10–24.
55. James-Todd T, Senie R, Terry MB. Racial/ethnic differences in hormonally-active hair product use: a plausible risk factor for health disparities. J Immigr Minor Health 2012;14(3):506–11.
56. Blacks and Hispanics face extra challenges in getting home loans, Available at: https://www.pewresearch.org/fact-tank/2017/01/10/blacks-and-hispanics-face-extra-challenges-in-getting-home-loans/. Accessed January 15, 2024.
57. Yearby R. Racial disparities in health status and access to healthcare: the continuation of inequality in the United States due to structural racism. Am J Econ Sociol 2018;77(3–4):1113–52.
58. Burris HHYN, Riis V, Valeri L, et al. The role of neighborhood deprivation in the cervicovaginal microbiota. Am J Obstet Gynecol MFM 2024. https://doi.org/10.1016/j.ajogmf.2024.101291.
59. Dixon M, Dunlop AL, Corwin EJ, et al. Joint effects of individual socioeconomic status and residential neighborhood context on vaginal microbiome composition. Front Public Health 2023;11:1029741.
60. Wright ML, Dunlop AL, Dunn AB, et al. Factors associated with vaginal lactobacillus predominance among African American women early in pregnancy. J Womens Health (Larchmt) 2022;31(5):682–9.
61. Virtanen S, Rantsi T, Virtanen A, et al. Vaginal microbiota composition correlates between pap smear microscopy and next generation sequencing and associates to socioeconomic status. Sci Rep 2019;9(1):7750.
62. Kindschuh WF, Baldini F, Liu MC, et al. Preterm birth is associated with xenobiotics and predicted by the vaginal metabolome. Nat Microbiol 2023;8(2):246–59.
63. Fiume MM, Heldreth B, Bergfeld WF, et al. Safety assessment of decyl glucoside and other alkyl glucosides as used in cosmetics. Int J Toxicol 2013;32(5 Suppl): 22s–48s.
64. Waters B, Nakano R, Hara K, et al. A validated method for the separation of ethyl glucoside isomers by gas chromatography-tandem mass spectrometry and quantitation in human whole blood and urine. J Chromatogr B Analyt Technol Biomed Life Sci 2022;1188:123074.
65. Fiume MM, Heldreth B, Bergfeld WF, et al. Safety Assessment of diethanolamine and its salts as used in cosmetics. Int J Toxicol 2017;36(5_suppl2):89s–110s.
66. Cherpes TL, Hillier SL, Meyn LA, et al. A delicate balance: risk factors for acquisition of bacterial vaginosis include sexual activity, absence of hydrogen peroxide-producing lactobacilli, black race, and positive herpes simplex virus type 2 serology. Sex Transm Dis 2008;35(1):78–83.

67. Brotman RM, He X, Gajer P, et al. Association between cigarette smoking and the vaginal microbiota: a pilot study. BMC Infect Dis 2014;14:471.

68. Nelson TM, Borgogna JC, Michalek RD, et al. Cigarette smoking is associated with an altered vaginal tract metabolomic profile. Sci Rep 2018;8(1):852.

69. Orr ST, James SA, Casper R. Psychosocial stressors and low birth weight: development of a questionnaire. J Dev Behav Pediatr 1992;13(5):343–7.

70. Amabebe E, Anumba DOC. Psychosocial stress, cortisol levels, and maintenance of vaginal health. Front Endocrinol 2018;9:568.

71. Tipton MJ, Wagner SA, Dixon A, et al. Association of living in a food desert with pregnancy morbidity. Obstet Gynecol 2020;136(1):140–5.

72. Salow AD, Pool LR, Grobman WA, et al. Associations of neighborhood-level racial residential segregation with adverse pregnancy outcomes. Am J Obstet Gynecol 2018;218(3):351.e1–7.

73. Mandal S, Godfrey KM, McDonald D, et al. Fat and vitamin intakes during pregnancy have stronger relations with a pro-inflammatory maternal microbiota than does carbohydrate intake. Microbiome 2016;4(1):55.

74. Barrett HL, Gomez-Arango LF, Wilkinson SA, et al. A vegetarian diet is a major determinant of gut microbiota composition in early pregnancy. Nutrients 2018; 10(7):890.

75. Crusell MKW, Hansen TH, Nielsen T, et al. Gestational diabetes is associated with change in the gut microbiota composition in third trimester of pregnancy and postpartum. Microbiome 2018;6(1):89.

76. Ponzo V, Fedele D, Goitre I, et al. Diet-gut microbiota interactions and gestational diabetes mellitus (GDM). Nutrients 2019;11(2):330.

77. Sugino KY, Hernandez TL, Barbour LA, et al. A maternal higher-complex carbohydrate diet increases bifidobacteria and alters early life acquisition of the infant microbiome in women with gestational diabetes mellitus. Front Endocrinol 2022; 13:921464.

78. Wang J, Li W, Wang C, et al. Enterotype bacteroides is associated with a high risk in patients with diabetes: a pilot study. J Diabetes Res 2020;2020:6047145.

79. Ferrocino I, Ponzo V, Gambino R, et al. Changes in the gut microbiota composition during pregnancy in patients with gestational diabetes mellitus (GDM). Sci Rep 2018;8(1):12216.

80. France M, Alizadeh M, Brown S, et al. Towards a deeper understanding of the vaginal microbiota. Nat Microbiol 2022;7(3):367–78.

81. Manuck TA, Esplin MS, Biggio J, et al. The phenotype of spontaneous preterm birth: application of a clinical phenotyping tool. Am J Obstet Gynecol 2015; 212(4):487.e1–11.

82. O'Callaghan JL, Willner D, Buttini M, et al. Limitations of 16S rRNA gene sequencing to characterize lactobacillus species in the upper genital tract. Front Cell Dev Biol 2021;9:641921.

83. Bashiardes S, Zilberman-Schapira G, Eran E. Use of metatranscriptomics in microbiome research. Bioinform Biol Insights 2016;10:19–25.

84. Aguiar-Pulido V, Huang W, Suarez-Ulloa V, et al. Metagenomics, metatranscriptomics, and metabolomics approaches for microbiome analysis. Evol Bioinform Online 2016;12(Suppl 1):5–16.

85. Kim D-E, Kim J-K, Han S-K, et al. Lactobacillus plantarum NK3 and bifidobacterium longum nk49 alleviate bacterial vaginosis and osteoporosis in mice by suppressing NF-κB-linked TNF-α expression. J Medicinal Food 2019;22(10):1022–31.

86. Macklaim JM, Clemente JC, Knight R, et al. Changes in vaginal microbiota following antimicrobial and probiotic therapy. Microb Ecol Health Dis 2015;26: 27799.
87. Husain S, Allotey J, Drymoussi Z, et al. Effects of oral probiotic supplements on vaginal microbiota during pregnancy: a randomised, double-blind, placebo-controlled trial with microbiome analysis. BJOG 2020;127(2):275–84.
88. Oerlemans EFM, Bellen G, Claes I, et al. Impact of a lactobacilli-containing gel on vulvovaginal candidosis and the vaginal microbiome. Sci Rep 2020;10(1):7976.
89. Marcotte H, Larsson PG, Andersen KK, et al. An exploratory pilot study evaluating the supplementation of standard antibiotic therapy with probiotic lactobacilli in South African women with bacterial vaginosis. BMC Infect Dis 2019;19(1):824.
90. Bohbot JM, Daraï E, Bretelle F, et al. Efficacy and safety of vaginally administered lyophilized Lactobacillus crispatus IP 174178 in the prevention of bacterial vaginosis recurrence. J Gynecol Obstet Hum Reprod 2018;47(2):81–6.
91. Stapleton AE, Au-Yeung M, Hooton TM, et al. Randomized, placebo-controlled phase 2 trial of a Lactobacillus crispatus probiotic given intravaginally for prevention of recurrent urinary tract infection. Clin Infect Dis 2011;52(10):1212–7.
92. Reid G, Beuerman D, Heinemann C, et al. Probiotic Lactobacillus dose required to restore and maintain a normal vaginal flora. FEMS Immunol Med Microbiol 2001;32(1):37–41.
93. Bayar E, MacIntyre DA, Sykes L, et al. Safety, tolerability, and acceptability of Lactobacillus crispatus CTV-05 (LACTIN-V) in pregnant women at high-risk of preterm birth. Benef Microbioms 2023;14:45–55.
94. Cohen CR, Wierzbicki MR, French AL, et al. Randomized trial of lactin-v to prevent recurrence of bacterial vaginosis. N Engl J Med 2020;382(20):1906–15.
95. Juul FE, Garborg K, Bretthauer M, et al. Fecal microbiota transplantation for primary Clostridium difficile infection. N Engl J Med 2018;378(26):2535–6.
96. Leffler DA, Lamont JT. Clostridium difficile infection. N Engl J Med 2015;372(16): 1539–48.
97. Lev-Sagie A, Goldman-Wohl D, Cohen Y, et al. Vaginal microbiome transplantation in women with intractable bacterial vaginosis. Nat Med 2019;25(10):1500–4.

Predicting Spontaneous Preterm Birth Using the Immunome

Dorien Feyaerts, PhD, MSc[a], Ivana Marić, PhD[b], Petra C. Arck, MD[c],
Jelmer R. Prins, MD, PhD[d], Nardhy Gomez-Lopez, PhD[e,f],
Brice Gaudillière, MD, PhD[a,g], Ina A. Stelzer, PhD, MSc[h,*]

KEYWORDS

- Spontaneous preterm birth • Spontaneous preterm labor • Maternal immune system
- Maternal blood • Multiomics modeling • Single-cell cytometry
- Whole blood transcriptome

KEY POINTS

- Maternal blood displays characteristic immune dynamics across pregnancy.
- The peripheral immune clock of pregnancy likely reflects immune processes in reproductive tissues.
- Leveraging the cellular immune clock in pregnant individuals for early risk assessment and prediction of spontaneous preterm birth (sPTB) is in its infancy.
- Integration of multiple biological data modalities promises to identify clinically actionable biomarkers and improve our understanding of sPTB pathobiology.

INTRODUCTION

Preterm birth (PTB) - delivery before 37 weeks of gestation - is a complex disorder with multiple etiologies.[1,2] Around 60% to 70% of PTB cases occur spontaneously in

[a] Department of Anesthesiology, Perioperative and Pain Medicine, Stanford University, Stanford, CA 94305, USA; [b] Division of Neonatal and Developmental Medicine, Department of Pediatrics, Stanford University School of Medicine, 453 Quarry Road, Palo Alto, CA 94304, USA; [c] Department of Obstetrics and Fetal Medicine and Hamburg Center for Translational Immunology, University Medical Center Hamburg-Eppendorf, Martinistrasse 52, 20251 Hamburg, Germany; [d] Department of Obstetrics and Gynecology, University of Groningen, University Medical Center Groningen, Postbus 30.001, 9700RB, Groningen, The Netherlands; [e] Department of Obstetrics and Gynecology, Washington University School of Medicine, 425 S. Euclid Avenue, St. Louis, MO 63110, USA; [f] Department of Pathology and Immunology, Washington University School of Medicine, 425 S. Euclid Avenue, St. Louis, MO 63110, USA; [g] Division of Neonatal and Developmental Medicine, Department of Pediatrics, Stanford University School of Medicine, 300 Pasteur Drive, Palo Alto, CA 94304, USA; [h] Department of Pathology, University of California San Diego, 9500 Gilman Drive, La Jolla, CA 92093, USA
* Corresponding author.
E-mail address: istelzer@health.ucsd.edu

Clin Perinatol 51 (2024) 441–459
https://doi.org/10.1016/j.clp.2024.02.013
0095-5108/24/© 2024 Elsevier Inc. All rights reserved.

asymptomatic pregnant individuals, while 30% to 40% cases are medically indicated (ie, iatrogenic) due to complications such as pre-eclampsia, fetal growth restriction, acute fetal distress, symptomatic placenta previa, or triggered by environmental adversities (eg, heat stress), among others.[1,3,4] Spontaneous PTB (sPTB) follows either spontaneous preterm labor with intact membranes (sPTL) or preterm prelabor rupture of the membranes (PPROM). sPTB is associated with intra-amniotic infection, sterile intra-amniotic inflammation, and fetal immune activation.[2] However, for a significant subset of sPTB (20%–30%), the cause remains unidentified (ie, idiopathic).[2,3,5] To date, sPTB remains unpredictable due to a lack of reliable biomarkers and an incomplete understanding of the underlying pathobiological mechanisms.[6]

Significant immune cell alterations occur at the maternal–fetal interface (comprising decidua and intervillous space) over the course of a healthy pregnancy (reviewed by PrabhuDas et al.,[7] Yang and colleagues,[8] and Gomez-Lopez et al.[9]), contributing to the reproductive processes of decidualization, implantation, placentation, maternal–fetal tolerance, pregnancy homeostasis, and parturition.[7–13] These local immunologic adaptations are reflected in the circulating maternal immune system, which adapts to the pregnancy-induced hormonal and metabolic changes during pregnancy,[14–27] making blood draws an accessible tool for clinical assessment of pregnancy progression. Recent advances in high-content technologies have enabled investigating this maternal peripheral "immune clock" systematically and with high temporal resolution. These studies have shed light on the dynamics of the maternal immune system from preconception, throughout gestation until labor, and into the postpartum period.[15,16,19,20,24–28] The peripheral immune dynamics have informed computational models to predict gestational age (GA) and the time to labor in uncomplicated pregnancies based on immune cell frequencies, intracellular signaling activities, and gene expression signatures relating to immune responses, leukocyte activation, inflammation, and development.[16,19,20,24,25,27,28]

The pathobiology of sPTB involves disruptions in immune cell populations in various reproductive tissues and at the maternal–fetal interface.[2] Various studies have thoroughly described the peripheral immune profile of sPTB during sPTL or PPROM compared with healthy pregnancies carrying to term and matched for GA at sampling; and/or with term cases that are in labor or are not in labor, indicating an overall exaggerated inflammatory response in preterm cases that is distinct from term labor.[12,20,24,29–35] In addition, local processes of sPTL are reflected in the peripheral maternal blood immune profile,[19,25,29,36,37] and already identifiable during the second trimester.[20,22,24,37] As such, leveraging the maternal peripheral immune profile could inform the development of models to predict sPTB.

This review summarizes the currently available immunome studies for the prediction of sPTB. Focusing exclusively on immunologic, cytometric, and transcriptomics studies on the cellular level, we aim to provide a knowledge base to inform the design of future investigations into single-cell immune correlates and mechanisms preceding sPTB in the maternal peripheral circulation.

LEVERAGING THE MATERNAL IMMUNE CLOCK FOR THE PREDICTION OF SPONTANEOUS PRETERM BIRTH

Several clinical scenarios would benefit from sPTB prediction (**Fig. 1**). First, pregnant individuals presenting in the clinic before 37 weeks' GA with regular uterine contractions must be assessed and monitored for sPTL. Only a fraction (~10%) of these cases will culminate in sPTB and those patients with continued pregnancies are considered as having experienced an episode of threatened sPTL.[38] Current

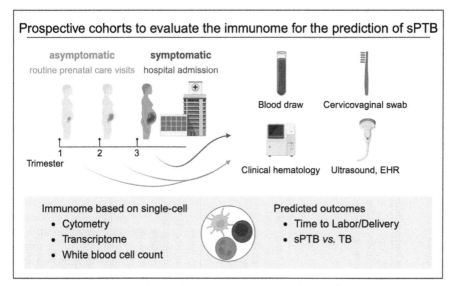

Fig. 1. Cohort design to evaluate the immunome as a predictor of spontaneous preterm birth. (Created with BioRender.com.).

predictive tools to distinguish threatened sPTL are inaccurate,[39,40] although optimized multifactorial integration might improve risk assessment.[41] Predicting time to delivery during threatened sPTL could significantly improve clinical management, including need for hospitalization, referral to a tertiary center with neonatal intensive care unit availability, medication (eg, need for antenatal corticosteroids), and/or tocolysis, while avoiding unnecessary hospitalization and treatment for those with remitting contractions who will carry to term.

A second scenario are asymptomatic pregnancies in early pregnancy who would benefit from a prospective risk assessment for sPTB. Despite established clinical risk factors (eg, shortened cervix, history of PTB[1]) and recent efforts to develop plasma proteome- and cell-free (cf) RNA-based tools,[42,43] no prospective predictive tests are currently clinically available to monitor ongoing pregnancies for their healthy progression to term. Providing an accurate prospective risk assessment for sPTB is an important tool to identify those at risk. Simultaneously, such tool has the potential to advance the development of preventive strategies and medications. A predictive test for sPTB in asymptomatic individuals would be administered during their pregnancy-confirming visits in the first trimester or at the mid-pregnancy fetal organ screen (around 20 weeks' GA). Pregnancies at increased risk could be prescribed prophylactic medications, such as progesterone, where indicated, and closely monitored throughout their pregnancy.

Prediction of sPTB in symptomatic individuals with threatened PTL

The peripheral immune profile of pregnant individuals with regular uterine contractions admitted to the hospital for threatened PTL has facilitated the prediction of sPTB within 48 hours, 7 days, or before 34 or 37 weeks gestation.[44–49] **Table 1** displays the 6 current studies using single-cell protein and bulk transcriptomics signatures of blood immune cells to predict sPTB. Whole blood RNA gene expression data, a migration assay of peripheral blood mononuclear cells (PBMCs), and flow cytometry of single cells, at times in

Table 1
Studies analyzing blood immune cells in association with spontaneous preterm birth following threatened preterm labor

Authors, Year, Geographic Site	Method	n	GA at Sampling	Predicted Outcome	Model Performance	Informative Biology	References
Heng et al,[46] 2014, Australia	• Whole-blood RNA transcriptome (microarray) + clinical hematology data	• 48 sPTB within 48h • 27 sPTB after 48 h • 79 TB	• 24–36 wks	• sPTB within 48 h	• AUC: 0.79 • Sensitivity: 70.8% • Specificity: 75.5%	• 9 genes • Clinical blood data (total leukocyte, neutrophil, lymphocyte and monocyte counts, and hemoglobin levels)	Heng et al,[46] 2014, meta-analyzed in Vora et al,[37] 2018
Chim et al,[47] 2020, Hong Kong	• Whole-blood RNA-seq	• 10 sPTL with PTB <34 wk • 10 sPTL with TB > 37 wk • Validation in 119 subjects	• <34 wks	• sPTB <34 wk • Validated in sPTB <37 wk	• PUT1 and PUT2: • AUC: 0.75–0.91 • sensitivity: 63%–92.6% • specificity: 75.5%–85%	• 10 genes validated: positivity for 2 sets of identified preterm-upregulated transcripts (PUT1 and 2)	Chim et al,[47] 2020
Ran et al,[48] 2022, China	• Whole-blood RNA transcriptome (microarray) • qPCR	• Reanalysis of public data of Heng et al. 2014, then validated on 14 TPTL with PTB < 7 d, 10 TPTL without PTB	• 24 wks • 36 wks	• sPTB <37 wk	• AUC: 0.907 • sensitivity: 83.9% • specificity: 87.0% • PPV: 86.6% • NPV: 84.4%	• JOSD1 • IDNK • ZMYM3 • IL1B	Ran et al,[48] 2022
Ran et al,[49] 2023, China	• Whole-blood RNA transcriptome (RNASeq and microarray)	• 154 TPTL	• 28–34 wks	• PTB <37 wk • PTB within 7 d • PTB within 48h	AUC: • 0.761 • 0.829 • 0.836 • No other parameters reported	• Activity score of IL6-JAK-STAT3 signaling	Ran et al,[49] 2023

Study	Method	Population	Outcome	Results	Cut-off	Reference
Takeda et al,[44] 2017, Canada	PBMC migration assay	• 10 PTL • 11 TPTL • 8 PPROM • 16 PTNL (normal pregnancies sampled preterm, not-in-labor) controls	• Delivery within 7 d	• AUC: 0.83 • Sensitivity: 78.1% • Specificity: 88.9% • PPV: 91.4% • NPV: 72.7%	• Cut-off value of 37,082 leukocytes or more migrated within 90 min	Takeda et al,[44] 2017
Koucký et al,[45] 2014, Czech Republic	• Single-cell flow cytometry of PBMC + cervical length	• 60 with regular uterine contractions and/or cervical incompetence	• Delivery: • Within 48 h • <34 wk • >34 • <37 wk • Term >37 wk	• OR (95% CI): • 35.21 (13.3; 214) • 29.57 (15.1; 179) • 42.10 (4.3; 282)	• $CD4^+$ $CD25^{int/hi}$ $CD127^{lo}$ Treg count < 0.031 × 10^9/L + cervical length <17.50 mm	Koucký et al,[45] 2014

Abbreviations: AUC, area under the curve; CI, confidence interval; GA, gestational age; NPV, negative predictive value; OR, odds ratio; PBMC, peripheral blood mononuclear cells; PPROM, preterm prelabor rupture of membranes; PPV, positive predictive value; sPTB, spontaneous preterm birth; sPTL, spontaneous preterm labor; TB, term birth; TPTL, threatened preterm labor; wks, weeks.

combination with clinical data, show that the biology informing these predictions involves immune regulatory shifts with approaching delivery and enhanced immune cell migration as well as metabolic, epigenetic, and transcriptomics changes, the latter prominently in the innate compartment, associated with PTL.

Prospective prediction of sPTB in asymptomatic individuals

Plasma or serum is currently most frequently used in studies aimed at predicting sPTB before the onset of clinical symptoms.[50,51] Fewer studies analyze the cervicovaginal fluid to update the clinically applied, yet inefficient fetal fibronectin test.[52–54] A recent comprehensive systematic review specifically focused on blood-based predictive biomarkers of sPTL or PPROM resulting in sPTB found that, out of 77 eligible publications, 70 measured protein and gene expression levels in plasma or serum.[6] Early pregnancy omics profiles with predictive capacity for PTB have been generated using high-dimensional measurements of the plasma proteome, lipidome, and metabolome, within exosome cargo, and cfRNA.[55–61] Notably, the inclusion of maternal demographic and clinical factors strengthens PTB characterization.[62,63]

In contrast to plasma/serum-based analyses, fewer studies have included cell-based technologies to monitor the peripheral immune system during pregnancy, despite the central and cell-type specific role of innate and adaptive immune cells in the pathobiology of PTB.[2,12,20,34,35,64–66] **Table 2** displays 14 currently available prediction studies aimed at associating sPTB with single-cell protein, bulk transcriptomics signatures, and clinical laboratory parameters of immune cells in asymptomatic pregnancies.[25,27,49,67–77] The majority of the 14 studies uses whole blood RNA gene expression data, while fewer look at either clinical hematology parameters, micro (mi)RNA expression in PBMCs, or flow/mass cytometry of single cells.

A common approach has been to identify biomarkers unique to PTB via testing potential marker performance in predicting sPTB in a classification task (case–control setting) and reporting the area under the receiver-operator curve (AUROC) or by estimating odds ratios. Informative biology of gene expression studies, conducted across various time points during pregnancy, include expected increased inflammation gene sets in sPTB pregnancies,[25,49,68,71] as well as dysregulated markers of the epigenetic machinery (miRNA, long non-coding [lnc]RNA, histone modification) that can distinguish preterm from term deliveries.[69,70,76] Clinical laboratory blood parameters such as the neutrophil–lymphocyte ratio (NLR) could be a cost-effective tool to assess the risk for PTB.[67,74] While its predictive capacity for PPROM remains to be definitively determined,[67,74] in retrospective studies, the NLR was associated with histologic chorioamnionitis at the time of sPTB in asymptomatic pregnancies.[78]

Another approach for the predictive modeling of sPTB uses a regression method to estimate the time between blood sampling and the occurrence of spontaneous labor from longitudinal immunome data.[22] Two proof-of-concept studies successfully predicted time (in days or weeks) to sPTB, informed by longitudinal transcriptomic (first [T1], second [T2], and third [T3] trimesters) and single-cell proteomic (T2, T3) prelabor immune dynamics in asymptomatic pregnancies.[25,27] In both studies, the prediction error was higher for sPTB compared with term cases, indicative of processes unique to PTB and emphasizing the immunologic heterogeneity of the PTL syndrome. In addition, model performance benefitted from integrating multiple layers of biological information (proteome, metabolome), thereby improving prediction accuracy.[27]

The majority of PTB prediction studies assess peripheral immune cells mid-pregnancy (from 20–36 weeks' GA). A limitation of this design is the potential inclusion of individuals who have already developed disease, albeit subclinically, leading to overestimation of the model performance for earlier GA. Tarca and colleagues[25] report

Table 2
Studies analyzing blood immune cells in association with spontaneous preterm birth in asymptomatic pregnancies

Authors, Year, Geographic Site	Method	N	GA at Sampling	Predicted Outcome	Model Performance	Informative Biology	Reference
Heng et al,[68] 2016, Canada	• Whole-blood RNA transcriptome (microarray)	• 51 sPTB (15 sPTL, 36 PPROM) • 114 TB	• T2: 17–23 wks • T3: 27–33 wks	• sPTB <37 wks	• AUC: 0.84 for T2/T3 difference • sensitivity: 64.7% • specificity: 88.3%	• Transcripts • LOC100128908 • MIR3691 • LOC101927441 • CST13P • ACAP2 • ZNF324 • SH3PXD2B • TBX21 • history of abortion and anemia • GSEA: upregulated pathways of inflammation	Heng et al,[68] 2016, meta-analyzed in Vora et al,[37] 2018
Zhou et al,[69] 2020, Canada (re-analysis of Heng et al,[68] 2016)	• Whole-blood mRNA transcriptome (microarray)	• 51 sPTB (15 sPTL, 36 PPROM) • 106 TB	• T2: 17–23 wks • T3: 27–33 wks	• sPTB <37 wks	• T2: OR: 2.86 (95% CI 1.08, 7.58) • T3: OR: 4.43 (95% CI 1.57, 12.50)	• mRNA levels of EBF1 and associated enriched gene sets	Zhou et al,[69] 2020
Zhou et al,[70] 2021, Canada (re-analysis of Heng et al,[68] 2016)	• Whole-blood mRNA and lncRNA transcriptome (microarray)	• 51 sPTB (15 sPTL, 36 PPROM) • 106 TB	• T2: 17–23 wks • T3: 27–33 wks	• sPTB <37 wks	• T3: highest tertile of LINC00870 OR:4.08 (95% CI: 1.60, 10.40) • lowest tertile of LINC00094 (OR: 5.16 (95% CI:1.96, 13.61)	• EBF1-correlated long non-coding RNA (lncRNA) expression	Zhou et al,[70] 2021

(continued on next page)

Table 2
(continued)

Authors, Year, Geographic Site	Method	N	GA at Sampling	Predicted Outcome	Model Performance	Informative Biology	Reference
Manuck et al,[71] 2021, USA	• Whole blood mRNA and miRNA transcripts (custom microarray)	• 68 sPTB (36 sPTL, 24 PPROM, 2 fetal indication, 10 placental abruption, 11 intra-amniotic infection) • 68 TB	• <28 wks	• sPTB <37 wks • sPTB <34 wks	• <37 wk: • AUC: 0.79 (95% CI: 0.0.71–0.87) • sensitivity: 69.1% • specificity: 77.9% • PPV: 75.8% • NPV: 71.6%	• <37 wk: • 14 genes of NO-pathway, including RUNX3, B2M gene expression	Manuck et al,[71] 2021
Tarca et al,[25] 2021, USA/Canada	• Whole-blood RNA transcriptome (microarray)	• 37 PPROM • 34 sPTL • 11 TL	• T1: <12 wks • T2: 12–24 wks • T3: 24–37 wks	• Time to sPTB	• R: 0.75 • RMSE: 5.6 wk	• Pregnancy age and parturition biology • PPROM associated with leukocyte (myeloid and lymphocyte) mediated immunity gene sets at 27–33 wk	Tarca et al,[25] 2021
Ran et al,[49] 2023, China	• Whole-blood RNA transcriptome (RNASeq and microarray)	• T1: • 47 sPTL • 37 TL • T2 • 180 sPTL • 101 TL • T3 • 128 sPTL • 95 TL	• T1: 9–13 + 6 wks • T2: 14–27 + 6 wks • T3: 28–36 + 6 wks	• sPTB <37 wks	• AUC: • T1: 0.810 • T2: 0.695 • T3: 0.779 • no other parameters reported	• Enhanced IL6 gene expression signature	Ran et al,[49] 2023

Study	Parameters	Sample size	Gestational age	Outcome	Results	Features	Reference
Ma et al,[72] 2020, China	• Complete blood count parameters	• 105 PTB (68 PPROM) • 1529 TB (210 propensity score-matched)	• 20–30 wks	• sPTB <37 wks	• AUC: 0.672 (95% CI: 0.62–0.72) • sensitivity: 88.6% • specificity: 40.5% • PPV: 10.2% • NPV: 97.9%	• Combined neutrophil-to-lymphocyte ratio (NLR) • hemoglobin (Hb) • platelet distribution width (PDW)	Ma et al,[72] 2020, meta-analysis of NLR in Vakili et al,[67] 2021
Park et al,[73] 2022, South Korea	• White blood cell count + vaginal microbiome and cervical length	• 54 PTB • 96 TB	• 17–32 wks	• PTB <37 wks	• AUC: 0.85 • sensitivity: 79% • specificity: 83% • precision: 77% • recall: 71%	• Top 5 features: • Cervical length • Lactobacillus crispatus • Peptoniphilus lacrimalis • WBC • *Ruminococcus bromii*	Park et al,[73] 2022
Morisaki et al,[74] 2021, Japan	• NLR • platelet-to-lymphocyte ratio (PLR) • lymphocyte-to-monocyte ratio (LMR)	• 76,853 total pregnancies, of which 3358 all-cause PTB (808 PPROM)	• 8–11 wks • 12–17 wks • 18–21 wks	• PPROM	• AUC: 0.5–0.52	N/A	Morisaki et al,[74] 2021
Winger et al,[75] 2017, USA	• 30 microRNA of PBMC	• 7 sPTB (4 PPROM) • 25 TB	• 8 ± 3 wks	• PTB <37 wks	• AUC: 0.98 (95% CI 0.86–1)	• miR1267 • miR148a • miR181a • miR210 • miR223 • miR301 • miR 340 • miR671	Winger et al,[75] 2017

(continued on next page)

Table 2
(continued)

Authors, Year, Geographic Site	Method	N	GA at Sampling	Predicted Outcome	Model Performance	Informative Biology	Reference
Winger et al,[76] 2020, USA	• 45 microRNA of PBMC	• 18 sPTB • 139 TB	• 6.6–12.9 wks	• sPTB <35 wks	• AUC: 0.80 (95% CI: 0.69, 0.88) - sensitivity: 89% - specificity: 71%	• miR-181a-3p • miR-221-3p • miR-33a-5p • miR-6752-3p • miR-1244 • miR-148a-3p • miR-1-3p • miR-1267 • miR-223-5p • miR-199b-5p • miR-133b • miR-144-3p	Winger et al,[76] 2020
Akoto et al,[77] 2020, South Africa	• PBMC flow cytometry	• 25 PTB (spontaneous + iatrogenic) • 20 TB	• 8–14 wks • 20–27 wks • 30–39 wks	• PTB at <37, 32–36, 28–31, or 16–28 wks	N/A	• T1 circulating ILC2 and ILC3 frequencies are lower in sPTB vs TB	Akoto et al,[77] 2020
Stelzer et al,[27] 2021 USA	• Whole blood mass cytometry (CyTOF) + proteome, metabolome	• 5 sPTL • 58 sTL	• 26–34 wks	• Time to sPTL (days)	• R: 0.67, 95%CI (0.21, 0.86) • $P = 8.8 \times 10^{-3}$ • RMSE: 27.3 d	• Dampened signaling activity in NK, dendritic, and monocytic cells upon stimulation	Stelzer et al,[27] 2021

Abbreviations: AUC, area under the curve; CI, confidence interval; GA, gestational age; NK, natural killer; NPV, negative predictive value; OR, odds ratio; PBMC, peripheral blood mononuclear cells; PPROM, preterm prelabor rupture of membranes; PPV, positive predictive value; sPTB, spontaneous preterm birth; sPTL, spontaneous preterm labor; T1, 1st trimester; T2, 2nd trimester; T3, 3rd trimester; TB, term birth; wks, weeks.

that excluding data from greater than 33 weeks' GA, to ensure that only asymptomatic samples are considered, limited the predictive capacity of models built from transcriptomic data to predict PPROM (AUC ~0.6), while a plasma proteomic model had a better performance.

While distinct T1[49,76,77] and T2[49,69] immune profiles have been described, the most informative immunologic window for the prediction of sPTB and its GA range (early vs late sPTB) remains to be determined. To our knowledge, there is currently only one available longitudinal characterization of immune features using flow cytometry throughout pregnancies ending with sPTB. This study reports decreased frequencies of innate lymphoid cell (ILC2 and ILC3) populations in T1 compared with term births.[77] This emphasizes a significant knowledge gap in our basic understanding of immune dynamics preceding PTB and indicates that sPTB peripheral signatures might be detectable at the outset of pregnancy.

Overall, monitoring of immune cell responses during pregnancy for the risk assessment of sPTB is in its infancy. Single-cell proteomic or transcriptomic approaches are transforming our ability to understand the cellular basis of sPTL pathobiology, a prerequisite for the identification of biologically plausible predictive biomarkers that can be translated into actionable clinical interventions (see **Tables 1** and **2**).

OUTLOOK ON IDENTIFYING ACTIONABLE CLINICAL BIOMARKERS

Several important considerations are necessary to address the knowledge gaps in our understanding of the immune mechanisms underlying preterm pregnancies and to identify actionable clinical biomarkers for the prediction and, ultimately, prevention of sPTB.

Reporting of sPTB subtypes and interventions

Subclassifying sPTL according to known etiologies (ie, intra-amniotic infection, sterile intra-amniotic inflammation, fetal immune activation, or idiopathic)[2,5] during predictive modeling has important implications for the implementation of sPTB prediction in the clinical setting for asymptomatic individuals. In the studies reported in **Table 2**, the majority only reports the presence of sPTL or PPROM, with only one study co-reporting the presence of intra-amniotic infection.[71] As such, enhancing our ability to predict sPTB requires an improvement in the reporting of its subtypes in future assessments. For instance, a recent single-cell investigation suggested that placental single-cell signatures in the maternal circulation of pregnancies who ultimately underwent sPTL or PPROM involved both shared and distinct signatures, depending on the sPTB subset.[24] This observation highlights the importance of distinguishing between sPTB subsets, which may involve differing underlying mechanisms, when generating predictive models. Another important consideration is reporting of sampling timing alongside administered intervention protocols in the case of symptomatic threatened sPTL. Blood samples should be collected upon hospital admission before any medications are administered as certain medications such as betamethasone could alter the maternal peripheral immune system.[79] In addition, tocolytics, vaginal progesterone, antibiotics, or cervical cerclage interventions in the case of threatened sPTL are potential confounders for the prediction of sPTB.

Cross-tissue analysis to improve understanding of pathobiology

In the quest for novel predictive clinical biomarkers, peripheral immunity plays a foundational role. While the fetal–maternal interface is largely inaccessible during pregnancy for routine prognostic assessments, its phenotype at birth serves as a valuable indicator of pregnancy health, offering retrograde predictive insights. It is conceivable that integrating peripheral immunity with local immunity of the maternal–fetal interface holds the key to identifying therapeutic targets. The various sPTB subtypes exhibit distinct differences at the maternal–fetal interface, including placenta and cervix (cervicovaginal fluid), offering crucial information on the underlying pathobiology.[2,80,81] Recent data-mining studies have demonstrated that monitoring of maternal circulation throughout pregnancy can reveal placental cell type-specific gene expression signatures identified by single-cell placental transcriptomics at birth.[20,22,24,37] In addition, highly multiplexed single-cell imaging approaches such as imaging mass cytometry can add spatial complexity to the study of the immune landscape of the maternal–fetal interface.[82,83] Investigating the association between placental pathology and PTB also holds promise for unveiling subtype-specific pathobiology.[50,84] While all 4 patterns of placental injury (maternal vascular malperfusion, fetal vascular malperfusion, acute inflammation, and chronic inflammation)[85] can be seen in preterm placentas, maternal vascular malperfusion, and acute inflammation, alone or in combination, are the most common patterns,[86] although chronic inflammation is most commonly associated with recurrent[87] or late[88] PTB. Overall, identifying sPTB subtypes and their distinct differences at the maternal–fetal interface will dictate specific intervention approaches.[2] For instance, patients with intra-amniotic infection will typically benefit from treatment with appropriate antibiotic regimens, while anti-inflammatory medications may be more appropriate for sterile inflammation. Recent advances in computational drug repurposing leveraging transcriptomics data derived from maternal blood could pave the way for identifying compounds that could be effective in preventing sPTB subtypes.[89]

Multiomics integration to improve predictive performance and identify reliable biomarkers

Integrative approaches that combine multiple omic modalities have been instrumental in simultaneously characterizing multiple biological systems implicated in the progression of healthy pregnancy and the pathogenesis of sPTB.[27,90,91] Profiling peripheral immune cell dynamics, together with cervicovaginal immunity and plasma/serum analytes, can enhance multiomics prediction performance.[25,27,63,73,90] However, the main challenges that occur when dealing with multiomics data are (1) the curse of dimensionality, and (2) the integration of multiple omics datasets into one predictive model.

The first challenge is the selection of sparse (a limited number) and reliable biomarkers among thousands of measured omics features, many of them highly correlated.[91] Sparsity promoting regularization methods such as lasso and elastic net have been used very efficiently on high-dimensional omics data to develop predictive models based on a subset of selected omics features.[92] However, biological interpretation and clinical translation is often impeded as high sensitivity to small perturbations of the input data causes drastic changes in the selected predictors.[93] This problem is especially pronounced when the sample sizes are small, as is often the case in clinical settings. When training these algorithms on small cohorts, slight changes in the training set can result in very different sets of selected features, leaving the discovery of the truly informative features uncertain. A novel machine learning framework, Stabl, overcomes this challenge.[94] Stabl builds on sparsity-promoting regularization methods to perform both predictive modeling of high accuracy and selection of reliable candidate biomarkers. Stabl achieves this by adding artificial noise into the data to obtain a data-driven threshold that separates true biomarkers from noise. It comes with a theoretic performance guarantee of reduced number of false discoveries. The use of this and similar machine learning frameworks to profile immune dynamics during pregnancy, together with plasma/serum analytes, has been shown to enhance multiomics prediction performance and to select an interpretable signature of biomarkers of pregnancy outcomes.[25,27,63,90,94]

Additionally, the integration of data coming from multiple datasets poses a layer of difficulty as the data vary in size, signal-to-noise ratio, and correlation structures depending on the technology that is utilized.[90] Analytical approaches for multiomics integration need to account for the high dimensionality of data as well as the hetero-geneity of the different omics platforms. This can be performed using a variety of ma-chine learning approaches, including Bayesian modeling and deep learning.[95,96] In addition to biological data, various maternal clinical and demographic characteris-tics—such as comorbidities and pregnancy history—can be risk factors for adverse pregnancy outcomes.[3] Including data from several modalities in the modeling approach can further improve predictive performance.[63,97] Here, Stabl can prove to be an advantageous strategy as it provides multiomics integration based on the iden-tified biomarkers of each omics set.[94]

CONCLUSION

The cellular immune clock of pregnancy remains underexplored. Monitoring the cellular immune profile emerges as a promising strategy for early risk assessment of sPTB in asymptomatic individuals and threatened sPTL in symptomatic individuals as highlighted in **Tables 1** and **2**. Leveraging current data from single-cell high-dimen-sional approaches provides a foundation for modeling the progression of pregnancy, differentiating cases from controls, and predicting the time to delivery. To bridge the knowledge gaps in the immune clock of preterm pregnancy and identify actionable clinical biomarkers for sPTB prediction and prevention, careful consideration of sPTB subtypes and intervention reporting, cross-tissue analyses, and multiomic inte-gration—including demographic, behavioral, and environmental factors[98–100]—is imperative in the design of new study cohorts.

FUNDING SOURCES

This work was supported by the following entities: Society for Reproductive Investi-gation and Bayer Innovation/Discovery Grant (D. Feyaerts); Stanford Maternal and Child Health Research Institute Postdoctoral Support Award (D. Feyaerts); Next Gen-eration Partnership Grant, provided by the State Ministry of Education and Research, Germany (P.C. Arck); ZonMw, Netherlands (Netherlands Organisation for Health Research and Development) Grant 09032212110019 (J.R. Prins); the March of Dimes Prematurity Research Center at Stanford University (22-FY-169–12; I. Marić); NIH P01HD106414 (B. Gaudillière, D. Feyaerts); and NIH R00HD105016 (I.A. Stelzer). The funders had no role in study design, data collection and analyses, decision to publish, or preparation of the manuscript.

ACKNOWLEDGMENTS

The authors thank Julien J. Hedou MSc, Jose Galaz MD, Jakob F. Einhaus MD, Masaki Sato MD, Kazuo Ando MD, Maïgane Diop BSc, Dyani Gaudilliere MD/MPH, Ronald J. Wong PhD, Martin S. Angst MD, Nima Aghaeepour PhD, David K. Stevenson MD, Vir-ginia D. Winn MD/PhD, Anke Diemert MD, Mana M. Parast MD/PhD, and Cynthia Gyamfi-Bannerman MD/MSc, for their contribution to conceptualization, writing, and editing of this review.

DISCLOSURE

The authors indicate no conflict of interest regarding a financial or non-financial interest in the subject matter discussed in this article.

Best Practices

What is the current practice for preterm birth?

Currently, there is no best practice for the prediction of preterm birth (PTB) based on cellular immune profiles.

What changes in current practice are likely to improve outcomes?

Profiling the immune system in the maternal circulation, a sample easily accessible during pregnancy, promises to enable the identification of biomarkers and potential therapeutic targets for the prediction and prevention of PTB, respectively.

To establish the usefulness of the immunome for such purposes, prospective cohorts are needed to profile the immunome in two clinically relevant scenarios (see **Fig. 1**), the screening of (1) symptomatic pregnancies with threatened PTB at the time of hospitalization and (2) asymptomatic pregnancies at low- or high-risk for spontaneous PTB at routine prenatal care visits. Integration of the cervicovaginal immunome, hematologic parameters, routine pregnancy care parameters (eg, ultrasound), and electronic health records promises to improve predictive performance. Besides PTB risk assessment, the immunome contains valuable clues into pathobiological mechanisms, the basis for developing treatment strategies.

REFERENCES

1. Romero R, Dey SK, Fisher SJ. Preterm labor: one syndrome, many causes. Science 2014;345(6198):760–5.
2. Gomez-Lopez N, Galaz J, Miller D, et al. The immunobiology of preterm labor and birth: intra-amniotic inflammation or breakdown of maternal-fetal homeostasis. Reproduction 2022;164(2):R11–45.
3. Goldenberg RL, Culhane JF, Iams JD, et al. Epidemiology and causes of preterm birth. Lancet 2008;371(9606):75–84.
4. Yüzen D, Graf I, Tallarek AC, et al. Increased late preterm birth risk and altered uterine blood flow upon exposure to heat stress. EBioMedicine 2023;93:104651.
5. Barros FC, Papageorghiou AT, Victora CG, et al. The distribution of clinical phenotypes of preterm birth syndrome: implications for prevention. JAMA Pediatr 2015;169(3):220–9.
6. Hornaday KK, Wood EM, Slater DM. Is there a maternal blood biomarker that can predict spontaneous preterm birth prior to labour onset? A systematic review. PLoS One 2022;17(4):e0265853.
7. PrabhuDas M, Bonney E, Caron K, et al. Immune mechanisms at the maternal-fetal interface: perspectives and challenges. Nat Immunol 2015;16(4):328–34.
8. Yang F, Zheng Q, Jin L. Dynamic function and composition changes of immune cells during normal and pathological pregnancy at the maternal-fetal interface. Front Immunol 2019;10:2317.
9. Gomez-Lopez N, StLouis D, Lehr MA, et al. Immune cells in term and preterm labor. Cell Mol Immunol 2014;11(6):571–81.
10. Zhou JZ, Way SS, Chen K. Immunology of the uterine and vaginal mucosae. Trends Immunol 2018;39(4):302–14.
11. Peterson LS, Stelzer IA, Tsai AS, et al. Multiomic immune clockworks of pregnancy. Semin Immunopathol 2020;42(4):397–412.

12. Miller D, Garcia-Flores V, Romero R, et al. Single-cell immunobiology of the maternal-fetal interface. J Immunol 2022;209(8):1450–64.
13. Erlebacher A. Immunology of the maternal-fetal interface. Annu Rev Immunol 2013;31(1):387–411.
14. Gomez-Lopez N, Guilbert LJ, Olson DM. Invasion of the leukocytes into the fetal-maternal interface during pregnancy. J Leukoc Biol 2010;88(4):625–33.
15. Chen D, Wang W, Wu L, et al. Single-cell atlas of peripheral blood mononuclear cells from pregnant women. Clin Transl Med 2022;12(5):e821.
16. Aghaeepour N, Ganio EA, McIlwain D, et al. An immune clock of human pregnancy. Sci Immunol 2017;2(15):eaan2946.
17. Robinson DP, Klein SL. Pregnancy and pregnancy-associated hormones alter immune responses and disease pathogenesis. Horm Behav 2012;62(3):263–71.
18. Monteiro C, Kasahara T, Sacramento PM, et al. Human pregnancy levels of estrogen and progesterone contribute to humoral immunity by activating TFH/B cell axis. Eur J Immunol 2021;51(1):167–79.
19. Tarca AL, Romero R, Xu Z, et al. Targeted expression profiling by RNA-Seq improves detection of cellular dynamics during pregnancy and identifies a role for T cells in term parturition. Sci Rep 2019;9(1):848.
20. Pique-Regi R, Romero R, Tarca AL, et al. Single cell transcriptional signatures of the human placenta in term and preterm parturition. Elife 2019;8:e52004.
21. Sharma S, Rodrigues PRS, Zaher S, et al. Immune-metabolic adaptations in pregnancy: a potential stepping-stone to sepsis. EBioMedicine 2022;86:104337.
22. Gomez-Lopez N, Romero R, Galaz J, et al. Transcriptome changes in maternal peripheral blood during term parturition mimic perturbations preceding spontaneous preterm birth. Biol Reprod 2022;106(1):185–99.
23. Pique-Regi R, Romero R, Garcia-Flores V, et al. A single-cell atlas of the myometrium in human parturition. JCI Insight 2022;7(5):e153921.
24. Garcia-Flores V, Romero R, Tarca AL, et al. Deciphering maternal-fetal cross-talk in the human placenta during parturition using single-cell RNA sequencing. Sci Transl Med 2024;16(729):eadh8335.
25. Tarca AL, Pataki BÁ, Romero R, et al. Crowdsourcing assessment of maternal blood multi-omics for predicting gestational age and preterm birth. Cell Rep Med 2021;2(6):100323.
26. Apps R, Kotliarov Y, Cheung F, et al. Multimodal immune phenotyping of maternal peripheral blood in normal human pregnancy. JCI Insight 2020;5(7):e134838.
27. Stelzer IA, Ghaemi MS, Han X, et al. Integrated trajectories of the maternal metabolome, proteome, and immunome predict labor onset. Sci Transl Med 2021;13(592):eabd9898.
28. Gomez-Lopez N, Romero R, Hassan SS, et al. The cellular transcriptome in the maternal circulation during normal pregnancy: a longitudinal study. Front Immunol 2019;10:2863.
29. Bukowski R, Sadovsky Y, Goodarzi H, et al. Onset of human preterm and term birth is related to unique inflammatory transcriptome profiles at the maternal fetal interface. PeerJ 2017;5:e3685.
30. Xu Y, Romero R, Miller D, et al. An M1-like macrophage polarization in decidual tissue during spontaneous preterm labor that is attenuated by rosiglitazone treatment. J Immunol 2016;196(6):2476–91.
31. Arenas-Hernandez M, Romero R, Xu Y, et al. Effector and activated t cells induce preterm labor and birth that is prevented by treatment with progesterone. J Immunol 2019;202(9):2585–608.

32. Gomez-Lopez N, Garcia-Flores V, Chin PY, et al. Macrophages exert homeostatic actions in pregnancy to protect against preterm birth and fetal inflammatory injury. JCI Insight 2021;6(19):e146089.

33. Gomez-Lopez N, Arenas-Hernandez M, Romero R, et al. Regulatory T cells play a role in a subset of idiopathic preterm labor/birth and adverse neonatal outcomes. Cell Rep 2020;32(1):107874.

34. Yuan M, Jordan F, McInnes IB, et al. Leukocytes are primed in peripheral blood for activation during term and preterm labour. Mol Hum Reprod 2009;15(11):713–24.

35. Gomez-Lopez N, Estrada-Gutierrez G, Jimenez-Zamudio L, et al. Fetal membranes exhibit selective leukocyte chemotaxic activity during human labor. J Reprod Immunol 2009;80(1–2):122–31.

36. Couture C, Brien ME, Boufaied I, et al. Proinflammatory changes in the maternal circulation, maternal-fetal interface, and placental transcriptome in preterm birth. Am J Obstet Gynecol 2023;228(3):332.e1–17.

37. Vora B, Wang A, Kosti I, et al. Meta-analysis of maternal and fetal transcriptomic data elucidates the role of adaptive and innate immunity in preterm birth. Front Immunol 2018;9:993.

38. Waks AB, Martinez-King LC, Santiago G, et al. Developing a risk profile for spontaneous preterm birth and short interval to delivery among patients with threatened preterm labor. Am J Obstet Gynecol MFM 2022;4(6):100727.

39. FIGO Working Group on Good Clinical Practice in Maternal-Fetal Medicine. Good clinical practice advice: prediction of preterm labor and preterm premature rupture of membranes. Int J Gynaecol Obstet 2019;144(3):340–6.

40. Jun SY, Lee JY, Kim HM, et al. Evaluation of the effectiveness of foetal fibronectin as a predictor of preterm birth in symptomatic preterm labour women. BMC Pregnancy Childbirth 2019;19(1):241.

41. Carter J, Seed PT, Watson HA, et al. Development and validation of predictive models for QUiPP App v.2: tool for predicting preterm birth in women with symptoms of threatened preterm labor. Ultrasound Obstet Gynecol 2020;55(3):357–67.

42. Khanam R, Fleischer TC, Boghossian NS, et al. Performance of a validated spontaneous preterm delivery predictor in South Asian and Sub-Saharan African women: a nested case control study. J Matern Fetal Neonatal Med 2022;35(25):8878–86.

43. Camunas-Soler J, Gee EPS, Reddy M, et al. Predictive RNA profiles for early and very early spontaneous preterm birth. Am J Obstet Gynecol 2022;227(1):72.e1–16.

44. Takeda J, Fang X, Olson DM. Pregnant human peripheral leukocyte migration during several late pregnancy clinical conditions: a cross-sectional observational study. BMC Pregnancy Childbirth 2017;17(1):16.

45. Koucký M, Malíčková K, Cindrová-Davies T, et al. Low levels of circulating T-regulatory lymphocytes and short cervical length are associated with preterm labor. J Reprod Immunol 2014;106:110–7.

46. Heng YJ, Pennell CE, Chua HN, et al. Whole blood gene expression profile associated with spontaneous preterm birth in women with threatened preterm labor. PLoS One 2014;9(5):e96901.

47. Chim SSC, Chan TF, Leung TY. Whole-transcriptome analysis of maternal blood for identification of RNA markers for predicting spontaneous preterm birth among preterm labour women: abridged secondary publication. Hong Kong Med J 2020;26(Suppl 6):20–3.

48. Ran Y, He J, Peng W, et al. Development and validation of a transcriptomic signature-based model as the predictive, preventive, and personalized medical strategy for preterm birth within 7 days in threatened preterm labor women. EPMA J 2022;13(1):87–106.

49. Ran Y, Huang D, Yin N, et al. Predicting the risk of preterm birth throughout pregnancy based on a novel transcriptomic signature. Maternal Fetal Med 2023;5(4): 213–22.

50. Sun B, Parks WT, Simhan HN, et al. Early pregnancy immune profile and preterm birth classified according to uteroplacental lesions. Placenta 2020;89:99–106.

51. Denney JM, Nelson E, Wadhwa P, et al. Cytokine profiling: variation in immune modulation with preterm birth vs. uncomplicated term birth identifies pivotal signals in pathogenesis of preterm birth. J Perinat Med 2021;49(3):299–309.

52. Abbott DS, Chin-Smith EC, Seed PT, et al. Raised trappin2/elafin protein in cervico-vaginal fluid is a potential predictor of cervical shortening and spontaneous preterm birth. PLoS One 2014;9(7):e100771.

53. Leow SM, Di Quinzio MKW, Ng ZL, et al. Preterm birth prediction in asymptomatic women at mid-gestation using a panel of novel protein biomarkers: the Prediction of PreTerm Labor (PPeTaL) study. Am J Obstet Gynecol MFM 2020;2(2): 100084.

54. Heng YJ, Liong S, Permezel M, et al. Human cervicovaginal fluid biomarkers to predict term and preterm labor. Front Physiol 2015;6:151.

55. Ngo TTM, Moufarrej MN, Rasmussen MH, et al. Noninvasive blood tests for fetal development predict gestational age and preterm delivery. Science 2018; 360(6393):1133–6.

56. Saade GR, Boggess KA, Sullivan SA, et al. Development and validation of a spontaneous preterm delivery predictor in asymptomatic women. Am J Obstet Gynecol 2016;214(5):633.e1–24.

57. D'Silva AM, Hyett JA, Coorssen JR. Proteomic analysis of first trimester maternal serum to identify candidate biomarkers potentially predictive of spontaneous preterm birth. J Proteomics 2018;178:31–42.

58. Morillon AC, Yakkundi S, Thomas G, et al. Association between phospholipid metabolism in plasma and spontaneous preterm birth: a discovery lipidomic analysis in the cork pregnancy cohort. Metabolomics 2020;16(2):19.

59. Liang L, Rasmussen MLH, Piening B, et al. Metabolic dynamics and prediction of gestational age and time to delivery in pregnant women. Cell 2020;181(7): 1680–92.e15.

60. McElrath TF, Cantonwine DE, Jeyabalan A, et al. Circulating microparticle proteins obtained in the late first trimester predict spontaneous preterm birth at less than 35 weeks' gestation: a panel validation with specific characterization by parity. Am J Obstet Gynecol 2019;220(5):488.e1–11.

61. Menon R, Debnath C, Lai A, et al. Circulating exosomal miRNA profile during term and preterm birth pregnancies: a longitudinal study. Endocrinology 2019;160(2): 249–75.

62. Jelliffe-Pawlowski LL, Rand L, Bedell B, et al. Prediction of preterm birth with and without preeclampsia using mid-pregnancy immune and growth-related molecular factors and maternal characteristics. J Perinatol 2018;38(8):963–72.

63. Espinosa CA, Khan W, Khanam R, et al. Multiomic signals associated with maternal epidemiological factors contributing to preterm birth in low- and middle-income countries. Sci Adv 2023;9(21):eade7692.

64. Pawelczyk E, Nowicki BJ, Izban MG, et al. Spontaneous preterm labor is associated with an increase in the proinflammatory signal transducer TLR4 receptor on maternal blood monocytes. BMC Pregnancy Childbirth 2010;10:66.

65. Paquette AG, Shynlova O, Kibschull M, et al. Comparative analysis of gene expression in maternal peripheral blood and monocytes during spontaneous preterm labor. Am J Obstet Gynecol 2018;218(3):345.e1–30.

66. Paquette AG, Shynlova O, Wu X, et al. MicroRNA-transcriptome networks in whole blood and monocytes of women undergoing preterm labour. J Cell Mol Med 2019;23(10):6835–45.

67. Vakili S, Torabinavid P, Tabrizi R, et al. The association of inflammatory biomarker of neutrophil-to-lymphocyte ratio with spontaneous preterm delivery: a systematic review and meta-analysis. Mediators Inflamm 2021;2021:6668381.

68. Heng YJ, Pennell CE, McDonald SW, et al. Maternal whole blood gene expression at 18 and 28 weeks of gestation associated with spontaneous preterm birth in asymptomatic women. PLoS One 2016;11(6):e0155191.

69. Zhou G, Holzman C, Heng YJ, et al. EBF1 gene mRNA levels in maternal blood and spontaneous preterm birth. Reprod Sci 2020;27(1):316–24.

70. Zhou G, Holzman C, Chen B, et al. EBF1-correlated long non-coding RNA transcript levels in 3rd trimester maternal blood and risk of spontaneous preterm birth. Reprod Sci 2021;28(2):541–9.

71. Manuck TA, Eaves LA, Rager JE, et al. Mid-pregnancy maternal blood nitric oxide-related gene and miRNA expression are associated with preterm birth. Epigenomics 2021;13(9):667–82.

72. Ma M, Zhu M, Zhuo B, et al. Use of complete blood count for predicting preterm birth in asymptomatic pregnant women: a propensity score-matched analysis. J Clin Lab Anal 2020;34(8):e23313.

73. Park S, Moon J, Kang N, et al. Predicting preterm birth through vaginal microbiota, cervical length, and WBC using a machine learning model. Front Microbiol 2022;13:912853.

74. Morisaki N, Piedvache A, Nagata C, et al. Maternal blood count parameters of chronic inflammation by gestational age and their associations with risk of preterm delivery in the Japan Environment and Children's Study. Sci Rep 2021;11(1):15522.

75. Winger EE, Reed JL, Ji X. Early first trimester peripheral blood cell microRNA predicts risk of preterm delivery in pregnant women: proof of concept. PLoS One 2017;12(7):e0180124.

76. Winger EE, Reed JL, Ji X, et al. MicroRNAs isolated from peripheral blood in the first trimester predict spontaneous preterm birth. PLoS One 2020;15(8):e0236805.

77. Akoto C, Chan CYS, Tshivuila-Matala COO, et al. Innate lymphoid cells are reduced in pregnant HIV positive women and are associated with preterm birth. Sci Rep 2020;10(1):13265.

78. Ridout AE, Horsley V, Seed PT, et al. The neutrophil-to-lymphocyte ratio: a low-cost antenatal indicator of placental chorioamnionitis in women who deliver preterm without clinical signs and symptoms of infection. Eur J Obstet Gynecol Reprod Biol 2023;280:34–9.

79. Hensleigh PA, Herzenberg LA, Lipman SH, et al. Transient immunologic effects of betamethasone in human pregnancy after suppression of preterm labor. Am J Reprod Immunol 1983;4(2):83–7.

80. Stranik J, Kacerovsky M, Andrys C, et al. Intra-amniotic infection and sterile intra-amniotic inflammation are associated with elevated concentrations of

cervical fluid interleukin-6 in women with spontaneous preterm labor with intact membranes. J Matern Fetal Neonatal Med 2022;35(25):4861–9.

81. Hunter PJ, Sheikh S, David AL, et al. Cervical leukocytes and spontaneous preterm birth. J Reprod Immunol 2016;113:42–9.

82. Giesen C, Wang HA, Schapiro D, et al. Highly multiplexed imaging of tumor tissues with subcellular resolution by mass cytometry. Nat Methods 2014;11(4): 417–22.

83. Greenbaum S, Averbukh I, Soon E, et al. A spatially resolved timeline of the human maternal-fetal interface. Nature 2023;619(7970):595–605.

84. Layden AJ, Bertolet M, Parks WT, et al. Latent class analysis of placental histopathology: a novel approach to classifying early and late preterm births. Am J Obstet Gynecol 2022;227(2):290.e1–21.

85. Redline RW, Ravishankar S, Bagby CM, et al. Four major patterns of placental injury: a stepwise guide for understanding and implementing the 2016 Amsterdam consensus. Mod Pathol 2021;34(6):1074–92.

86. Freedman AA, Keenan-Devlin LS, Borders A, et al. Formulating a meaningful and comprehensive placental phenotypic classification. Pediatr Dev Pathol 2021; 24(4):337–50.

87. Suresh SC, Freedman AA, Hirsch E, et al. A comprehensive analysis of the association between placental pathology and recurrent preterm birth. Am J Obstet Gynecol 2022;227(6):887.e1–15.

88. Lee J, Kim JS, Park JW, et al. Chronic chorioamnionitis is the most common placental lesion in late preterm birth. Placenta 2013;34(8):681–9.

89. Le BL, Iwatani S, Wong RJ, et al. Computational discovery of therapeutic candidates for preventing preterm birth. JCI Insight 2020;5(3):e133761.

90. Ghaemi MS, DiGiulio DB, Contrepois K, et al. Multiomics modeling of the immunome, transcriptome, microbiome, proteome and metabolome adaptations during human pregnancy. Bioinformatics 2019;35(1):95–103.

91. Jehan F, Sazawal S, Baqui AH, et al. Multiomics characterization of preterm birth in low- and middle-income countries. JAMA Netw Open 2020;3(12):e2029655.

92. Hastie T, Tibshirani R, Wainwright M. Statistical learning with sparsity: the lasso and generalizations. 1st ed. New York: Chapman and Hall/CRC; 2015.

93. Huan X, Caramanis C, Mannor S. Sparse algorithms are not stable: a no-free-lunch theorem. IEEE Trans Pattern Anal Mach Intell 2012;34(1):187–93.

94. Hédou J, Marić I, Bellan G, et al. Discovery of sparse, reliable omic biomarkers with Stabl. Nat Biotechnol 2024. https://doi.org/10.1038/s41587-023-02033-x.

95. Espinosa C, Becker M, Marić I, et al. Data-driven modeling of pregnancy-related complications. Trends Mol Med 2021;27(8):762–76.

96. Leng D, Zheng L, Wen Y, et al. A benchmark study of deep learning-based multi-omics data fusion methods for cancer. Genome Biol 2022;23(1):171.

97. Marić I, Contrepois K, Moufarrej MN, et al. Early prediction and longitudinal modeling of preeclampsia from multiomics. Patterns (NY) 2022;3(12):100655.

98. Ravindra NG, Espinosa C, Berson E, et al. Deep representation learning identifies associations between physical activity and sleep patterns during pregnancy and prematurity. NPJ Digit Med 2023;6(1):171.

99. Becker M, Dai J, Chang AL, et al. Revealing the impact of lifestyle stressors on the risk of adverse pregnancy outcomes with multitask machine learning. Front Pediatr 2022;10:933266.

100. De Francesco D, Reiss JD, Roger J, et al. Data-driven longitudinal characterization of neonatal health and morbidity. Sci Transl Med 2023;15(683):eadc9854.

Computational Approaches for Predicting Preterm Birth and Newborn Outcomes

David Seong, BA[a,b,c,d], Camilo Espinosa, MPhil[a,d,e,f],
Nima Aghaeepour, PhD[d,e,f],*, Aghaeepour Laboratory[a,b,c,d,e,f,g,1]

KEYWORDS

- Preterm birth • Computational modeling • Multimodal • Neonatal outcomes

KEY POINTS

- The use of electronic health records allows accurate predictive modeling of preterm birth (PTB)-associated morbidities, a clinically complex phenotype.
- Application of artificial intelligence (AI)-based models using biological data generates new knowledge regarding the pathogenesis of PTB.
- Social determinants of health are an important component of predictive models for PTB.
- The successful deployment of predictive models for PTB will require careful consideration of ethical issues including bias, generalizability, and interpretability.

INTRODUCTION

Globally, preterm birth (PTB) is the leading cause of infant morbidity and mortality among children under the age of 5 years[1] and its rates have not decreased significantly in the past decade ($\sim$10%).[2] However, the proportion of deaths caused by

[a] Immunology Program, Stanford University School of Medicine, 300 Pasteur Drive, Grant S280, Stanford, CA 94305-5117, USA; [b] Medical Scientist Training Program, Stanford University School of Medicine, 300 Pasteur Drive, Grant S280, Stanford, CA 94305-5117, USA; [c] Department of Microbiology and Immunology, Stanford University School of Medicine, 300 Pasteur Drive, Grant S280, Stanford, CA 94305-5117, USA; [d] Department of Anesthesiology, Perioperative and Pain Medicine, Stanford University, School of Medicine, 300 Pasteur Drive, Grant S280, Stanford, CA 94305-5117, USA; [e] Department of Pediatrics, Stanford University School of Medicine, 300 Pasteur Drive, Grant S280, Stanford, CA 94305-5117, USA; [f] Department of Biomedical Data Science, Stanford University, 300 Pasteur Drive, Grant S280, Stanford, CA 94305-5117, USA; [g] Department of Pathology, Stanford University School of Medicine, 300 Pasteur Drive, Grant S280, Stanford, CA 94305-5117, USA
[1] The members of the Aghaeepour Laboratory that contributed as co-authors to the writing of various sections throughout this manuscript are listed in the acknowledgment section.
* Corresponding author. 300 Pasteur Drive, Grant S280, Stanford, CA 94305-5117.
E-mail address: naghaeep@stanford.edu

PTB complications has increased from 14.5% in 2000 to 17.7% in 2019.[1] Those who survive PTB are at a greater risk of long-term morbidities, including brain injury,[3] cognitive impairments,[4] cardiovascular diseases, and more. Identifying PTB outcomes and early interventions are critical to mitigating these morbidities.

Traditionally, single risk factors, such as maternal age or medical history, or simple rule-based calculators incorporating these clinical variables, were used to estimate the likelihood of adverse outcomes or to identify high-risk pregnancies. One of the oldest and frequently used metrics is the APGAR score that focuses on various aspects of the neonate to determine health status.[5] More recently developed risk scores such as the Extremely Preterm Birth Outcomes Tool developed by the Eunice Kennedy Shriver National Institute of Child Health and Development in the early 2000s use both maternal and fetal measurements combined with logistic regression to generate predictive values for infant morbidity and mortality.[6] While such parameters and simple scoring methods provide clinicians with an estimated risk for neonatal morbidity and mortality, there is growing acknowledgment that these data are relatively ineffective in predicting such outcomes.[7,8] For example, around 60% to 70% of PTB newborns survived without any major morbidities compared with those born extremely preterm despite being technically classified as being PTB.[9,10] This paradox highlights the potential contribution of confounding factors as well as modifying factors that result in individual heterogeneity for neonatal outcomes and the limitations of simple gestational age (GA)-based metrics.[11,12]

A multimodal approach may be required to fully grasp the clinical progression of the pathogenesis of PTB due to its high complexity. With artificial intelligence (AI), large multimodal data sets can be seamlessly processed, integrated, and digested. For example, the increasing popularity and availability of electronic health records (EHRs) has created a rich source of data for AI-based predictive models. Unlike traditional risk scores that utilize very limited clinical data, EHRs are a much more complete representation of the mother's medical history, including longitudinal information throughout the course of her pregnancy. These advantages of using EHRs have already begun to show superior predictive ability compared with traditional GA-based risk scores.[13–19] Second, recent advancements in high-throughput omics assays have decreased the cost, time, and sample size needed for generating biological datasets. These datasets range from multidimensional flow cytometry-based immunomics to mass spectrometry-based metabolomics.

Incorporating biological data into AI models can capture the complex dynamics involved in PTB and therefore potentially identify key biological pathways or biomarkers[14] that may ultimately lead to novel therapeutic targets and approaches. Finally, social determinants of health (SDOH) such as race and socioeconomic status have been shown to impact adverse outcomes of pregnancy, including PTB.[20] For example, Black women in the United States have a 2-fold greater risk for PTB compared with White women.[21] Being able to integrate SDOH into predictive models may not only improve their accuracy but also identify nonpharmacologic strategies capable of modulating PTB morbidities.

In this review, we provide an overview of different data modalities that can be used to predict, understand, and derive a more accurate taxonomy for PTB and associated adverse outcomes. These include phenotypical, biological, and social determinant data (**Table 1**). We then conclude with an overview on ethical considerations of using AI models for PTB-associated morbidities. To develop more accurate and socially equitable predictive models for PTB and its associated morbidities, it is necessary to understand how to leverage AI appropriately and ethically.

Table 1
Key papers by data type and computational methodology

Data Type	Methodology	Goal	Citations
Electronic Health Record	Use EHR data from neonatal intensive care unit (NICU) patients and classification/regression tree models	Predict probabilities of severe neonatal morbidities	Hamilton, et al,[23] 2020.
	Use EHR data from NICU patients and 8 different classification models optimized using a nested crossvalidation meth	Predict occurrence of sepsis at least 4 h before using EHR records	Masino, et al,[24] 2019.
	Use EHR data of prenatal visits and elastic net/gradient boosting algorithms	Predict preeclampsia from early pregnancy information	Marić, et al,[18] 2020
Biological	Use metabolomic, proteomic, and immune data to build a single stacked generalization model	Predict labor onset independent of gestational age	Stelzer, et al.[31] 2021
	Use urinary metabolites with random forest algorithm	Predict gestational age using urinary metabolites in both healthy and pathologic pregnancies	Contrepois, et al,[32] 2022
	Use mass cytometry-based immune data and modified elastic net algorithm	Model immunological events during pregnancy	Aghaeepour, et al,[33] 2017
Social Determinants of Health	Use both maternal and newborn EHR data including SDOH features in a long short-term memory (LSTM) neural network	Predict 24 different neonatal outcomes	De Francesco, et al,[15] 2023
	Use maternal plasma analytes and covariates (including SDOHs) with cross-validated gradient-boosted tree model (XGBoost)	Profile biological and epidemiological signatures of pregnancy	Espinosa, et al.[44] 2023

DISCUSSION
Use of Electronic Health Records to Predict Maternal and Neonatal Health

Clinical decision support systems for predicting maternal and neonatal health outcomes have evolved significantly over the past decade. To diagnose PTB, the oldest methods used a few parameters, such as GA and/or birthweight. Newer clinical risk scores followed, derived from phenotypical (ie, laboratory measurements, medical history) and epidemiologic (ie, maternal age, race) analyses of PTB to better delineate the risk of associated morbidities, further advancing our understanding of PTB. These advances were made by using concurrent advances in AI that allowed clinicians and scientists to fully leverage the large and increasingly available phenotypic data available in EHRs to predict maternal and neonatal complications.

With the increasing availability of EHR data through efforts such as the Meaningful Use initiative,[22] the field has incorporated more sophisticated risk calculators and machine learning based systems that leverage comprehensive phenotypic data. For instance, predictive models incorporating EHR data into regularized linear regressions have been shown to be predictive of early preeclampsia, a major cause of PTB, and a maternal morbidity that has a complex clinical etiology.[18] A second study used EHR data and machine learning to predict severe neonatal morbidities, including intraventricular hemorrhage and necrotizing enterocolitis, and was demonstrated to be more accurate compared with traditional multivariable analyses.[23] Such studies show the effectiveness of leveraging the enormity of EHR data to increase the predictive accuracy for clinically multifaceted phenomena such as PTB.

Second, machine learning algorithms can also aid in determining the optimal timing of treatment of PTB-associated morbidities. A machine learning model based on EHR data was able to identify septic infants at least 4 hours prior to clinical presentation and confirmation, enabling rapid and timely treatment, such as administration of antibiotics.[24] Other machine learning based tools such as the Bhutani nomogram and the subsequent development of the interactive BiliTool application have enabled the identification of treatment thresholds for infants with hyperbilirubinemia, recommending when phototherapy or more intensive interventions should be initiated.[25] Predictive AI models will become increasingly accurate as pipelines to incorporate EHR data continue to evolve, providing clinicians with rapid and useful real-time recommendations.

Finally, generalizability is an important characteristic for any EHR-based AI model because these models often perform variably across different health systems. In one example, a model trained to predict PTB on a cohort of patients from Vanderbilt performed nearly as accurately on a similar-sized cohort from the University of California, San Francisco.[26] However, it is important to consider that this generalizability may not always hold, especially across 2 settings with extremely different patient populations. Therefore, other studies have begun to examine methods of fine-tuning models to fit a particular context. A study on the early prediction of COVID-19 infections showed that techniques such as transfer learning were effective at increasing the predictive power of EHR-based AI models.[27] However, transfer learning requires the availability of model architecture and pretrained weights from the original developing institution. However, the authors also discovered that fine-tuning models using site-specific thresholds, which do not require any prior knowledge of the model, were reasonably effective at discriminating COVID-19 infections. As similar studies are now being conducted for PTB, the generalizability of EHR-based models will further improve, making them a cost-effective and highly portable tool for predicting PTB and its associated morbidities.

Despite the accuracy and advantages of using EHR-derived AI prediction models, one drawback is the lack of "interpretability" compared with traditional rule-based systems. Interpretability, the degree to which a human can understand how the model works is important in the clinical setting where clinicians and hospital leadership need to trust a model's outputs before deployment. In addition, interpretability is beneficial during model development and maintenance for identifying errors and/or areas for improvement. Finally, interpretability is an important first step to "explainability" for clinicians where they must be able to explain their rationale for treatment to patients and other physicians before beginning treatment. Traditional scoring metrics incorporate small numbers of clinical risk factors with clear associations to the disease of interest, making their output scores more interpretable for clinicians. This is in contrast to EHR-based models, which sacrifice interpretability for accuracy in leveraging the full complexity of the EHR data. For example, one technique uses subclustering of patients by specific features and/or risk factors for post hoc analyses and reasoning. This technique was used in the cardiovascular field to predict drug-induced QT prolongation where the interpretable model revealed specific antiarrhythmic medications associated with higher risk while antiemetics decreased risk.[28] While much more research is needed in this area for EHR-based AI models in PTB, achieving interpretable models will be transformational for the field.

The shift from rule-based systems to machine learning models is beneficial for the field, as machine learning models often outperform rule-based systems that often fail to capture more subtle clinical nuances.[29,30] Despite their current imperfections, machine learning models utilizing EHR data have shown incredible promise in providing more accurate predictions, clinically useful metrics, and cost-effective generalizability, which were not previously possible at this scale using traditional PTB-scoring methods.

Utilization of High-Dimensional Biological Data in Predictive Models

In addition to EHRs, biological data are a second major source useful in deriving machine learning models for PTB and its morbidities. Technological advancements in high-throughput multidimensional analytical techniques are cheaper, faster, and easier to perform on a smaller volume of sample than ever before and have created an explosion of rich biological data sets. These include flow and mass cytometry, transcriptomics, genomics, proteomics, and metabolomics data sets. These omics data are at the single-cell resolution with some techniques capable of preserving spatial information or combining multiple omics analysis within a single cell. The distinguishing advantage of such biological data is its potential to reveal detailed molecular mechanisms of health and disease, especially in complex clinical states, such as PTB, likely driven by the interaction of multiple biological components rather than a single molecule or cell type.

A better understanding of how metabolites, for example, change throughout a healthy pregnancy may provide foundations for downstream identification of pathways and molecules that are part of the pathogeneses of various pregnancy-related diseases. One study used a combination of mass spectrometry, mass cytometry, and aptamer-based technology to measure the metabolites, immune cells, and proteins, respectively, in the blood of healthy pregnant women.[31] Integrating these biological data sets using an AI-based approach, the authors were able to predict time to labor and precisely track changes in metabolites, immune cells, and proteins, laying the foundation for future studies to identify disruptions in this "normal" cadence or profile. Another study analyzed urinary metabolites using a mass cytometry-based technique to predict GA while also establishing a reference for steroid hormones.[32] Such studies lay the groundwork for establishing a reference for multiple types of biological data during pregnancy, thereby allowing the identification of abnormal deviations from these references that may be exploited for therapeutic benefit.

Much effort has also been spent on using biological data and AI models to predict PTB-associated morbidities. In some cases, such models may additionally identify novel and/or potential disease-relevant pathways. For example, one study used cytometry by time-of-flight data combined with a modified elastic net model to predict immune events during pregnancy.[33] Importantly, the study identified a novel IL-2-dependent signaling mechanism in T-cell subsets that maintains progesterone levels during pregnancy. A second study, also using a modified elastic net model, integrated blood transcriptomics, proteomics, metabolomics and lipidomics, and vaginal microbiomics datasets to predict preeclampsia.[34] In addition to predicting preeclampsia, the model and subsequent downstream analyses revealed biological pathways important in the pathogenesis of preeclampsia, such as tryptophan, caffeine, and arachidonic acid metabolism. Finally, many studies have focused on analyzing the microbiome in relation to PTB. The microbiome is inherently complex since it is composed of an incredibly diverse set of bacterial species that act in concert rather than individually. This complexity makes AI an ideal tool for analyzing microbiome data. Indeed, one study that utilized 9 publicly available vaginal microbiome data sets was able to identify 3 metrics encompassing species diversity and bacterial community states that were particularly helpful in predicting PTB.[35] An increasing use of biological data in AI models will lead to new scientific discoveries that may be therapeutically beneficial. While such results will require individual follow-up studies for verification, they do provide a rich resource of new biological questions that may otherwise have gone undetected.

Despite the exciting advantages of using biological data in AI models for predicting PTB-associated morbidities, an important obstacle to overcome is often small sizes of biological data sets. While the technological advances have certainly increased the ease of generating high-throughput multidimensional data, these data are still not as readily available as routine laboratory tests or use in clinical examinations that are part of EHR data. The small sample sizes present challenges for traditional AI models that require large sample sizes. However, some studies have already begun to optimize models with limited numbers of sample. For example, one study used a deep learning model and cytometry data to synthetically simulate a patient's immune responses to various stimuli in a cell-type agnostic manner.[36] Their results showed that the in silico-generated cell responses were highly similar to ground-truth responses. In addition, studies like those abovementioned have already begun to successfully integrate multiple kinds of biological data (ie, proteomics, transcriptomics, and lipidomics[34]) for each patient sample, thereby increasing the depth of analysis per sample rather than the number of samples itself. The utilization of additional forms of biological data such as epigenetics or spatial transcriptomics, which have thus far not been extensively integrated into machine learning models for PTB, may further increase the predictive power of AI models for PTB despite limited sample sizes. Such techniques allow for a more profound understanding of biological data sets, even when working with limited sample sizes.

As multidimensional biological data become increasingly available, AI models for predicting PTB-associated morbidities will be able to make better predictions. In addition to showing effective predictive power, these models have also created new biological avenues for investigation. Even with the limitations discussed, the use of biological data in AI models for PTB will transform the bench-to-bedside process.

Importance of Considering Social Determinants of Health in Predictive Models

While EHR and biological data encompass a wide range of measurable features for building machine learning models, they do not account for the social context of the patient. SDOH are defined as conditions in the environments of individuals that affect a wide range of health and quality of life issues.[37] The US Department of Health and Human Services has largely grouped SDOH into 5 categories: access to health care, education, environment/neighborhood, economic stability, and social/community context.[37] Each of these categories can directly or indirectly impact biological and consequently, clinical outcomes in a patient. Unsurprisingly, one of the major drivers of PTB in addition to phenotypic and biological data is SDOH.[38,39] Thus, understanding the role of SDOH in PTB is not only necessary for a complete understanding of disease pathogenesis but also presents an opportunity for alternative "therapies" such as utilizing policies or social health initiatives to target PTB rather than pharmacologic therapies. Therefore, understanding the effect of SDOH on the universally important medical conditions of prenatal and perinatal-related complications is important for early treatment and intervention.

While SDOH can theoretically have positive and negative impacts on prenatal health for all, they have historically impacted racial/ethnic minority groups and the socially vulnerable population. First, minority groups have different levels of access to medical care. Compared to 80% of White women, only 50% to 70% of Black, Hispanic, or Native Hawaiian/Pacific Islander women receive prenatal care during their first trimester.[40] The cause for this difference is multifactorial, including health care coverage, the presence of physical hospitals/care facilities in the area, and transportation to care. The number of mothers on Medicaid in non-White racial groups is nearly double that of White mothers, especially in certain states where these discrepancies in numbers have further exacerbated the quality of prenatal care.[40,41] In rural underserved areas, there is an increasing loss of hospitals and care facilities for pregnant women leading to limited opportunities for prenatal care. Transportation to facilities with quality care adds to the burden of an already vulnerable population. Second, disparities in education also present implications for prenatal health. Women with lower education have been found to possess lower health literacy and knowledge of birth options throughout the various gestational stages.[42] These women are also prone to experience psychosocial stressors, such as lack of social support, support of the father, general anxiety, and lower happiness, all of which have been shown to have deleterious effects on prenatal health and increase the risk of PTB.[43] Third, economic instability exerts a strong influence on prenatal health. Unsurprisingly, moms from lower socioeconomic classes are less able to obtain adequate prenatal care. However, interestingly, the collective socioeconomic status of a neighborhood has been shown to influence prenatal health.[39] All of these SDOH factors cause delays in obtaining prenatal care or the inability to receive adequate care, resulting in greater rates of pregnancy-related mortality and complications in minority groups compared to Whites.[38] SDOH have also been found to influence disparities in perinatal care. The use of quantitative measures such as the Dhabhar Quick-Assessment Questionnaire for Stress and Psychosocial Factors has found that economic stress was a significant factor in assessing the risk of PTB.[43] A machine learning-based interdependency analysis followed by generation of a nonlinear support vector machine predictive model was conducted to find interdependencies between various features, including SDOH and PTB. The study revealed that a variety of deleterious factors associated with economic stability, including general anxiety, perceived risk of birth complications, self-rated health, and divorce play a role in the risk of PTB.[43] Economic instability is also tied to an increased likelihood of obesity, as well as the presence of food deserts, poor nutrition, and high blood pressure, all of which increase the risk of complications during pregnancy. These factors help index and control for other factors not addressed within the questionnaire and demonstrate that self-awareness of maternal health can itself be a strong predictor of risk assessment for PTB. The social environment also has been shown to buffer against the effects of chronic stress. Women with higher levels of support from parents, siblings, and the father show decreased risk for PTB.[43] Effectively assessing prematurity, PTB, and complications surrounding pregnancy will require a data-driven understanding of a patient's phenotype, SDOH, and a litany of biopsychosocial factors.

While not as commonly studied as other clinical or biological characteristics as predictive features of PTB, recent studies have begun incorporating SDOH into their models. For example, one study found that specific SDOH, such as homelessness and incarceration, have distinct effects on PTB even though they may share many superficial characteristics (ie, low socioeconomic status, stress).[15] Another verified that many of the associations between SDOH and PTB that we observe in the United States are also similarly associated with PTB in low- or middle-income countries.[44] Such studies demonstrate that incorporating SDOH into AI models is not only necessary to generate accurate models of PTB but may also additionally provide new insights into the complicated connections between SDOH and PTB, which were not previously evident.

Ethical Model Development and Deployment

The increasing adoption of AI approaches in health care has highlighted the need for a rigorous examination of how these technologies can be developed and implemented in an ethical fashion. Broadly, concerns surrounding AI include algorithmic bias,[45] prospects of unethical data collection and usage,[46] lack of transparency or interpretability and its impact on patient safety,[47] and possibilities of exploitation.[48] International organizations such as the World Health Organization have put forward recommendations for unified guidelines across fields, yet these have not been widely adopted. Critically, patient acceptance of the use of AI in their care is reliant on the existence of such protections,[49] emphasizing the need for these ethical frameworks.

Without a rigorous ethical framework to guide the development and deployment of AI methods in pregnancy and neonatology, these approaches can also exacerbate preexisting health disparities.[50] Algorithmic bias, arising from inadequate training data and model implementation, can reinforce racial inequities which already exist in pregnancy outcomes.[51] This can be further exacerbated by inadequate data collection with poor representation across different patient populations.[52] The result is an AI model that solidifies, rather than mitigates, racial inequalities in health care. Finally, the "black box" nature of AI, characterized by lack of interpretability, hinders transparency and can compromise informed decision-making in health care settings for both the clinician and patient.[53,54] The lack of interpretability may particularly be harmful in marginalized communities that are already struggling with mistrust of the health care system. To avoid harmful clinical decisions made from flawed AI output, thorough bias mitigation strategies are essential.

Comprehensive assessments at multiple stages in the development and deployment process of AI methods in health care are necessary to minimize the possibility of harm. First, it is essential that final clinical decisions be made by humans properly trained to interpret results with caution. AI models' potential for bias must be characterized and communicated to medical providers before deployment followed by continuous monitoring postdeployment. AI models must be created by diverse groups of developers to ensure thorough inspection and mitigation of potential bias.[55] Furthermore, transparency from developers about data sets and algorithms[55] used during model development should be required, so that relevant regulatory agencies can perform effective audits to evaluate the AI models for adequate representation of patient populations and communities. Ensuring that AI models are built and implemented ethically is critical to improve maternal and neonatal care and reduce outcome disparities in marginalized populations.

When these considerations are sufficiently implemented into the research and implementation process, AI models have the potential to reduce disparities and improve health equity in pregnancy and neonatology.[56] In research settings, AI has been used effectively to predict adverse pregnancy outcomes and neonatal complications across racially and socioeconomically diverse cohorts.[57,58] Furthermore, the deployment of AI methods to understand and address the needs of under-resourced communities has shown early promise.[44,59] These examples demonstrate the beneficial potential of AI models that can extend beyond scientific or therapeutic advancement.

SUMMARY

Prematurity, currently defined as birth before 37 weeks of gestation, encompasses a heterogenous population of infants. The exclusive reliance on GA and birth weight as the principal measures of prematurity fails to account for neonates who, despite being born well before the arbitrary 37-week demarcation, do not manifest any adverse health complications. Here, we have presented studies that have utilized a combination of EHR, biological, and SDOH data to generate more holistic and accurate models of PTB. As more data are incorporated from newer sources such as wearable health technologies, diet tracking, and parsed clinical notes, AI-driven approaches will continue to open new avenues not only for discovering new therapeutic targets or pathways but also for continuous risk assessment and real-time risk recalibration, providing clinicians with dynamic insights for timely interventions.[60] Despite the technological and organizational hurdles that still exist, machine learning models will no doubt provide valuable clinical and biological information to physicians and scientists alike for the understanding of PTB and its associated morbidities.

ACKNOWLEDGMENTS

The authors listed here are part of the Aghaeepour Laboratory that contributed to the writing of this manuscript: Eloise Berson, Dipro Chakraborty, Alan L. Chang, Will Haberkorn, Natasha Harrison, Debapriya Hazra, Tomin James, Yeasul Kim, Ivana Marić, Samson Mataraso, Neshat Mohammadi, Thanaphong Phongpreecha, S Momsen Reincke, Jonathan Reiss, Geetha Saarunya, Sayane Shome, Nolan Shu, Yuqi Tan, Feng Xie, and Lei Xue from Stanford University.

DISCLOSURE

The authors have nothing to disclose.

FUNDING

This study was supported by the NIH (R35GM138353), Burroughs Wellcome Fund (1019816), the March of Dimes, the Robertson Foundation, Alfred E. Mann Foundation, and the Bill and Melinda Gates Foundation (INV-037517).

Best Practices

What is the current practice for predicting preterm birth and associated morbidities?

Best Practice/Guideline/Care Path Objective(s).
- Improve accuracy of prediction models using multimodal data
- Generate new biological and clinical knowledge using multimodal data
- Maintain interpretability of predictive models
- Be conscious of potential biases in predictive model development and deployment

What changes in current practice are likely to improve outcomes?

- Integrate social determinants of health into predictive models

- Use strategies for bias mitigation and increase interpretability

Bibliographic Source(s)

He J, Baxter SL, Xu J, Xu J, Zhou X, Zhang K. The practical implementation of artificial intelligence technologies in medicine. Nat Med 2019;25(1):30-6.

Marić I, Contrepois K, Moufarrej MN, et al. Early prediction and longitudinal modeling of preeclampsia from multiomics. Patterns (NY) 2022;3(12):100,655.

Becker M, Mayo JA, Phogat NK, et al. Deleterious and protective psychosocial and stress-related factors predict risk of spontaneous preterm birth. Am J Perinatol 2023;40(1):74 to 88.

Thomasian NM, Eickhoff C, Adashi EY. Advancing health equity with artificial intelligence. J Public Health Policy 2021;42(4):602-11.

REFERENCES

1. Blencowe H, Krasevec J, de Onis M, et al. National, regional, and worldwide estimates of low birthweight in 2015, with trends from 2000: a systematic analysis. Lancet Glob Health 2019;7(7):e849-60.
2. Lawn JE, Ohuma EO, Bradley E, et al. Small babies, big risks: global estimates of prevalence and mortality for vulnerable newborns to accelerate change and improve counting. Lancet 2023;401(10389):1707-19.
3. Reiss JD, Peterson LS, Nesamoney SN, et al. Perinatal infection, inflammation, preterm birth, and brain injury: a review with proposals for future investigations. Exp Neurol 2022;351:113988.
4. Doyle LW, Spittle A, Anderson PJ, et al. School-aged neurodevelopmental outcomes for children born extremely preterm. Arch Dis Child 2021;106(9):834-8.
5. Simon LV, Hashmi MF, Bragg BN. APGAR score. Available at:. In: StatPearls. StatPearls Publishing; 2023 http://www.ncbi.nlm.nih.gov/books/NBK470569/. [Accessed 13 July 2023].
6. Rysavy MA, Horbar JD, Bell EF, et al. Assessment of an updated neonatal research network extremely preterm birth outcome model in the Vermont oxford network. JAMA Pediatr 2020;174(5):e196294.
7. Tyson JE, Parikh NA, Langer J, et al, National Institute of Child Health and Human Development Neonatal Research Network. Intensive care for extreme prematurity – moving beyond gestational age. N Engl J Med 2008;358(16):1672-81.
8. Stoll BJ, Hansen NI, Bell EF, et al. Trends in care practices, morbidity, and mortality of extremely preterm neonates, 1993-2012. JAMA 2015;314(10):1039-51.

9. Lee HC, Liu J, Profit J, et al. Survival without major morbidity among very low birth weight infants in California. Pediatrics 2020;146(1):e20193865.

10. Jiang S, Huang X, Zhang L, et al. Estimated survival and major comorbidities of very preterm infants discharged against medical advice vs treated with intensive care in China. JAMA Netw Open 2021;4(6):e2113197.

11. Blencowe H, Cousens S, Oestergaard MZ, et al. National, regional, and worldwide estimates of preterm birth rates in the year 2010 with time trends since 1990 for selected countries: a systematic analysis and implications. Lancet 2012;379(9832):2162–72.

12. Lynch CD, Zhang J. The research implications of the selection of a gestational age estimation method. Paediatr Perinat Epidemiol 2007;21(Suppl 2):86–96.

13. Espinosa C, Becker M, Marić I, et al. Data-driven modeling of pregnancy-related complications. Trends Mol Med 2021;27(8):762–76.

14. De Francesco D, Blumenfeld YJ, Marić I, et al. A data-driven health index for neonatal morbidities. iScience 2022;25(4):104143.

15. De Francesco D, Reiss JD, Roger J, et al. Data-driven longitudinal characterization of neonatal health and morbidity. Sci Transl Med 2023;15(683):eadc9854.

16. Yeo KT, Safi N, Wang YA, et al. Prediction of outcomes of extremely low gestational age newborns in Australia and New Zealand. BMJ Paediatr Open 2017; 1(1):e000205.

17. Ge WJ, Mirea L, Yang J, et al. Prediction of neonatal outcomes in extremely preterm neonates. Pediatrics 2013;132(4):e876–85.

18. Marić I, Tsur A, Aghaeepour N, et al. Early prediction of preeclampsia via machine learning. Am J Obstet Gynecol MFM 2020;2(2):100100.

19. Jaskari J, Myllärinen J, Leskinen M, et al. Machine learning methods for neonatal mortality and morbidity classification. IEEE Access 2020;8:123347–58.

20. Stevenson DK, Wong RJ, Aghaeepour N, et al. Towards personalized medicine in maternal and child health: integrating biologic and social determinants. Pediatr Res 2021;89(2):252–8.

21. Manuck TA. Racial and ethnic differences in preterm birth: a complex, multifactorial problem. Semin Perinatol 2017;41(8):511–8.

22. Blumenthal D, Tavenner M. The "meaningful use" regulation for electronic health records. N Engl J Med 2010;363(6):501–4.

23. Hamilton EF, Dyachenko A, Ciampi A, et al. Estimating risk of severe neonatal morbidity in preterm births under 32 weeks of gestation. J Matern Fetal Neonatal Med 2020;33(1):73–80.

24. Masino AJ, Harris MC, Forsyth D, et al. Machine learning models for early sepsis recognition in the neonatal intensive care unit using readily available electronic health record data. PLoS One 2019;14(2):e0212665.

25. Bahr TM, Henry E, Christensen RD, et al. A new hour-specific serum bilirubin nomogram for neonates ≥35 weeks of gestation. J Pediatr 2021;236:28–33.e1.

26. Abraham A, Le B, Kosti I, et al. Dense phenotyping from electronic health records enables machine learning-based prediction of preterm birth. BMC Med 2022;20: 333–x.

27. Yang J, Soltan AAS, Clifton DA. Machine learning generalizability across healthcare settings: insights from multi-site COVID-19 screening. NPJ Digit Med 2022; 5(1):1–8.

28. Simon ST, Trinkley KE, Malone DC, et al. Interpretable machine learning prediction of drug-induced QT prolongation: electronic health record analysis. J Med Internet Res 2022;24(12):e42163.

29. Yalçın N, Kaşıkcı M, Çelik HT, et al. Development and validation of machine learning-based clinical decision support tool for identifying malnutrition in NICU patients. Sci Rep 2023;13(1):5227.

30. Hsu JF, Yang C, Lin CY, et al. Machine learning algorithms to predict mortality of neonates on mechanical intubation for respiratory failure. Biomedicines 2021; 9(10):1377.

31. Stelzer IA, Ghaemi MS, Han X, et al. Integrated trajectories of the maternal metabolome, proteome, and immunome predict labor onset. Sci Transl Med 2021; 13(592):eabd9898.

32. Contrepois K, Chen S, Ghaemi MS, et al. Prediction of gestational age using urinary metabolites in term and preterm pregnancies. Sci Rep 2022;12(1):8033.

33. Aghaeepour N, Ganio EA, Mcilwain D, et al. An immune clock of human pregnancy. Sci Immunol 2017;2(15):eaan2946.

34. Marić I, Contrepois K, Moufarrej MN, et al. Early prediction and longitudinal modeling of preeclampsia from multiomics. Patterns (NY) 2022;3(12):100655.

35. Golob JL, Oskotsky TT, Tang AS, et al. Microbiome Preterm Birth DREAM Challenge: crowdsourcing machine learning approaches to advance preterm birth research. medRxiv 2023;2023:23286920.

36. Fallahzadeh R, Bidoki NH, Stelzer IA, et al. In-silico generation of high-dimensional immune response data in patients using a deep neural network. Cytometry 2023;103(5):392–404.

37. Brach C, Harris LM. Healthy People 2030 health literacy definition tells organizations: make information and services easy to find, understand, and use. J Gen Intern Med 2021;36(4):1084–5.

38. Petersen EE, Davis NL, Goodman D, et al. Vital signs: pregnancy-related deaths, United States, 2011-2015, and strategies for prevention, 13 states, 2013-2017. MMWR Morb Mortal Wkly Rep 2019;68(18):423–9.

39. Dench D, Joyce T, Minkoff H. United States preterm birth rate and COVID-19. Pediatrics 2022;149(5). e2021055495.

40. Martin JA, Hamilton BE, Osterman MJK, et al. Births: final data for 2017. Natl Vital Stat Rep 2018;67(8):1–50.

41. Marcin JP, Shaikh U, Steinhorn RH. Addressing health disparities in rural communities using telehealth. Pediatr Res 2016;79(1–2):169–76.

42. Murugesu L, Damman OC, Derksen ME, et al. Women's participation in decision-making in maternity care: a qualitative exploration of clients' health literacy skills and needs for support. Int J Environ Res Publ Health 2021;18(3):1130.

43. Becker M, Mayo JA, Phogat NK, et al. Deleterious and protective psychosocial and stress- related factors predict risk of spontaneous preterm birth. Am J Perinatol 2023;40(1):74–88.

44. Espinosa CA, Khan W, Khanam R, et al. Multiomic signals associated with maternal epidemiological factors contributing to preterm birth in low- and middle-income countries. Sci Adv 2023;9(21):eade7692.

45. Thomasian NM, Eickhoff C, Adashi EY. Advancing health equity with artificial intelligence. J Publ Health Pol 2021;42(4):602–11.

46. Price WN, Cohen IG. Privacy in the age of medical big data. Nat Med 2019;25(1): 37–43.

47. He J, Baxter SL, Xu J, et al. The practical implementation of artificial intelligence technologies in medicine. Nat Med 2019;25(1):30–6.

48. Martinez-Martin N. What are important ethical implications of using facial recognition technology in health care? AMA J Ethics 2019;21(2):E180–7.

49. Richardson JP, Smith C, Curtis S, et al. Patient apprehensions about the use of artificial intelligence in healthcare. NPJ Digit Med 2021;4(1):140–1.
50. Pammi M, Aghaeepour N, Neu J. Multiomics, artificial intelligence, and precision medicine in perinatology. Pediatr Res 2023;93(2):308–15.
51. O'Reilly-Shah VN, Gentry KR, Walters AM, et al. Bias and ethical considerations in machine learning and the automation of perioperative risk assessment. Br J Anaesth 2020;125(6):843–6.
52. Topol EJ. High-performance medicine: the convergence of human and artificial intelligence. Nat Med 2019;25(1):44–56.
53. Luxton DD. Should Watson be consulted for a second opinion? AMA J Ethics 2019;21(2):E131–7.
54. Anderson M, Anderson SL. How should AI be developed, validated, and implemented in patient care? AMA J Ethics 2019;21(2):E125–30.
55. Solanki P, Grundy J, Hussain W. Operationalising ethics in artificial intelligence for healthcare: a framework for AI developers. AI Ethics 2023;3(1):223–40.
56. Wahl B, Cossy-Gantner A, Germann S, et al. Artificial intelligence (AI) and global health: how can AI contribute to health in resource-poor settings? BMJ Glob Health 2018;3(4):e000798.
57. Jehan F, Sazawal S, Baqui AH, et al. Multiomics characterization of preterm birth in low- and middle-income countries. JAMA Netw Open 2020;3(12):e2029655.
58. Moufarrej MN, Vorperian SK, Wong RJ, et al. Early prediction of preeclampsia in pregnancy with cell-free RNA. Nature 2022;602(7898):689–94.
59. Dey A, Hay K, Afroz B, et al. Understanding intersections of social determinants of maternal healthcare utilization in Uttar Pradesh, India. PLoS One 2018;13(10):e0204810.
60. Kwok TC, Henry C, Saffaran S, et al. Application and potential of artificial intelligence in neonatal medicine. Semin Fetal Neonatal Med 2022;27(5):101346.

Etiologically Based Functional Taxonomy of the Preterm Birth Syndrome

Jose Villar, MD[a],*, Paolo Ivo Cavoretto, MD, PhD[b],
Fernando C. Barros, PhD[c], Roberto Romero, MD[d,e,f],
Aris T. Papageorghiou, MD[a], Stephen H. Kennedy, MD[a]

KEYWORDS

- Preterm birth • Preterm labor • PPROM • Preterm prelabor rupture of membranes
- Etiology • Phenotype • Taxonomy

KEY POINTS

- Preterm birth (PTB) can no longer be defined by GA alone since this approach fails to provide any pathophysiologic insights or assessment of specific risks.
- A robust conceptual, functional PTB taxonomy is presented, based upon maternal, placental, fetal/neonatal conditions, and signs of parturition initiation, defining major clinical phenotypes.
- Prenatal assessment of the phenotype should be followed by postnatal confirmation and refinement, if necessary, to complete the classification of each specific case.
- The conceptual model has been validated showing dynamic adaptation to different population risk profiles, confirming its validity, strength, reproducibility and applicability.
- Global implementation of this taxonomy model will favour research on homogeneous subpopulations, facilitating identification of etiologically-specific screening and diagnostic methods, and effective prevention and treatment.

[a] Nuffield Department of Women's & Reproductive Health, Oxford Maternal & Perinatal Health Institute, Green Templeton College, University of Oxford, Oxford OX3 9DU, UK; [b] Department of Obstetrics and Gynaecology, Vita-Salute San Raffaele University and IRCCS San Raffaele Scientific Institute, Milan 20132, Italy; [c] Post-Graduate Program in Health in the Life Cycle, Catholic University of Pelotas, Rua Félix da Cunha, Pelotas, Rio Grande do Sul 96010-000, Brazil; [d] Pregnancy Research Branch, Division of Obstetrics and Maternal-Fetal Medicine, Division of Intramural Research, Eunice Kennedy Shriver National Institute of Child Health and Human Development, National Institutes of Health, United States Department of Health and Human Services, Bethesda, MD, USA; [e] Department of Obstetrics and Gynecology, University of Michigan, L4001 Women's Hospital, 1500 East Medical Center Drive, Ann Arbor, MI 48109-0276, USA; [f] Department of Epidemiology and Biostatistics, Michigan State University, East Lansing, MI, USA
* Corresponding author. Nuffield Department of Women's & Reproductive Health, Level 3 Women's Centre, John Radcliffe Hospital, Headington, Oxford, OX3 9DU.
E-mail address: jose.villar@wrh.ox.ac.uk

Clin Perinatol 51 (2024) 475–495
https://doi.org/10.1016/j.clp.2024.02.014
0095-5108/24/© 2024 Elsevier Inc. All rights reserved.
perinatology.theclinics.com

INTRODUCTION

Preterm birth (PTB) is a major public health issue, which substantially impacts lifelong health and childhood development. However, despite extensive research, its etiologic complexities remain poorly understood, with limited progress in prevention and treatment, a global prevalence of 10%, and local rates as high as 13% to 16%.[1]

Maternal illnesses, including infectious diseases and nutritional deficiencies, which are still frequent in many regions of the world, significantly influence PTB risks, as does poor access to medical care.[2,3]

In the last 40 years, different factors have contributed to rising PTB rates, including increased provider-initiated delivery of sick mothers and/or compromised fetuses, societal shifts in maternal age and obesity rates, and multiple pregnancies associated with assisted reproductive technologies.[4–7] In contrast, the PTB rate can be as low as 5% among adequately nourished, healthy, educated women who are not exposed to infections and environmental contaminants.[8–11] This sets an evidence-based population target, but a major conceptual issue must first be considered.

PTB has traditionally been defined purely in terms of gestational age (GA) at birth, that is, less than 37 completed weeks' of gestation.[12] However, PTB is a complex, highly heterogeneous syndrome with multiple risk factors and etiologically associated conditions that contribute to distinct pregnancy, postnatal, and early childhood phenotypic outcomes.[13–19] A precise taxonomy of these phenotypes, that distinguishes clearly between risk factors, causal conditions, and mechanisms of action, is required to achieve effective, cause-specific PTB prevention and treatment strategies.

The authors previously proposed a new phenotypic taxonomy of PTB based on known etiologic factors, which acknowledges that multiple causal factors interact dynamically with biological mechanisms, and the environment—the *"pregnancy exposome"*[20] Uniquely, the authors have shown distributions of PTB phenotypes and their interrelation (**Fig. 1**A) as a proportion of total PTB in multinational populations.[17,18] Measured against international standards,[21] these phenotypes are associated with different neurodevelopmental outcomes in early childhood (**Fig. 1**B).

Here, the authors provide an update and add new elements that have emerged in the last decade to promote an etiologically based PTB taxonomy in epidemiologic, clinical, and research activities.

THE LIMITATIONS OF AN EXCLUSIVELY GESTATIONAL AGE–BASED PRETERM BIRTH CLASSIFICATION

The traditional definition of PTB as a single clinical entity demarcated by GA alone does not acknowledge its syndromic characteristics.[19] Such a limited definition would be akin to defining premature adult death based solely on an arbitrary age (eg, 40 years), which would inevitably fail to include the diverse range of possible causes, such as cancer, cardiovascular disease, accidents, infections, and suicide. Similarly, the older an individual is, the higher the risk of disease owing to cumulative insults experienced during life; so the aim is to prevent the factors related to the process of aging rather than treat senescence.

Clearly, research and preventive strategies focused on the biology, genetics, prediction, prevention, or treatment of syndromes are bound to be unsuccessful if age is the sole defining parameter. Similarly, PTB should be classified based on the understanding of its causes, clinical presentation, nutritional status, and laboratory features; moreover, setting an upper limit of 36 + 6 weeks' gestation for defining PTB suggests there is a strong biological reason for doing so, which is not the case.

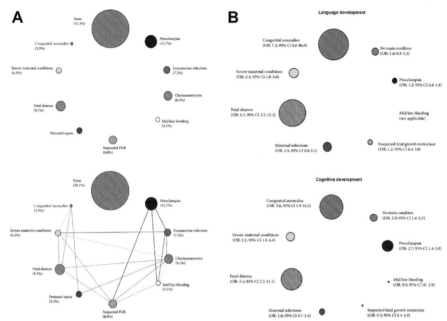

Fig. 1. (*A, upper panel*) Frequencies (proportions) of the etiologically linked conditions (phenotypes) for PTB, in a specific population. (*lower panel*) Frequencies (proportions) and interrelationships of the etiologically linked conditions (phenotypes) for PTB. Each line connecting the phenotypes represents the interrelationship and overlap between different categories, in a specific population. Please note that each circle with different color represents a different phenotype, and each circle size is proportional to the frequency (proportion) of each category in the population in analysis. Color legend: gray, no major phenotype detectable; black, preeclampsia; red, extrauterine, infection; orange, chorioamnionitis; yellow, mid-/late-pregnancy bleeding; light green, suspected FGR; dark green, perinatal sepsis; pink, fetal distress; light blue, severe maternal conditions; dark blue, congenital anomalies. (*B, upper panel*) Odds ratios (ORs) of risk of abnormal neurodevelopment in language domain according to PTB phenotypes using the term newborn population as a reference (OR = 1), in a specific population. (*lower panel*) ORs of risk of abnormal neurodevelopment in cognitive domain according to PTB phenotypes using the term newborn population as a reference (OR = 1), in a specific population. Please note that each circle with different color represents a different phenotype, and each circle size is proportional to the OR of each category in the population in analysis for the abnormal outcome in object (*upper panel*: language domain and lower panel: cognitive domain). Color legend: gray, no major phenotype detectable; black, preeclampsia; red, extrauterine, infection; orange, chorioamnionitis; yellow, mid-/late-pregnancy bleeding; light green, suspected FGR; dark green, perinatal sepsis; pink, fetal distress; light blue, severe maternal conditions; dark blue, congenital anomalies. (*Reproduced from* Frenquelli and colleagues[19] with data from Barros and colleagues[18])

Although GA alone is insufficient for defining PTB phenotypically, it remains a crucial summary marker for neonatal outcomes because it reflects organ immaturity, that is, increased risk of death, as well as short- and long-term complications.[22] In summary, PTB morbidity and mortality encompass both the consequences on the fetus of the underlying pathologic processes leading to PTB, plus the newborn organ-specific immaturity that relates to the timing of birth.[22]

It has been argued that a pragmatic definition (such as low birthweight) is more appropriate in many parts of the world where reliable means of estimating GA are not available.[23–25] However, accurate estimation of GA, in accordance with World Health Organization (WHO) recommendations, is essential.[26] Relying only on menstrual history is subject to recall bias; often not possible because of unavailable or poorly recorded information, and inaccurate if there has been menstrual irregularity because of normal variation, malnutrition, anemia, recent discontinuation of oral contraceptives, recent birth, miscarriage, or breastfeeding. Presently, ultrasound is the least biased and most practical method to determine GA at individual and population levels. GA should be recorded based on equations that consider early and late pregnancy antenatal care attendance.[27–29]

Unfortunately, all existing equations that rely on fetal anthropometric parameters can result in very wide confidence intervals and poor estimates in late pregnancy, in the presence of fetal growth restriction (FGR), or when the quality of ultrasound imaging is poor.[27,29–40] Recent machine-learning strategies to estimate GA based on repeat fetal measurements between 20 and 30 weeks' gestation have been shown to have a 3-day accuracy, improving GA estimation 3 to 5 times compared with previous methods.[28] Promising, deep-learning methods for GA estimation based on image characteristics alone, without the need for any fetal measurements, also open the door to widen use of deep-learning enabled ultrasound.[41]

Finally, the lower limit for defining PTB varies from 20 to 28 weeks' gestation, depending on the context. However, risk factors for births between 14 to 23 and 20 to 25 weeks' gestation are similar, suggesting shared mechanisms. There is also a strong case for redefining term birth as $\geq$39 weeks' gestation (instead of $\geq$37) as children born at 39 to 41 weeks' gestation have better respiratory, metabolic, and long-term outcomes, including cognitive development[42] compared with those born at "early term" (37–38 weeks' gestation). Therefore, the authors propose that PTB should be defined, both clinically and for research purposes, as birth between 16 and less than 39 weeks' gestation.[43,44]

Specific Issues for Classifying Preterm Births

Multiple pregnancy

Multiple pregnancy is strongly associated with PTB. In 2020–2021, twin births in the United States accounted for 18.4% and 22.5% of all PTBs at less than 37 and less than 34 weeks' of gestation, respectively.[45] Thus, multiple pregnancy, which presents specific challenges, should be treated as a distinct phenotype within the PTB syndrome with subcategories (eg, following infertility treatment, with or without embryo reduction). Reporting criteria for multiple pregnancy should include accurate assessment of the number of fetuses, chorionicity, amnionicity, and diagnosis of specific complications, such as twin-to-twin transfusion syndrome, twin anemia-polycythemia sequence, vanishing twin or co-twin fetal demise, intertwin birthweight differences, selective FGR, and structural anomalies.

Preterm prelabor rupture of membranes and cervical insufficiency with or without bleeding

When spontaneous labor does not follow preterm prelabor rupture of membranes (PPROM), induction of labor is recommended after a variable waiting period or if evidence of infection is documented. To standardize the approach in regard to timing of induction and individual operator decisions, all pregnancies affected by PPROM should be categorized and defined as PTB, irrespective of whether labor eventually occurs spontaneously or after induction.

Cervical insufficiency usually presents as spontaneous, painless dilatation of the cervix with or without bleeding in the second trimester, resulting in PTB. Determination of responsible underlying factors is often challenging. Similarly, bleeding can involve many factors, such as uterine contractions, cervical changes, placental abruption, and placenta previa. Every effort should be made to define the anatomic origin of the bleeding.

Fetal death and termination of pregnancy

Most studies exclude stillbirths from the estimation of PTB rates, but this practice should be reconsidered. Stillbirths constitute about 5% of PTBs and share causal factors, such as poor fetal growth and placental dysfunction.[46–48] Because stillbirth data may not be consistently recorded everywhere, the authors recommend including stillbirth in PTB assessment.[24] This approach also extends to late pregnancy terminations owing to fetal anomalies, which, depending on data documentation, may be categorized as stillbirths in the late second or third trimester. Therefore, a research recommendation is to include all births greater than 16 weeks' gestation as PTBs, including terminations, and incorporate a pregnancy termination phenotype at the level of any other PTB, avoiding confusion and discrepancies across different studies.[24]

The placenta and preterm birth

Prenatal ultrasound with gray-scale and Doppler studies of the uterine and umbilical circulation can provide valuable information about placental anatomy and function and fetal well-being. Altered maternal serum marker levels, such as pregnancy-associated plasma protein-A (PAPP-A), placental growth factor (PlGF), soluble fms-like tyrosine kinase-1 (sFlt-1), and their ratio are often associated with obstetric syndromes, such as preeclampsia.[49,50] Recent work has shown an association between increasing first-trimester risk of preterm preeclampsia (according to the Fetal Medicine Foundation screening method) and rates of spontaneous birth, at term or preterm, in women without preeclampsia, reinforcing the link between placental dysfunction and spontaneous labor.[51]

Globally, histopathologic examination of the placenta has been limited by the scarcity of specialized perinatal pathologists and late reporting of results. Nevertheless, with the appropriate training, quality control, and resources in place, macroscopic and microscopic histopathologies can provide retrospective, indirect evidence of placental function and disease during pregnancy. Hence, placental pathology, including inflammation, should be part of refining the phenotypic characterization of PTB after delivery. In particular, maternal vascular malperfusion and related placental lesions should be noted because of their association with FGR and stillbirth.[48] Recent work recommended a novel taxonomy of perinatal syndromes related to placental lesions of maternal vascular malperfusion, enhancing the connection between placental dysfunction (PlGF/sFlt-1 <20th centile) and preterm labor and producing hopes for prediction and prevention.[49]

Fetal abnormalities and preterm birth

Congenital and genetic abnormalities, and their fetal surgical interventions, are associated with PTB risk. Congenital anomalies can result in spontaneous or medically indicated PTB owing primarily to the effect of polyhydramnios complicating many congenital anomalies or secondarily to placental dysfunction that occurs with major congenital heart defects.[52] Open or percutaneous fetal surgery increases the risk of membrane rupture, preterm labor, bleeding, and medical indications for delivery.[53,54] Finally, confined placental mosaicism is associated with increased risk of small for gestational age and FGR, and possible provider-indicated PTB.[55]

Beyond Spontaneous and Medically Indicated Preterm Birth: An Etiologically Based Taxonomy

Distinguishing between spontaneous and medically indicated PTBs represents a conceptual problem for a PTB taxonomy. A medically initiated PTB by definition occurs when a clinical condition is judged to be severe and the likelihood of spontaneous delivery in the coming days is considered to be minimal. Obviously, these 2 conditions are very difficult to evaluate, document, and standardize.

Therefore, it is evident that a PTB taxonomy based on this dichotomy cannot satisfy the broad scope of a complex syndrome such as PTB. Confronted with this dilemma in both clinical practice and large epidemiologic studies, in which this classification is used,[16] 20 years ago the authors started a consultation process to create an etiologically based classification.

The first output of this process was a set of 3 reports presenting the issues and challenges to be considered in defining a classification system, followed by a prototype of an etiologically based classification.[29,32,56] Subsequently, the authors explored in a large multicountry, population-based study, the phenotypic structure of PTB using cluster analysis based on the conceptual framework presented above. The authors were able to identify a set of phenotypes with clear epidemiologic descriptions and related conditions.[27] More recently, to make a comprehensive phenotypic characterization of PTB, the authors incorporated neonatal morbidity, postnatal growth, and developmental patterns of identified PTB phenotypes up to 2 years of age.[26] A detailed description of the sample selection, variables definitions, statistical strategy, and limitations appears in the conceptual papers cited above.[29,32,56] In short, based on standardized information collected in multipopulation studies, the authors have assessed how known causal factors and their related complications classify PTBs. They identified 8 to 12 PTB phenotypes (depending on sample size and the statistical strategy for cluster identification and cluster number restrictions) that share the GA at birth definition. They represent distinct clinical entities with specific predominant causes, known clinically related complications, and both short- and long-term patterns of growth, morbidity, and neurodevelopment.

The authors tested these clusters based on etiologic conditions empirically in a medium- to high-risk population.[17] These phenotypes comprised infections, preeclampsia, fetal distress (defined as abnormal fetal heart rate pattern in labor or prelabor, indicating the need to expedite delivery), FGR, bleeding (early and late), and congenital anomalies with no observable common factor.

Understanding these phenotypes, their associated maternal risk factors, and their impact on neonatal and childhood health is crucial for interventions, prevention, and overall clinical management to be effective.[17,18,57,58] Nevertheless, 30% to 35% PTBs could not be associated with any main maternal, fetal, or placental conditions based on current clinical and routine laboratory criteria. Even in these cases, a preterm newborn faces a higher risk of growth and developmental issues in early childhood than a term newborn.[17] All this work supports the concept that PTB is a complex syndrome and that etiologically and postnatally based phenotypes can be characterized, far beyond clinical presentation, mode of early delivery and GA.

Deciding which characteristics should be included in the etiologically based phenotypic taxonomy of PTB is complicated by the need to differentiate between risk factors or markers and those etiologically related to PTB's phenotypic features. In addition, prenatal interventions for women at risk (or with symptoms) are expected to influence (at least in principle) the natural history of the PTB phenotype significantly.

Therefore, prospective adjustment of the taxonomy would be useful, considering the clinical evolution of each condition prenatally and postnatally. The phenotype should be assessed prenatally with the results of all investigations available (as part of medical care) and then reassessed postnatally to complete the description by incorporating all maternal, fetal, placental, and neonatal features.

The strength of the etiologically based PTB phenotype model lies in its comprehensiveness and adaptability to both (1) the epidemiologic transition, that is, different population risk profiles or geographic settings; and (2) new pathophysiological insights, that is, discovering the mechanisms underlying the etiologic conditions so as to refine the phenotypes by creating more homogeneous subgroups.

Reproducibility across various circumstances and populations demonstrates dynamic readaptation to different risk profiles and characteristics.[18,59] Local populations may exhibit variations in specific phenotypes influenced by referrals for specialist care, lower risk of the population characteristics, or legal considerations (for example, influencing the likelihood of multiple pregnancy after assisted conception, management of fetal anomalies, or early delivery for maternal request) (Appendix 1).

A practical example of the new taxonomy purpose is the infection with the SARS-CoV-2 virus and its principal variant, omicron, which emerged as a new cause during the COVID-19 pandemic. The INTERCOVID Consortium reported the effect of this extrauterine infection on the risk of PTB, as compared with noninfected pregnant women, with its distinct maternal, fetal, and neonatal outcomes.[59–63] This demonstrates how a new underlying cause, in the taxonomy extrauterine infection, can be secondarily associated with different phenotypes (effect modification) based on its clinical manifestations, such as severe pneumonitis causing maternal hypoxia, or placental damage leading to FGR or preeclampsia necessitating provider-initiated delivery.

Limitations

Like any classification model, the authors' proposed taxonomy has some limitations. First, it is difficult to implement it prospectively in pregnancy, owing to post hoc acquisition of several important components after birth, for example, placental histology, initiation of labor, and complications during and after birth. In this update of the conceptual background, the authors recommend overcoming this limitation by postnatal reassessment of the prenatal, prospective phenotyping as a form of retrospective review and refinement.

Second, the presence of phenotypic overlap between different coexisting categories may introduce an unwanted degree of subjectivity in the assessment and definition of the main component of the phenotype, that is, the leading causal factor (see **Fig. 1**). This complexity is not an intrinsic limitation rather an expression of the unique characteristics of PTB that are associated with (1) changes in the etiologic profiles according to GA; (2) a combination of pregnancy-related conditions, socioeconomic, lifestyle factors, the environment, and non-Mendelian genetics, that are not completely understood or quantified; and (3) the fact that after birth, a newborn has phenotypic characteristics that influence their immediate health, growth, and development, as well as longer-term clinical conditions.[19]

Standardized Prenatal Assessment of the Preterm Birth Phenotypes

Prenatal PTB phenotyping involves assessment of maternal characteristics as well as the fetus and placenta. Fetal assessment involves ultrasound for fetal biometry and morphology. Importantly, fetal size and other parameters should be compared with international standards,[34,36] which helps identify and compare deviations from optimal growth trajectories that could contribute to PTB phenotypes. The use of these international standards differentiates a normal intrauterine environment from one in which placental dysfunction is part of the clinical spectrum defining a PTB phenotype.

Prenatal assessment of placental function may start in the first trimester with measurement of hormones reflecting placental mass and function, such as PAPP-A and PIGF.[64,65] In the second and third trimesters, Doppler studies of uterine and umbilical arteries[66] and measurement of sFlt-1/PIGF[67] also contribute to placental functional assessment, particularly in the presence of coexisting FGR and/or a hypertensive disorder.[56,68,69] Clinical presentation of PTB onset within each phenotype should be considered.

Standardized Postnatal Assessment of the Preterm Birth Phenotypes

Understanding the skewed distribution of GAs in PTB is essential, as about 90% occur after 32 weeks' gestation. The remaining 10%, which constitute very early PTBs, represent a relatively small but high-risk group that requires, according to the etiologic phenotype, considerable intensive care. It is important to emphasize that, contrary to the belief that moderate and late preterm infants are low risk and require only routine care after discharge, substantial evidence shows they face significant risks (even those without a recognized phenotype) in relation to growth, morbidity, and development compared with term newborns.[70,71]

Prenatal corticosteroid use is a GA-specific intervention that has significantly improved survival for those born before 30 weeks' gestation.[25] A recent systematic review and meta-analysis showed that a single course of prenatal steroids was associated with a significantly lower risk of neurodevelopmental impairment in children born extremely preterm; however, in children born late-preterm or at term, who constituted approximately half those exposed to prenatal steroids, there was a significantly higher risk of adverse neurocognitive and/or psychological outcomes.[72] This is another example of the profound heterogeneity of PTB and the combined effect of GA and etiologic factors.

In the recent study of 6529 infants, of whom 1381 were born preterm, 8 PTB phenotypes were identified.[17] Certain phenotypes, such as FGR, bleeding, and congenital anomaly, were associated with delayed achievement of the WHO gross motor development milestone for walking alone. Using the INTERGROWTH-21st Neurodevelopment Assessment (INTER-NDA) tool to assess the preterm infants at 2 years of age,[21] those born with the congenital anomaly and fetal distress phenotypes had the highest risk of cognitive, fine- and gross-motor, and language development issues, whereas those with the preeclampsia phenotype had a high risk of cognitive and fine- and gross-motor development problems.[17] Those with the fetal distress and congenital anomaly phenotypes also had a significantly higher risk of scoring below the 10th centile in the fine-motor domain of the INTER-NDA. This showed clearly that PTB phenotypes affect the outcome, independently of GA (see **Fig. 1**).

The authors offer as an example the manual of operation in use by the INTERGROWTH-21st global network to gather core outcomes for specific PTB phenotypes with a standardized checklist for the prenatal and postnatal assessment items included in the standardized data collection forms (Appendix 2).

Actions and Clinical Implementation

Addressing and correctly classifying PTB requires considerable proactive measures. Governments, international organizations, and donors are urged to strengthen prenatal care by ensuring that a health care professional evaluates women early in pregnancy. The importance of initiating prenatal care early cannot be underestimated: this entails using ultrasound to confirm GA or estimate GA in the absence of reliable menstrual dates; conducting a comprehensive risk assessment, including early identification of PTB etiologic conditions; initiating preventive measures promptly; and scheduling a comprehensive ultrasound examination of fetal anatomy around 20 weeks' gestation.[73,74] These evidence-based guidelines offer a specific, adaptable program target based on the varying distribution of causal factors.[75–85] A good understanding of the distribution of population-specific PTB phenotypes is of great benefit for planning resource distribution and referral systems.

The Future

The proposed PTB taxonomy provides a foundation for future research, public health planning, and clinical understanding. PTB phenotypes need reconciliation with emerging risk factors, such as fetal surgical techniques, assisted reproduction, maternity with advanced maternal age, chronic morbidities or after reproductive surgery, and lessons from the COVID-19 pandemic among others. Empirical validation at scale offers benefits, including defining the frequency of each phenotype in specific populations and identifying more homogeneous PTB groups for referral systems and research studies.

For screening and effectiveness studies, stratification in primary and secondary intervention analysis, meta-analyses of mechanisms or randomized clinical trials, and subgroup level interventions based on etiologically based phenotypes, the impact on sample size estimation will be significant.

Understanding the full range of PTB taxonomy means that interventions can be targeted toward specific phenotypes and possible causes. For example, delivery should be expedited in some cases of threatened preterm labor (eg, because of infection or placental dysfunction), as prolonging exposure to a hostile intrauterine environment may worsen the outcome for the baby owing to the association of spontaneous PTB and fetal hypoxia.[86] Conversely, when the intrauterine environment is favorable (eg, threatened preterm labor or mechanical PPROM with no infection, hemorrhage, or significant inflammation), delivery may be postponed for as long as possible with available treatments, to maximize fetal maturation. In other words, the concept of prolonging GA per se (the original single-factor definition) should be challenged based on the system of phenotypic taxonomy presented here.

The authors suggest that if this line of epidemiologic and clinical reasoning is systematically implemented, the understanding of neonatal morbidity and mortality related to PTB would be improved. Consequently, predicting outcomes more accurately based on the phenotypes and their subgroups, particularly encompassing placental histology, should be achievable.[49] Future studies based on this phenotypic-based research strategy and clinical taxonomy should explore the extent and timing of varied interventions and clinical protocols as compared with GA-single parameter care.

DISCLOSURE

A.T. Papageorghiou is supported by the National Institute for Health and Care Research, United Kingdom (NIHR) Oxford Biomedical Research Centre (BRC) and is a Senior Scientific Advisor of Intelligent Ultrasound Ltd. All other authors declare they have no competing interests or other interests that might be perceived to influence the results and/or discussion reported in this paper.

Best Practices

What is the current practice for defining preterm birth?

- Current practice defines preterm birth as a condition based on gestational age alone (any delivery before a predefined threshold, eg, 37 weeks' gestation), which provides no insights into phenotype or cause. This definition makes preterm birth too heterogeneous a condition, which is a barrier to prediction, prevention, and treatment.

Best practice objective

- To provide a comprehensive taxonomy for preterm birth based on a sound conceptual framework, as well as high-quality experimental data showing generalizability potential of the model with postnatal trajectories of different phenotypes of preterm birth remaining present up to 2 years of age.

What changes in current practice are likely to improve outcomes?

- It is biologically plausible to hypothesize that wide implementation of the model for classifying preterm birth based on phenotypes/taxonomy, rather than gestational age alone, will lead to major improvements in maternal and neonatal outcomes. This will arise from research on more homogeneous study groups, leading to individualization of targeted screening and diagnostic methods as well as preventive strategies, monitoring, and treatment protocols.

Is there a clinical algorithm?

- The clinical algorithm includes a collection of clinical information with a predefined checklist and data collection form. The proposed taxonomy of preterm birth is based on 5 major domains (maternal, placental, and fetal/neonatal conditions; signs of parturition initiation; and path to delivery) that define 12 major phenotypes. Prospective prenatal assessment needs to be confirmed and refined, if necessary, postnatally to complete the phenotypic attribution of each specific case.

Pearls/pitfalls at the point-of-care

- Any case that pertains to more than one phenotype category should not be forced into a specific group. When all data are available, the major component from a qualitative or quantitative perspective will define the phenotype.

Major recommendations

- The use of gestational age or estimated fetal/neonatal size alone to define and classify preterm birth should be avoided. Gestational age and fetal/neonatal size are major moderators of preterm birth outcomes; however, they are insufficient to define the phenotype, assign a prognosis, plan surveillance protocols, or design prophylactic or therapeutic interventions. Clinical implementation of preterm birth phenotypes will lead to individualized preventive and treatment protocols, both prenatally and postnatally, with great potential to improve outcomes.

REFERENCES

1. Ohuma EO, Moller AB, Bradley E, et al. National, regional, and global estimates of preterm birth in 2020, with trends from 2010: a systematic analysis. Lancet 2023;402(10409):1261–71.
2. Englund-Ogge L, Brantsaeter AL, Sengpiel V, et al. Maternal dietary patterns and preterm delivery: results from large prospective cohort study. BMJ 2014;348: g1446.
3. Bloomfield FH. How is maternal nutrition related to preterm birth? Ann Rev Nutr 2011;31:235–61.

4. Cavoretto P, Candiani M, Giorgione V, et al. Risk of spontaneous preterm birth in singleton pregnancies conceived after IVF/ICSI treatment: meta-analysis of cohort studies. Ultrasound Obstet Gynecol 2018;51(1):43–53.

5. Cavoretto PI, Giorgione V, Sotiriadis A, et al. IVF/ICSI treatment and the risk of iatrogenic preterm birth in singleton pregnancies: systematic review and meta-analysis of cohort studies. J Matern Fetal Neonatal Med 2022;35(10):1987–96.

6. Cavoretto PI, Candiani M, Farina A. Fertility and mode of conception affect the risk of preterm birth related to both spontaneous and iatrogenic etiologies. Fertil Steril 2022;118(5):936–7.

7. Blondel B, Kogan MD, Alexander GR, et al. The impact of the increasing number of multiple births on the rates of preterm birth and low birthweight: an international study. Am J Pub Health 2002;92(8):1323–30.

8. Villar J, Papageorghiou AT, Pang R, et al. The likeness of fetal growth and newborn size across non-isolated populations in the INTERGROWTH-21st Project: the fetal growth longitudinal study and newborn cross-sectional study. Lancet Diabetes Endocrinol 2014;2(10):781–92.

9. Villar J, Cheikh Ismail L, Victora CG, et al. International standards for newborn weight, length, and head circumference by gestational age and sex: the Newborn Cross-Sectional Study of the INTERGROWTH-21st Project. Lancet 2014;384(9946):857–68.

10. Villar J, Giuliani F, Bhutta ZA, et al. Postnatal growth standards for preterm infants: the preterm postnatal follow-up study of the INTERGROWTH-21st project. Lancet Glob Health 2015;3(11):e681–91.

11. Villar J, Giuliani F, Fenton TR, et al. INTERGROWTH-21st very preterm size at birth reference charts. Lancet 2016;387(10021):844–5.

12. WHO. Manual of the international statistical classification of diseases, injuries, and causes of death: sixth revision of the International lists of diseases and causes of death. 1948.

13. Romero R, Espinoza J, Kusanovic JP, et al. The preterm parturition syndrome. BJOG 2006;113(Suppl 3):17–42.

14. Romero R, Mazor M, Munoz H, et al. The preterm labor syndrome. Ann NY Acad Sci 1994;734:414–29.

15. Romero R, Dey SK, Fisher SJ. Preterm labor: one syndrome, many causes. Science 2014;345(6198):760–5.

16. Villar J, Abalos E, Carroli G, et al. Heterogeneity of perinatal outcomes in the preterm delivery syndrome. Obstet Gynecol 2004;104(1):78–87.

17. Villar J, Restrepo-Mendez MC, McGready R, et al. Association between preterm-birth phenotypes and differential morbidity, growth, and neurodevelopment at age 2 years: results from the INTERBIO-21st Newborn Study. JAMA Pediatr 2021;175(5):483–93.

18. Barros FC, Papageorghiou AT, Victora CG, et al. The distribution of clinical phenotypes of preterm birth syndrome: implications for prevention. JAMA Pediatr 2015;169(3):220–9.

19. Frenquelli R, Ratcliff M, Villar de Onis J, et al. Complex perinatal syndromes affecting early human growth and development: issues to consider to understand their aetiology and postnatal effects. Front Neurosci 2022;16:856886.

20. Robinson O, Vrijheid M. The pregnancy exposome. Curr Environ Health Rep 2015;2(2):204–13.

21. Fernandes M, Villar J, Stein A, et al. INTERGROWTH-21st Project international INTER-NDA standards for child development at 2 years of age: an international prospective population-based study. BMJ Open 2020;10:e035258.

22. Villar J, Knight HE, de Onis M, et al. Conceptual issues related to the construction of prescriptive standards for the evaluation of postnatal growth of preterm infants. Arch Dis Child 2010;95(12):1034–8.

23. Kramer MS, Papageorghiou A, Culhane J, et al. Challenges in defining and classifying the preterm birth syndrome. Am J Obstet Gynecol 2012;206(2):108–12.

24. Goldenberg RL, Gravett MG, Iams J, et al. The preterm birth syndrome: issues to consider in creating a classification system. Am J Obstet Gynecol 2012;206(2):113–8.

25. Ashorn P, Ashorn U, Muthiani Y, et al. Small vulnerable newborns-big potential for impact. Lancet 2023;401(10389):1692–706.

26. WHO. WHO recommendations on antenatal care for a positive pregnancy experience. 2016.

27. Papageorghiou AT, Kemp B, Stones W, et al. Ultrasound-based gestational-age estimation in late pregnancy. Ultrasound Obstet Gynecol 2016;48(6):719–26.

28. Fung R, Villar J, Dashti A, et al. Achieving accurate estimates of fetal gestational age and personalised predictions of fetal growth based on data from an international prospective cohort study: a population-based machine learning study. Lancet Digit Health 2020;2(7):e368–75.

29. Cheikh Ismail L, Knight H, Ohuma E, et al. Anthropometric standardisation and quality control protocols for the construction of new, international, fetal and newborn growth standards: the INTERGROWTH-21st Project. BJOG 2013; 120(Suppl 2):48–55.

30. Sarris I, Ioannou C, Ohuma E, et al. Standardisation and quality control of ultrasound measurements taken in the INTERGROWTH-21st Project. BJOG 2013; 120(Suppl 2):33–7.

31. Papageorghiou A, Sarris I, Ioannou C, et al. Ultrasound methodology used to construct the fetal growth standards in the INTERGROWTH-21st Project. BJOG 2013;120(Suppl 2):27–32.

32. Ioannou C, Sarris I, Hoch L, et al. Standardisation of crown-rump length measurement. BJOG 2013;120(Suppl 2):38–41.

33. Papageorghiou AT, Kennedy SH, Salomon LJ, et al. International standards for early fetal size and pregnancy dating based on ultrasound measurement of crown-rump length in the first trimester of pregnancy. Ultrasound Obstet Gynecol 2014;44(6):641–8.

34. Papageorghiou AT, Ohuma EO, Altman DG, et al. International standards for fetal growth based on serial ultrasound measurements: the Fetal Growth Longitudinal Study of the INTERGROWTH-21st Project. Lancet 2014;384(9946):869–79.

35. Papageorghiou AT, Ohuma EO, Gravett MG, et al. International standards for symphysis-fundal height based on serial measurements from the Fetal Growth Longitudinal Study of the INTERGROWTH-21st Project: prospective cohort study in eight countries. BMJ 2016;355:i5662.

36. Stirnemann J, Villar J, Salomon LJ, et al. International estimated fetal weight standards of the INTERGROWTH-21st Project. Ultrasound Obstet Gynecol 2017; 49(4):478–86.

37. Cavallaro A, Ash ST, Napolitano R, et al. Quality control of ultrasound for fetal biometry: results from the INTERGROWTH-21st Project. Ultrasound Obstet Gynecol 2018;52(3):332–9.

38. Cheikh Ismail L, Knight H, Bhutta Z, et al. Anthropometric protocols for the construction of new international fetal and newborn growth standards: the INTERGROWTH-21st Project. BJOG 2013;120(Suppl 2):42–7.

39. Ohuma EO, Villar J, Feng Y, et al. Fetal growth velocity standards from the fetal growth longitudinal study of the INTERGROWTH-21st project. Am J Obstet Gynecol 2021;224(2):208 e1–e208 e18.

40. Napolitano R, Donadono V, Ohuma EO, et al. Scientific basis for standardization of fetal head measurements by ultrasound: a reproducibility study. Ultrasound Obstet Gynecol 2016;48(1):80–5.

41. Lee LH, Bradburn E, Craik R, et al. Machine learning for accurate estimation of fetal gestational age based on ultrasound images. NPJ Digit Med 2023;6(1):36.

42. Murray SR, Shenkin SD, McIntosh K, et al. Long term cognitive outcomes of early term (37-38 weeks) and late preterm (34-36 weeks) births: a systematic review. Wellcome Open Res 2017;2:101.

43. Donovan EF, Besl J, Paulson J, et al. Infant death among Ohio resident infants born at 32 to 41 weeks of gestation. Am J Obstet Gynecol 2010;203(1):58 e1–e5.

44. Yang S, Platt RW, Kramer MS. Variation in child cognitive ability by week of gestation among healthy term births. Am J Epidemiol 2010;171(4):399–406.

45. Conde-Agudelo A, Romero R, Rehal A, et al. Vaginal progesterone for preventing preterm birth and adverse perinatal outcomes in twin gestations: a systematic review and meta-analysis. Am J Obstet Gynecol 2023;229(6):599–616 e3.

46. Pedersen NG, Figueras F, Wojdemann KR, et al. Early fetal size and growth as predictors of adverse outcome. Obstet Gynecol 2008;112(4):765–71.

47. Zeitlin J, Ancel PY, Saurel-Cubizolles MJ, et al. The relationship between intrauterine growth restriction and preterm delivery: an empirical approach using data from a European case-control study. BJOG 2000;107(6):750–8.

48. Amodeo S, Cavoretto PI, Seidenari A, et al. Second trimester uterine arteries pulsatility index is a function of placental pathology and provides insights on stillbirth aetiology: a multicenter matched case-control study. Placenta 2022;121:7–13.

49. Romero R, Jung E, Chaiworapongsa T, et al. Toward a new taxonomy of obstetrical disease: improved performance of maternal blood biomarkers for the great obstetrical syndromes when classified according to placental pathology. Am J Obstet Gynecol 2022;227(4):615 e1–e615 e25.

50. Sovio U, Gaccioli F, Cook E, et al. Association between adverse pregnancy outcome and placental biomarkers in the first trimester: a prospective cohort study. BJOG 2023. https://doi.org/10.1111/1471-0528.17691.

51. Cavoretto P, Farina A, Salmeri N, et al. First trimester risk of preeclampsia and rate of spontaneous birth in patients without preeclampsia. Am J Obstet Gynecol 2024. https://doi.org/10.1016/j.ajog.2024.01.008.

52. Giorgione V, Fesslova V, Boveri S, et al. Adverse perinatal outcome and placental abnormalities in pregnancies with major fetal congenital heart defects: a retrospective case-control study. Prenat Diagn 2020;40(11):1390–7.

53. Johnson MP, Bennett KA, Rand L, et al. The Management of Myelomeningocele Study: obstetrical outcomes and risk factors for obstetrical complications following prenatal surgery. Am J Obstet Gynecol 2016;215(6):778 e1–e778 e9.

54. Sanz Cortes M, Chmait RH, Lapa DA, et al. Experience of 300 cases of prenatal fetoscopic open spina bifida repair: report of the International Fetoscopic Neural Tube Defect Repair Consortium. Am J Obstet Gynecol 2021;225(6):678 e1–e678 e11.

55. Spinillo SL, Farina A, Sotiriadis A, et al. Pregnancy outcome of confined placental mosaicism: meta-analysis of cohort studies. Am J Obstet Gynecol 2022;227(5):714–727 e1.

56. Chaiworapongsa T, Espinoza J, Gotsch F, et al. The maternal plasma soluble vascular endothelial growth factor receptor-1 concentration is elevated in SGA

and the magnitude of the increase relates to Doppler abnormalities in the maternal and fetal circulation. J Matern Fetal Neonatal Med 2008;21(1):25–40.

57. Kennedy S, Victora C, Craik R, et al. Deep clinical and biological phenotyping of the preterm birth and small for gestational age syndromes: the INTERBIO-21st Newborn Case-Control Study protocol. Gates Open Res 2019;2:49.

58. Villar J, Papageorghiou AT, Knight HE, et al. The preterm birth syndrome: a prototype phenotypic classification. Am J Obstet Gynecol 2012;206(2):119–23.

59. Villar J, Ariff S, Gunier RB, et al. Maternal and neonatal morbidity and mortality among pregnant women with and without COVID-19 infection: the INTERCOVID Multinational Cohort Study. JAMA Pediatr 2021;175(8):817–26.

60. Papageorghiou AT, Deruelle P, Gunier RB, et al. Preeclampsia and COVID-19: results from the INTERCOVID prospective longitudinal study. Am J Obstet Gynecol 2021;225(3):289 e1–e289 e17.

61. Eskenazi B, Rauch S, Iurlaro E, et al. Diabetes mellitus, maternal adiposity, and insulin-dependent gestational diabetes are associated with COVID-19 in pregnancy: the INTERCOVID study. Am J Obstet Gynecol 2022;227(1):74 e1–e74 e16.

62. Giuliani F, Oros D, Gunier RB, et al. Effects of prenatal exposure to maternal COVID-19 and perinatal care on neonatal outcome: results from the INTERCOVID Multinational Cohort Study. Am J Obstet Gynecol 2022;227(3):488 e1–e488 e17.

63. Villar J, Soto Conti CP, Gunier RB, et al. Pregnancy outcomes and vaccine effectiveness during the period of omicron as the variant of concern, INTERCOVID-2022: a multinational, observational study. Lancet 2023;401(10375):447–57.

64. Tan MY, Wright D, Syngelaki A, et al. Comparison of diagnostic accuracy of early screening for pre-eclampsia by NICE guidelines and a method combining maternal factors and biomarkers: results of SPREE. Ultrasound Obstet Gynecol 2018;51(6):743–50.

65. O'Gorman N, Wright D, Poon LC, et al. Multicenter screening for pre-eclampsia by maternal factors and biomarkers at 11-13 weeks' gestation: comparison with NICE guidelines and ACOG recommendations. Ultrasound Obstet Gynecol 2017;49(6):756–60.

66. Drukker L, Staines-Urias E, Villar J, et al. International gestational age-specific centiles for umbilical artery Doppler indices: a longitudinal prospective cohort study of the INTERGROWTH-21st Project. Am J Obstet Gynecol 2020;222(6):602 e1–e602 e15.

67. Chen W, Wei Q, Liang Q, et al. Diagnostic capacity of sFlt-1/PlGF ratio in fetal growth restriction: a systematic review and meta-analysis. Placenta 2022;127:37–42.

68. Erez O, Romero R, Espinoza J, et al. The change in concentrations of angiogenic and anti-angiogenic factors in maternal plasma between the first and second trimesters in risk assessment for the subsequent development of preeclampsia and small-for-gestational age. J Matern Fetal Neonatal Med 2008;21(5):279–87.

69. Romero R, Nien JK, Espinoza J, et al. A longitudinal study of angiogenic (placental growth factor) and anti-angiogenic (soluble endoglin and soluble vascular endothelial growth factor receptor-1) factors in normal pregnancy and patients destined to develop preeclampsia and deliver a small for gestational age neonate. J Matern Fetal Neonatal Med 2008;21(1):9–23.

70. Liotto N, Gianni ML, Taroni F, et al. Is fat mass accretion of late preterm infants associated with insulin resistance? Neonatology 2017;111(4):353–9.

71. Gianni ML, Roggero P, Piemontese P, et al. Is nutritional support needed in late preterm infants? BMC Pediatr 2015;15:194.

72. Ninan K, Liyanage SK, Murphy KE, et al. Evaluation of long-term outcomes associated with preterm exposure to antenatal corticosteroids: a systematic review and meta-analysis. JAMA Pediatr 2022;176(6):e220483.

73. Papageorghiou AT, Kennedy SH, Salomon LJ, et al. The INTERGROWTH-21st fetal growth standards: toward the global integration of pregnancy and pediatric care. Am J Obstet Gynecol 2018;218(2S):S630–40.

74. Drukker L, Staines-Urias E, Papageorghiou AT. The INTERGROWTH-21st Doppler centile charts: complementing tools for monitoring of growth and development from pregnancy to childhood. Am J Obstet Gynecol 2020;224(2):249–50.

75. Chatfield A, Caglia JM, Dhillon S, et al. Translating research into practice: the introduction of the INTERGROWTH-21st package of clinical standards, tools and guidelines into policies, programmes and services. BJOG 2013;120(Suppl 2):139–42.

76. Roseman F, Knight HE, Giuliani F, et al. Implementation of the INTERGROWTH-21st project in the UK. BJOG 2013;120(Suppl 2):117–22.

77. Purwar M, Kunnawar N, Deshmukh S, et al. Implementation of the INTER-GROWTH-21st project in India. BJOG 2013;120(Suppl 2):94–9.

78. Pan Y, Wu M, Wang J, et al. Implementation of the INTERGROWTH-21st project in China. BJOG 2013;120(Suppl 2):87–93.

79. Giuliani F, Bertino E, Oberto M, et al. Implementation of the INTERGROWTH-21st project in Italy. BJOG 2013;120(Suppl 2):100–4.

80. Carvalho M, Vinayak S, Ochieng R, et al. Implementation of the INTERGROWTH-21st project in Kenya. BJOG 2013;120(Suppl 2):105–10.

81. Silveira MF, Barros FC, Sclowitz IK, et al. Implementation of the INTERGROWTH-21st project in Brazil. BJOG 2013;120(Suppl 2):81–6.

82. Millar K, Patel S, Munson M, et al. INTERGROWTH-21st gestational dating and fetal and newborn growth standards in peri-urban Nairobi, Kenya: quasi-Experimental Implementation Study Protocol. JMIR Res Protoc 2018;7(6):e10293.

83. Jones RM, Vesel L, Kimenju G, et al. Implementation of the INTERGROWTH-21st gestational dating and fetal and newborn growth standards in Nairobi, Kenya: women's experiences with ultrasound and newborn assessment. Glob Health Action 2020;13(1):1770967.

84. Jaffer YA, Al Abri J, Abdawani J, et al. Implementation of the INTERGROWTH-21st project in Oman. BJOG 2013;120(Suppl 2):111–6.

85. Dighe MK, Frederick IO, Andersen HF, et al. Implementation of the INTER-GROWTH-21st project in the United States. BJOG 2013;120(Suppl 2):123–8.

86. Romero R, Soto E, Berry SM, et al. Blood pH and gases in fetuses in preterm labor with and without systemic inflammatory response syndrome. J Matern Fetal Neonatal Med 2012;25(7):1160–70.

APPENDIX 1: PROPORTION OF PRETERM BIRTHS CORRESPONDING TO THE ETIOLOGICALLY BASED PHENOTYPES IN 2 MULTICOUNTRY POPULATIONS (2015–2021). THE VARIABILITY IN THE DISTRIBUTION OF PTB PHENOTYPES ACROSS POPULATIONS REFLECTS THE EFFECT OF THE RISK PROFILE OF THE UNDERLYING POPULATIONS.

Phenotype	Proportional Contribution of a Phenotype to the Total PTB	Most Frequent Associated Conditions
None[a,b]	30.0–35.1	None
Preeclampsia[a,b]	11.8	Perinatal sepsis, late bleeding, extrauterine infection, suspected FGR
Multiple births[a]	10.4	Extrauterine infection, suspected FGR
Extrauterine infection[a,b]	7.7	Mid-pregnancy bleeding, chorioamnionitis, severe maternal conditions
Chorioamnionitis[b]	7.6	Multiple births, perinatal sepsis, suspected FGR
Any infection[b]	20.9	Chorioamnionitis, extrauterine infection, perinatal sepsis
Early vaginal bleeding[a]	4.8	Multiple births, extrauterine infection, mid-/late-pregnancy bleeding
Mid-late vaginal bleeding[a]	6.2	Chorioamnionitis, perinatal sepsis, multiple births
Any bleeding[b]	5.1	Severe maternal condition, perinatal sepsis, chorioamnionitis, extrauterine infection
Suspected FGR[a,b]	5.5–8.0	Severe maternal condition, preeclampsia, perinatal sepsis, extrauterine infection, mid-/late-pregnancy bleeding
Congenital anomaly[a,b]	3.5–5.5	Perinatal sepsis, chorioamnionitis, extrauterine infection, suspected FGR, early bleeding
Antepartum stillbirth[a]	3.7	Severe maternal condition, extrauterine infection, mid-/late-pregnancy bleeding
Fetal distress[a,b]	3.4–9.5	Preeclampsia, extrauterine infection, suspected FGR, severe maternal condition, perinatal sepsis, mid-/late-pregnancy bleeding
Severe maternal conditions[a,b]	3.1–6.2	Multiple births, early bleeding, extrauterine infection, mid-/late-pregnancy bleeding, suspected FGR

Abbreviation: FGR, fetal growth restriction.

[a] From Barros et al., 2015.[18] Population from Brazil, Italy, Oman, England, United States, China, India, and Kenya. The 27 participating institutions (41% tertiary, 52% secondary, and 7% primary care) covered more than 80% of all deliveries in each urban area.

[b] From Villar et al., 2021.[17] Population from Brazil, Kenya, Pakistan, South Africa, Thailand, and the United Kingdom. Twins were excluded due to low sample size. Stillbirths were excluded, as the study incorporated postnatal follow-up.

APPENDIX 2: STANDARD DATA COLLECTION FORM FOR RESEARCH AND CLINICAL USE. ANY LIVEBIRTH OR STILLBIRTH, SINGLETON OR MULTIPLE, INCLUDING TERMINATIONS AND CONGENITAL MALFORMATIONS, FROM 16 + 0 TO 38 + 6 WEEKS GESTATION, MAY BE INCLUDED IN THIS ASSESSMENT. THE CLINICAL RECORD SHOULD BE THE PRIMARY SOURCE OF INFORMATION TO CAPTURE INTRAPARTUM AND POSTPARTUM DATA, AND THE RELEVANT OBSTETRIC AND MEDICAL HISTORY. THIS SHOULD BE SUPPLEMENTED BY QUESTIONING THE MOTHER AND OBSTETRICIAN IF THE PTB HAS BEEN SCHEDULED AND THE REASON FOR DELIVERY IS NOT CLEAR. FINALLY, PLACENTAL HISTOLOGY AND, FOR STILLBIRTHS, AN AUTOPSY OR PATHOLOGY REPORT ARE OPTIMAL REQUIREMENTS. RISK FACTORS AND MODE OF DELIVERY ARE NOT INCLUDED. ALL PRENATAL FEATURES SHOULD BE PRESENT BEFORE INITIATION OF DELIVERY.

(1) Substantial Maternal Conditions

Phenotype Category	Clinical Features and Diagnostic Investigations	
	Prenatal	*Postnatal*
Extrauterine infection	Pyrexia due to viremia, bacteremia, malaria, pyelonephritis, sexually transmitted disease (including syphilis and HIV), abscess, inflammatory indices (leukocyte count, CRP)	Persisting pyrexia or sepsis, cultures with etiologic definition of microbes involved, detailed imaging, inflammatory indices (leukocyte count, CRP)
Clinical chorioamnionitis	Pyrexia, ROM plus 2 of the following: maternal tachycardia, uterine tenderness, purulent amniotic fluid, fetal tachycardia, inflammatory indices (leukocyte count, CRP)	Persistent pyrexia or sepsis, inflammatory indices (leukocyte count, CRP)
Preeclampsia/eclampsia	Gestational hypertension with either proteinuria (300 mg/24 h or 20 mg/dL) or with organ dysfunction (doubling transaminase, increasing creatinine, angiogenic factors imbalance, or increased uterine artery pulsatility index), HELLP syndrome	Evolution including extent of organ damage and treatment
Maternal trauma	Severe or critical injury, wound or shock diagnosed by inspection, ultrasound, X-ray, and imaging	Procedures required to treat the trauma and outcome
Worsening maternal disease	Uncontrolled diabetes mellitus (increased HbA$_{1c}$ and capillary glucose, ketosis), endocrine disease (dysthyroidism), cardiac insufficiency (reduced ejection fraction at cardiac US), respiratory insufficiency (reduced oxygen saturation; eg, COVID-19), liver disease (increased enzymes and bile acids), renal disease (increased serum creatinine), progression of cancer, epilepsy, coagulopathy, or life-threatening hemodynamic instability with immediate risk to mother/fetus	Course of the disease, treatment modification
Uterine rupture	Bleeding and abnormal contractility due to uterine wall defect developing in pregnancy, fetal bradycardia, hypovolemic shock	Conservative vs demolitive surgical approach, DIC, hemorrhage, placenta accreta spectrum

(2) Substantial fetal or neonatal conditions

Phenotype Category	Clinical Features and Diagnostic Investigations	
	Fetal	Neonatal
Intrauterine fetal death	US fetal biometry, detection of fetal abnormalities, definition of onset: before labor vs intrapartum	Macroscopic assessment and postmortem pathologic report
FGR	EFW < 10th centile with Doppler evidence of abnormally increased umbilical or uterine pulsatility index; EFW or AC drop of 40 centiles on trajectory, EFW < 3rd centile	Birth weight, length, head circumference, postnatal course
Abnormal FHR/abnormal biophysical profile	CTG with pathologic pattern (FIGO 2015) or antepartum persistently reduced short-term variability or decelerations, ultrasound with BPP≤6	APGAR scores, neonatal blood gas analysis with pH and base excess, evidence of birth asphyxia
Fetal infection/fetal inflammatory response syndrome	CTG: fetal tachycardia, amniocentesis: increased amniotic IL-6, reduced glucose concentration	Neonatal sepsis or inflammatory indices (leukocyte count, CRP), any organ damage
Fetal anomaly	Any minor or major fetal defect	Any minor or major neonatal defect
Multiple pregnancy	Two or more fetuses, chorionicity, amnionicity, and specific features such as TTTS, TOPS, TAPS, selective FGR, and death of one fetus	Chorionicity assessment, presence of anastomoses

Phenotype Category	Prenatal	Postnatal
Fetal anemia	MCA Doppler peak systolic velocity (Hb reduced by 2 SD or MCA PSV increased by 1.5 SD). Alloimmune (Rhesus disease or antibodies), fetal hemorrhage (vasa previa), fetomaternal hemorrhage; CTG abnormality with sinusoidal pattern, positive Kleihauer-Betke test	Hemoglobin levels and differences, extent of hemotransfusions, signs of hypoxia, evidence of vasa previa
Polyhydramnios/Oligohydramnios	Deepest pool >8 cm (95th centile)/<2 cm (5th centile)	Associated defects (GE obstructions, renal failure, and so forth)

(3) Placental pathologic conditions related to PTB

Clinical Features and Diagnostic Investigations

Phenotype Category	Prenatal	Postnatal
Chorioamnionitis	Maternal fever, inflammatory indices (leukocyte count, CRP), fetal tachycardia, offensive vaginal discharge, US evidence of abnormal placental structure, thickness, and edema	Histology showing vasculitis (infiltration of neutrophils into the connective tissue of the chorionic plate), infarction, necrosis. villitis, funisitis, thrombosis
Placental abruption	US evidence of retroplacental or amniochorial clot, vaginal bleeding, maternal abdominal pain, hypovolemic shock	Retroplacental blood clot at delivery, parenchymal hemorrhage at histology, coagulopathy
Placenta previa	Placental location on US, myometrial invasion assessment, US structure, asymptomatic or vaginal bleeding	Postpartum hemorrhage, association to placenta accreta spectrum and amniotic fluid embolism
Placental dysfunction	US showing small placental volume, increased pulsatility index at uterine arteries, and/or umbilical artery	Small placental weight, placental infarctions, fibrosis, and necrosis

(continued on next page)

(continued)

	Doppler, low PAPP-A and PlGF, increased sFlt-1/PlGF ratio
Other placental abnormalities	US evidence of placental chorioangioma, jelly-like placenta (excess of placental lakes or lacunae), circumvallate placenta, vasa previa	Pathology with placental anomalies, evidence of amniotic, placental infection due to local or systemic process (eg, malaria); culture for bacteria
(4) Signs of parturition initiation		
Phenotype category		*Clinical features (existing before onset of delivery)*
No evidence of initiation of parturition		—
Evidence of initiation of parturition		Cervical shortening, PPROM, uterine tenderness, regular uterine contractions, cervical effacement or dilation, bleeding from uterus or cervix, unknown factor of initiation

(5) Pathway to delivery

Clinical features and diagnostic investigations

Phenotype category	Prenatal	Postnatal
Provider-initiated (iatrogenic):	Clinically mandatory (eg, severe preeclampsia), clinically optional or discretionary (eg, severe intrahepatic cholestasis), pregnancy termination (maternal request or fetal anomaly), social reasons or no discernible reason	APGAR scores, birth weight (define appropriateness indications and timing of interventions based on fetal weight estimation)
Spontaneous	Labor with intact membranes, PPROM, regular uterine contractions, pharmacologic augmentation with oxytocin	Course of labor (define appropriateness of interventions in labor)

Abbreviations: AC, abdominal circumference; IL-6, interleukin-6; CRP, serum C-reactive protein concentration; CTG, cardiotocography; DIC, disseminated intravascular coagulation; EFW, estimated fetal weight; FIGO, International Federation of Gynecology and Obstetrics; GE, gastroenteric; Hb, hemoglobin; HbA$_{1c}$, maternal serum glycosylated hemoglobin concentration; HELLP, hemolysis, elevated liver enzymes, low platelets; MCA, middle cerebral artery; pH, potential of hydrogen, defined as concentration of hydrogen ions; PSV, peak systolic velocity; ROM, rupture of membranes; TAPS, twin anemia polycythemia sequence; TOPS, twin oligohydramnios-polyhydramnios sequence; TTTS, twin-to-twin transfusion syndrome; US, ultrasound imaging; X-ray, conventional diagnostic radiograms.

Preventing Preterm Birth
Exploring Innovative Solutions

Tiffany Habelrih, BS[a,b], Béatrice Ferri, BS[a,b], France Côté, BS[a,b],
Juliane Sévigny[c], Thalyssa-Lyn Augustin[a,b], Kevin Sawaya[b,d],
William D. Lubell, PhD[e], David M. Olson, PhD, DSc[f],
Sylvie Girard, PhD[g], Sylvain Chemtob, MD, PhD[a,b],*

KEYWORDS

- Preterm birth • Therapeutics • Tocolytics • Inflammation • Pathophysiology
- Preterm labor • Neonatal outcome

KEY POINTS

- The pathogenesis of preterm labor is initiated and upregulated by inflammation.
- The prophylactic interventions preventing preterm labor are ineffective and involve antibiotics, progesterone analogs, mechanical approaches, nonsteroidal anti-inflammatory drugs, and nutritional supplementation.
- Tocolytic agents target preterm labor but do not prevent preterm birth as they do not tackle uteroplacental inflammation.
- Emerging therapies specifically target inflammation and show promise to effectively prevent preterm birth and neonatal tissue injury.

INTRODUCTION

Preterm birth (PTB) affects over 15 million births every year and is the primary cause of perinatal mortality and morbidity.[1] Premature survivors are subject to developing

[a] Université de Montréal, Pavillion Roger-Gaudry, 2900 boul Edouard-Montpetit, H3T 1J4, Montréal, Québec, Canada; [b] Centre de recherche du CHU Sainte-Justine, 3175 ch de la Côte-Sainte-Catherine, H3T 1C5, Montréal, Québec, Canada; [c] Département de Biologie, Université de Sherbrooke, Voie 9, J1X 2X9, Sherbrooke, Québec, Canada; [d] Department of Microbiology and Immunology, McGill University, 3775 Rue University, Room 511, H3A 2B4, Montréal, Québec, Canada; [e] Département de Chimie, Université de Montréal, Complexe des Sciences, 1375 avenue Thérèse-Lavoie-Roux, Montréal, Québec, H2V 0B3, Canada; [f] Departments of Obstetrics and Gynecology, Pediatrics, and Physiology, University of Alberta, 220 HMRC, T6G 2S2, Edmonton, Alberta, Canada; [g] Department of Obstetrics and Gynecology, Department of Immunology, Mayo Clinic, 200 First Street SW, Guggenheim Building 3rd floor, Rochester, MN 55905, USA

* Corresponding author. Centre de Recherche du CHU Sainte-Justine, 3175 ch de la Côte-Sainte-Catherine, H3T1C5, Montreal, Quebec, Canada.
E-mail address: sylvain.chemtob@umontreal.ca

Clin Perinatol 51 (2024) 497–510
https://doi.org/10.1016/j.clp.2024.02.006
0095-5108/24/© 2024 Elsevier Inc. All rights reserved.

grave short- and long-term complications affecting their neurologic, gastrointestinal, and respiratory systems due to the immaturity of their organs and to the exposure to a hostile intrauterine milieu.[2] The annual societal cost of PTB was determined to surpass \$26 billion in the United States as complications caused by PTB require neonatal intensive care as well as medical interventions.[3,4] Spontaneous preterm labor (PTL) occurs before 37 weeks of gestation and is ultimately triggered by an aberrant inflammatory response during pregnancy, leading to the activation of uteroplacental complex and subsequent premature expulsion of the fetus.[5,6] Actual interventions preventing and/or targeting the onset of labor have been shown to have a limited efficacy in prolonging gestation and preventing neonatal morbidity.[4] This review summarizes the effects of available clinical interventions on the prevention of PTB and presents promising emerging solutions.

RISK FACTORS FOR PRETERM BIRTH

Although the etiologies of PTB remain unknown, they are associated with numerous risk factors. Intrauterine infection accounts for 25% to 40% of PTBs.[2,7] The presence of pathogens and related noninfectious by-products in the placenta and the fetal space induce a fetal inflammatory response, leading to the release of cytokines.[8] Moreover, chronic inflammatory placental lesions (eg, villitis, chorioamnionitis, and deciduitis) involving the infiltration of maternal T cells to the placenta can disrupt fetomaternal tolerance.[9] Premature decidual senescence is linked to increased levels of cyclooxygenase-2 (COX-2) and prostaglandin (PG) F synthase, which are involved in myometrial contractility.[10] Abnormal placentation is associated with vascular resistance in the placental bed and reduced blood flow to the intervillous space,[11] which also participates in inflammation. Other known risk factors for PTB include genetic predispositions, cervical insufficiency, resistance to progesterone (P4), oxidative stress, preeclampsia, multiparous pregnancies, maternal history of PTB, increased maternal age, extreme maternal body mass index, smoking, stress, and low socioeconomic status among others.[10,12]

PATHOGENESIS OF PRETERM BIRTH: A PROMINENT ROLE OF INFLAMMATION

Parturition commences several days before fetal expulsion and is mediated by gradual changes occurring in gestational tissues as the quiescent uterus transitions toward a proinflammatory state. The phases of parturition are shared by term and PTL, which are both proinflammatory processes regardless of the presence of infection or other causative factors.

During gestation, P4, prostacyclin, relaxin, and other mediators inactivate the myometrium and promote uterine quiescence, allowing for physiologic intrauterine fetal development.[13] These mediators maintain a noncontractile uterus by increasing intracellular levels of cyclic nucleotides that decrease intracellular calcium (Ca^{2+}) concentrations, inhibiting the enzymatic activity of myosin light-chain kinase (MLCK) that is essential for uterine contractions.[14] P4 also downregulates the gene expression of uterine activating proteins (UAPs) such as COX-2, connexin-43, oxytocin receptor (OXTR) as well as proinflammatory mediators.[15,16] As gestation progresses, uterine stretch associated with fetal growth induces the production of UAPs that aids the uterus to transition to an active state.[5] The maturation of the fetal hypothalamic–pituitary–adrenal axis induces a decrease in P4 activity to favor the prolabor actions of estrogen. Estrogen promotes the production of OXTR and PG synthases, which synthesize PGs associated with myometrial stimulation such as prostaglandin E_2 (PGE_2) and prostaglandin F_2-α (PGF_2-α).[17] Cytokines, especially interleukin (IL)-1β, are significant contributors to the induction of UAPs and other inflammatory mediators as well as activating immune cells in gestational tissues. Smooth muscle contraction is induced when PGE_2 and PGF_2-α bind to their respective receptors EP_1, EP_3, and prostaglandin F2α (FP) and oxytocin binding to OXTR.[17] These receptors activate phospholipase C, leading to protein kinase C and inositol 1,4,5-triphosphate (IP_3) production and consequent increase of intracellular Ca^{2+} concentrations in the myometrium. Ca^{2+} forms a complex with calmodulin to activate MLCK that phosphorylates myosin to induce formation of a cross latch-bridge with actin to trigger smooth muscle contraction.[18] Other than signaling via Gαq, PGF_2-α elicits myometrial contraction through the $G_{\alpha 12}$-dependent Rho/Rho-associated protein kinase (Rho/ROCK) signaling pathway.[19] PGE_2 and PGF_2-α also possess proinflammatory actions and contribute to the production of inflammatory mediators and other UAPs such as matrix metalloproteinases (MMPs), which participate in cervical ripening by degrading the extracellular matrix of tissues to weaken and favor rupture of membranes, and ultimately triggering fetal expulsion.[13]

In pathologic conditions leading to PTL, the innate immune system is activated by pathogen-associated molecular patterns (PAMPs) in the context of infection and/or damage-associated molecular patterns (DAMPs).[5] DAMPs and PAMPs activate toll-like receptors (TLRs) that stimulate the production of proinflammatory mediators.[20] These receptors, more specifically TLR-2 and TLR-4, are highly expressed on gestational tissues and respond readily to mount an inflammatory response.[21] Functioning as proinflammatory agents, TLRs recruit and activate immune cell participation in the positive feed forward loop to parturition by secreting cytokines, MMPs, and chemokines. Inflammation is sufficient to initiate the parturition pathway, regardless of fetal maturation, thus leading to PTL and premature fetal expulsion.[5] Moreover, the infiltration of proinflammatory cytokines into the fetal space induces an immune reaction that leads to tissue injury to the immature fetus.[22] This damage predisposes a fragile infant to develop a plethora of lifelong complications involving the lungs, vascular system, brain, and/or retina.[23] A schematic diagram of mechanisms implicated in PTB is presented in **Fig. 1**.

CURRENT CLINICAL INTERVENTIONS TO PREVENT PRETERM BIRTH
Preventing Preterm Labor

Antibiotics
Infections participate in decidual activation through the stimulation of TLRs that generate an inflammatory response.[24] Antibiotic prophylaxis was proposed to contain infections to prevent PTL. Antibiotics reduced the occurrence of maternal infections, but did not significantly decrease the risk of PTB, perinatal mortality, or adverse neonatal outcomes in comparison with placebo.[24,25] Hence, although necessary for certain forms of chorioamnionitis and prevention of group B Streptococcus, antibiotics are ineffective in preventing PTB.

Progesterone analogs
Parturition is characterized by the withdrawal of circulating P4 that promotes myometrial quiescence to inhibit uterine activity.[26] The use of P4 analogs as a prophylaxis for PTL has been examined and shown to have only a few adverse maternal and neonatal outcomes.[27] For example, 17-hydroxyprogesterone caproate (administered intramuscular) was approved by the US Food and Drug Administration (FDA) in 2011 (accelerated phase 2 approval) but withdrawn after failing the Prevent Recurrent Preterm Birth in Singleton Gestations phase 3 clinical trial. No significant differences were observed with respect to the reduction in the rate of PTB, neonatal death, or

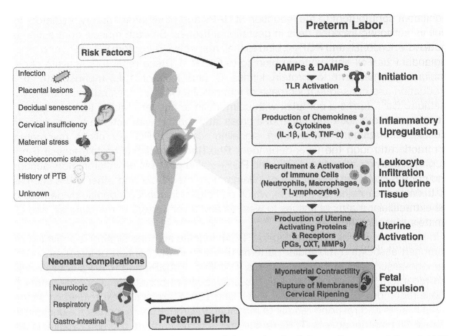

Fig. 1. Risk factors associated to the onset of the pathophysiology of preterm labor. DAMP, damage-associated molecular pattern; IL, interleukin; PAMP, pathogen-associated molecular pattern; PTB, preterm birth; TNF, tumor necrosis factor. (Created with BioRender.com.)

morbidity compared with placebo.[28] The efficacy of vaginal P4 and analogs to prevent PTB and improve neonatal outcomes remains inconsistent.[29]

Mechanical approaches
Women with a short cervix are at a higher risk for spontaneous PTB.[30] Mechanical approaches such as cervical cerclage and pessary both have been used to support the cervix to prevent PTB albeit without noteworthy improvements in rates, perinatal death, or fetomaternal outcomes.[25,30] Furthermore, cerclage has been associated with pregnancy and surgical complications.[31]

Nonsteroidal anti-inflammatory drugs: Aspirin
Nonsteroidal anti-inflammatory drugs (NSAIDs) inhibit COX-1 and COX-2, which are involved in PG synthesis.[32] Anti-inflammatory properties are believed to serve in the mechanism of NSAID action to prevent PTB.[33] Low-dose aspirin (<100 mg) reduces inflammation, trophoblast apoptosis, and oxidative stress.[34] Although a favorable safety profile was observed without significant differences from placebo in terms of mode of delivery and adverse neonatal and maternal outcomes, low-dose aspirin does not significantly reduce the rate of PTB.[35,36]

Nutritional supplementation
Nutritional supplementation including omega-3 fatty acids and vitamin D is used during pregnancy. The anti-inflammatory properties of omega-3 may decrease inflammation and myometrial activity. However, the efficacy of omega-3 intake during pregnancy has been inconsistent without significantly reducing the risk of PTB, perinatal death, or fetal complications.[25,37]

Vitamin supplements have been hypothesized to improve fetomaternal outcomes due in part to widespread deficiency of cholecalciferols (vitamin D) during pregnancy; however, no consistent evidence has revealed that vitamin supplementation during pregnancy can prevent either PTB or adverse maternal and neonatal outcomes.[38,39] Accordingly, nutritional vitamin D supplementation is ineffective to prevent PTL.

Interfering with Preterm Labor

Tocolytic agents are regularly administered to limit uterine activity and contractility. Yet, these drugs generally delay delivery for only a couple of days and are ineffective on short- and long-term neonatal outcomes. It is also troubling to point out that approximately 75% of the drugs used in obstetrics are off-label, as pharmaceutical companies have most often never established efficacy or safety in the context of PTL. Moreover, most tocolytics, except for OXTR antagonists, were developed for other medical indications and coincidentally discovered to have tocolytic properties.[40] An overview of mechanisms involved in myometrial contractions is presented in **Fig. 2**.

Magnesium sulfate

Although incompletely understood, the mechanism of action of magnesium sulfate is thought to implicate reduction of the influx of Ca^{2+} in smooth muscle cells to limit contractility. However, the administration of magnesium sulfate neither prevents PTB nor neonatal complications compared with placebo.[41] Given its reported benefit for fetal neurologic protection, magnesium sulfate is typically administered under close monitoring for treating adverse effects of pregnancy, including lethargy, weakness, flushing, or changes in heart rate. Of note, elevated doses of magnesium sulfate have been linked to increased risks of fetal and neonatal mortality.[42]

β2-adrenergic agonists/betamimetics

β2-adrenergic receptor agonists or betamimetics such as ritodrine, terbutaline, and salbutamol, confer actions by activating β2-adrenergic receptors on uterine smooth muscle cells. The activation of these receptors results in an increase in intracellular

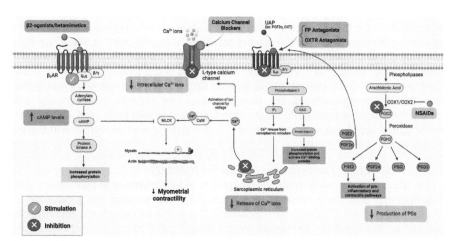

Fig. 2. Mechanism of action of tocolytic agents in inhibiting myometrial contractility. CaM, calmodulin; cAMP, cyclic adenosine monophosphate; COX, cyclooxygenase; DAG, diacylglycerol; FP, prostaglandin F2α receptor; IP3, inositol trisphosphate; MLCK, myosin light-chain kinase; PG, prostaglandin; OXT, oxytocin; OXTR, oxytocin receptor; UAP, uterine activating protein. (Created with BioRender.com.)

cyclic adenosine monophosphate levels that inactivate MLCK,[43] thus interfering with smooth muscle contraction. Betamimetic therapy allows, at best, a delay of 48 hours before parturition. Betamimetics can however induce adverse effects by acting on β2-adrenergic receptors in other organs, such as the lungs and blood vessels. A reduction in placental blood flow, increased heart rate, tremors, and pulmonary edema are common adverse effects associated with betamimetic tocolytics. Moreover, betamimetics can cross the placental barrier and can affect the fetus.[43]

Calcium channel blockers

Nicardipine and nifedipine are classified as calcium channel blockers and are the most frequently administrated tocolytics to prevent PTL. By interacting with voltage-gated Ca^{2+} channels, they inhibit Ca^{2+} influx into smooth muscle cells, thereby limiting interactions between Ca^{2+} and calmodulin and thus preventing uterine contractility.[44] Ca^{2+} channel blockers can delay preterm delivery for up to 5 to 7 days but are ineffective in preventing neonatal complications.[45] Although not officially approved by the FDA as a tocolytic agent, nifedipine is considered the tocolytic of choice due to affordability and safety profile. Nonetheless, Ca^{2+} channel blockers can cause cardiovascular complications, such as nausea, anxiety, and vomiting.[44]

Nonsteroidal anti-inflammatory drugs: Indomethacin and ibuprofen

As described, NSAIDs, such as indomethacin and ibuprofen, can inhibit PG synthesis by blocking the activity of COX-1 and COX-2, thereby limiting uterine contractility and cervical ripening during labor.[46] Although NSAIDs have initially displayed efficacy in prolonging parturition, comprehensive studies reveal that they are ineffective in preventing PTB when compared with placebo and other tocolytics.[47] Moreover, NSAIDs exert maternal side effects, which include gastrointestinal irritation, reduced renal blood flow, and hypertension. In addition, important fetal adverse effects have been associated with NSAIDs including oligohydramnios, premature constriction of the ductus arteriosus, necrotizing enterocolitis, and intraventricular hemorrhage.[48] Despite these concerns, NSAIDs are often used off-label to delay PTB.

Oxytocin receptor antagonists

Antagonists of the OXTR, such as atosiban, interfere with the prolabor actions of the peptide hormone oxytocin, which is a critical player in uterine contractility. The antagonism of OXTR prevents oxytocin from inducing an increase in intracellular Ca^{2+} levels, thereby limiting Ca^{2+}/calmodulin interactions and preventing uterine contractility.[49] Atosiban has been shown to delay PTB simply for a couple of days with limited fetomaternal adverse effects, but atosiban does not improve fetal/neonatal outcomes.[50] Maternal adverse effects are infrequent and limited to nausea, headaches, vomiting, and hypotension among others.[50,51] Atosiban is approved for use in Europe but not in the United States.

Prostaglandin receptor antagonists: Ebopiprant (OBE022)

During labor, PGF_2-α binds to the FP receptor to induce myometrial contractility, cervical ripening, and the rupture of membranes by upregulating the production of MMPs.[52] Ebopiprant (OBE022) reversibly antagonizes the FP receptor to limit myometrial contractility. Currently, in Phase II clinical trials,[53] OBE022 has been shown in preclinical studies to be most effective in decreasing myometrial contractility when combined with nifedipine or atosiban, but OBE022 did not prevent PTB.[53] Although no significant adverse effects were detected during the Phase I trials,[54] OBE022 may generate some side effects comparable to NSAIDs by perturbing PG function.[53] However, its safety profile on fetal/maternal health remains incomplete. Nonetheless, it should be noted that selective targeting of FP receptors may be beneficial in preventing PTB. Correspondingly, a separate drug candidate PDC31[55] has been found in a Phase 1b trial to safely reduce intrauterine pressure in healthy women treated for primary dysmenorrhea featuring PG-dependent excessive uterine contractility, leading to severe pain during menstruation.[56]

EMERGING INTERVENTIONS

A paucity of effective therapies exists in targeting PTL. As pointed out above current interventions, notably tocolytics, target the uterus by attempting to limit its activation and contractility. Tocolytics transiently delay parturition and preterm delivery, but do not act on the inflammation that triggers the uterine activation process and is involved in fetal tissue injury. It is imperative to target inflammation which is at the root of the pathophysiological cascade leading to PTB. An Accelerated Innovations for Mother (AIM) database analysis reports a number of compounds tested in single preclinical studies to exert potential efficacy in prolonging gestation.[57] The scarcity in rigorous reproducible documentation for drug candidates aimed at PTB highlights the fact that the development of safe therapies to effectively delay PTB and target the pathologic inflammation hindering fetal development remains a major unmet medical need. We hereby present the most promising drug candidates displaying reproducible results for preventing PTB.

Targeting Toll-like Receptors: Naloxone, a Toll-like Receptor-4 antagonist

Critical for activation of the immune system, TLRs are widely expressed on gestational tissues and immune cells. During labor, TLR-4 mediates the inflammatory response. The premature activation of TLR-4 may result in the induction of the PTL cascade. Recognizing DAMPs and PAMPs, TLR-4 acts as a central point of convergence in the activation of the PTL pathways.[58] (+)-Naloxone binds specifically to TLR-4, has anti-inflammatory properties, and does not interfere with opioid receptors.[59] Although studies regarding the effects of TLR-4 antagonists on neonatal development remain to be conducted, (+)-naloxone was shown to suppress the activation of the nuclear factor kappa B (NF-κB) signaling pathway, inhibit the production of proinflammatory mediators, and prevent PTB and fetal mortality.[59,60]

Targeting Chemokines: Broad-spectrum Chemokine Inhibitors

Chemokines play a key role in parturition by mediating the peripheral infiltration of leukocytes into uterine tissue, contributing to the fetomaternal inflammatory process. Broad-spectrum chemokine inhibitors (BSCIs) inhibit the action of multiple chemokines signaling pathways allegedly by specifically binding the cell-surface somatostatin receptor type 2 (SSTR2).[61] BSCIs act as partial agonists of SSTR2 and suppress chemokine signaling without affecting the classical receptor pathways.[16] Although the impact of BSCIs on neonates remains to be investigated, administration of the BSCI BN83470 in mice prevented PTB, blocked leukocyte infiltration, and mitigated inflammation.[62] In addition, the BSCI FX125 L was also found to inhibit the production of inflammatory cytokines and the onset of PTL in a nonhuman primate model induced by group B Streptococcus[63]; but lung injury to the fetus was not prevented by BSCIs.

Targeting Interleukin Receptors: Advantage of Allosteric Peptides

Orthosteric antagonists that target the native ligand binding site of IL receptors have proven efficient in suppressing inflammation.[64] For the prevention of PTB, hesitancy to administer such orthosteric antagonists, which are typically protein biologics, stems from their (1) increased half-life which is undesirable during pregnancy; (2) immunosuppressive actions that hinder fetomaternal immune vigilance; (3) large size; and (4) immunogenicity.[23] Specific inhibition of signaling pathways integral to the pathophysiology of PTL is desired to avoid drawbacks associated with the administration of orthosteric antagonists to pregnant women. Allosteric receptor modulation by ligands that bind to sites remote from the orthosteric binding site offers potential to modulate specific signaling pathways to achieve pharmacologic selectivity.[65] In this context, small peptide allosteric modulators offer attractive opportunity for prevention of PTB and associated neonatal complications.

Targeting the interleukin-1 receptor

IL-1 considerably amplifies the inflammatory response during PTL.[66] In humans and in animals, elevated levels of this cytokine have been quantified in the context of PTL. Sufficient to drive the PTL cascade alone, administration of IL-1 in pregnant animals results in preterm delivery.[23] Antagonism of the proinflammatory actions of the IL-1 system has acquired considerable interest to mitigate the induction and upregulation of the pathophysiology of PTL and to abate fetal tissue injury.

Kineret (Anakinra), canakinumab (Ilaris), and rilonacept (Arcalyst) are competitive inhibitors of the IL-1 system and intrinsically antagonize all signaling pathways associated to IL-1R. Neither of these biologics has been approved for use during pregnancy. Kineret, canakinumab, and rilonacept have been used to control chronic inflammatory diseases in pregnant women and were not linked to further undesirable obstetric or perinatal outcomes.[67] In preclinical studies, Kineret dampened the inflammatory response in models of PTL, but did not significantly prevent PTB or neonatal tissue injury.[66,68–70] Nonetheless, caution is warranted when administering these agents because total inhibition of the IL-1 system may predispose the fetus and the mother to opportunistic infections by blocking the immune response.

Rytvela is a small allosteric peptide that inhibits IL-1R. The peptide sequence (r-y-t-v-e-l-a) was derived from the extracellular domain of the IL-1R accessory protein and designed to bias IL-1R-associated signaling pathways. Rytvela was found to inhibit the activation of C-Jun N-terminal kinase/stress-activated protein kinase and p38 mitogen-activated protein kinase as well as the transcription factor c-jun and Rho/ROCK pathways.[66] Rytvela preserved the activation of the NF-kB pathway that is crucial to immune vigilance and cytoprotection. Preclinical studies reveal the efficacy of rytvela to inhibit fetomaternal inflammation and prevent PTB and neonatal tissue injury in numerous models of PTL.[66,69,71,72] By inhibiting specific IL-1R pathways, rytvela (and analogs[73]) represents a relevant and promising approach for preventing PTB and neonatal complications.

Targeting the interleukin-6 receptor

IL-6 is a proinflammatory cytokine that modulates immune cells such as regulatory T cells (Tregs) and helper T cells 17 (Th17).[74] IL-6 induces the transformation of cluster of differentiation 4 (CD4)$^+$ cells into proinflammatory Th17 cells while inhibiting the anti-inflammatory activity of Tregs, leading to an imbalance in the Th17/Treg ratio.[75] Contributing to the inflammatory state, IL-6 may affect pregnancy-related pathologies such as PTB. Women with higher levels of IL-6 were predisposed to delivering prematurely.[76–79] Moreover, IL-6 induces the expression of the gene for OXTR, which contributes to uterine contractility.[80]

Several IL-6R inhibitors exist. The antibody drug tocilizumab is the most frequently administered IL-6R inhibitor for the treatment of autoimmune diseases. Exhibiting orthosteric properties, tocilizumab, and related anti-IL-6R antibodies fully abrogate IL-6R signaling,[81] including pathways mediated by extracellular-regulated kinase and protein kinase B (or Akt), which play important roles in cell proliferation and survival.[82] Considering that inhibition of the latter signaling pathways is undesirable during pregnancy, allosteric ligands such as the peptide HSJ633 were conceived as anti-IL-6R agents. HSJ633 was shown to selectively inhibit the pathway implicating the signal transducer and activator of transcription 3 (STAT3), a transcription factor that predominantly activates proinflammatory genes.[83,84]

SUMMARY

PTB remains a multifactorial complication of pregnancy that represents the leading cause of neonatal mortality and morbidity. Although studies have unanimously demonstrated the indispensable role of inflammation in the PTL cascade leading to PTB, currently utilized prophylactic interventions and tocolytics do not tackle inflammation. An urgent need exists to develop safe and effective therapeutic agents that target inflammation to limit the initiation and the progression of the PTL cascade and improve neonatal outcomes. Causes of PTB remain to be fully elucidated; yet inflammation is clearly a major contributor. The scarcity of therapeutics to treat PTB stems in part from the lack of accurate and validated predictive models of PTB. The development of effective and safe therapeutics is also hindered by the reticence of governmental and pharmaceutical institutions to invest in fetomaternal research. A collaboration between researchers, clinicians, advocates, and regulatory institutions is necessary to bring to clinic therapeutic candidates that effectively prevent PTB and improve short- and long-term neonatal outcomes.

ACKNOWLEDGMENTS

T Habelrih is a Vanier scholar. F Côté and B Ferri are recipients of CIHR bursaries. S Chemtob holds a Canada Research Chair in vision science and the Leopoldine Wolfe Chair in translational research in vision health.

DISCLOSURE

S. Chemtob and W.D. Lubell hold a patent on composition of matter for the use of 101.10/rytvela (IL-1 receptor antagonists, compositions, and methods of treatment, United States patent no. USPTO8618054, May 5, 2005). S Chemtob, WD Lubell, DM Olson, and S Girard hold a patent on methods for reducing perinatal morbidity and/or mortality (US20210322509, March 9, 2016).

Best Practices

What is the current practice for preventing preterm birth?

- The prophylactic interventions preventing PTL involve antibiotics, P4 analogs, mechanical approaches, NSAIDs, and nutritional supplementation.
- Current tocolytic agents target PTL and consist of magnesium sulfate, betamimetics/β2-adrenergic receptor agonists, Ca^{2+} channel blockers, OXTRs, and NSAIDs.

What changes in current practice are likely to improve outcomes?

- The development of emerging therapies that specifically target inflammation shows promise to effectively prevent PTB and neonatal tissue injury.

Major recommendations

- A collaboration between researchers, clinicians, advocates, and regulatory institutions is necessary to bring to clinic promising therapeutic candidates that target inflammation to effectively prevent PTB and enhance neonatal outcomes.

Bibliographic sources

Coler BS, Shynlova O, Boros-Rausch A, et al. Landscape of preterm birth therapeutics and a path forward. J Clin Med 2021;10(13):2912.

Care A, Nevitt SJ, Medley N, et al. Interventions to prevent spontaneous preterm birth in women with singleton pregnancy who are at high risk: systematic review and network meta-analysis. BMJ 2022;376:e064547.

REFERENCES

1. Blencowe H, Cousens S, Chou D, et al. Born too soon: the global epidemiology of 15 million preterm births. Reprod Health 2013;10(Suppl 1):S2.
2. Goldenberg RL, Culhane JF, Iams JD, et al. Epidemiology and causes of preterm birth. Lancet 2008;371(9606):75–84.
3. Frey HA, Klebanoff MA. The epidemiology, etiology, and costs of preterm birth. Semin Fetal Neonatal Med 2016;21(2):68–73.
4. Miller FA, Sacco A, David AL, et al. Interventions for infection and inflammation-induced preterm birth: a preclinical systematic review. Reprod Sci 2022;30(2): 361–79.
5. Leimert KB, Xu W, Princ MM, et al. Inflammatory amplification: a central tenet of uterine transition for labor. Front Cell Infect Microbiol 2021;11:660983.
6. Prairie E, Cote F, Tsakpinoglou M, et al. The determinant role of IL-6 in the establishment of inflammation leading to spontaneous preterm birth. Cytokine Growth Factor Rev 2021;59:118–30.
7. Romero R, Dey SK, Fisher SJ. Preterm labor: one syndrome, many causes. Science 2014;345(6198):760–5.
8. Romero R, Gotsch F, Pineles B, et al. Inflammation in pregnancy: its roles in reproductive physiology, obstetrical complications, and fetal injury. Nutr Rev 2007; 65(12 Pt 2):S194–202.
9. Kim CJ, Romero R, Chaemsaithong P, et al. Chronic inflammation of the placenta: definition, classification, pathogenesis, and clinical significance. Am J Obstet Gynecol 2015;213(4 Suppl):S53–69, d.
10. Cha J, Bartos A, Egashira M, et al. Combinatory approaches prevent preterm birth profoundly exacerbated by gene-environment interactions. J Clin Invest 2013;123(9):4063–75.
11. Kim YM, Bujold E, Chaiworapongsa T, et al. Failure of physiologic transformation of the spiral arteries in patients with preterm labor and intact membranes. Am J Obstet Gynecol 2003;189(4):1063–9.
12. Phillips C, Velji Z, Hanly C, et al. Risk of recurrent spontaneous preterm birth: a systematic review and meta-analysis. BMJ Open 2017;7(6):e015402.
13. Institute of Medicine (US) Committee on Understanding Premature Birth and Assuring Healthy Outcomes. The national academies collection: reports funded by national institutes of health. In: Behrman RE, Butler AS, editors. Preterm birth: causes, consequences, and prevention. Washington, DC: National Academies Press (US) National Academy of Sciences; 2007. p. 169–76.

14. Challis JRG. Mechanism of parturition and preterm labor. Obstet Gynecol Surv 2000;55(10):650–60.
15. Soloff MS, Jeng YJ, Izban MG, et al. Effects of progesterone treatment on expression of genes involved in uterine quiescence. Reprod Sci 2011;18(8):781–97.
16. Coler BS, Shynlova O, Boros-Rausch A, et al. Landscape of preterm birth therapeutics and a path forward. J Clin Med 2021;10(13):2912.
17. Li WJ, Lu JW, Zhang CY, et al. PGE2 vs PGF2alpha in human parturition. Placenta 2021;104:208–19.
18. Ilicic M, Zakar T, Paul JW. The regulation of uterine function during parturition: an update and recent advances. Reprod Sci 2020;27(1):3–28.
19. Goupil E, Tassy D, Bourguet C, et al. A novel biased allosteric compound inhibitor of parturition selectively impedes the prostaglandin F2alpha-mediated Rho/ROCK signaling pathway. J Biol Chem 2010;285(33):25624–36.
20. Cook JL, Zaragoza DB, Sung DH, et al. Expression of myometrial activation and stimulation genes in a mouse model of preterm labor: myometrial activation, stimulation, and preterm labor. Endocrinology 2000;141(5):1718–28.
21. Youssef RE, Ledingham MA, Bollapragada SS, et al. The role of toll-like receptors (TLR-2 and -4) and triggering receptor expressed on myeloid cells 1 (TREM-1) in human term and preterm labor. Reprod Sci 2009;16(9):843–56.
22. Novak CM, Ozen M, Burd I. Perinatal brain injury: mechanisms, prevention, and outcomes. Clin Perinatol 2018;45(2):357–75.
23. Nadeau-Vallee M, Obari D, Quiniou C, et al. A critical role of interleukin-1 in preterm labor. Cytokine Growth Factor Rev 2016;28:37–51.
24. Flenady V, Hawley G, Stock OM, et al. Prophylactic antibiotics for inhibiting preterm labour with intact membranes. Cochrane Database Syst Rev 2013;12:CD000246.
25. Care A, Nevitt SJ, Medley N, et al. Interventions to prevent spontaneous preterm birth in women with singleton pregnancy who are at high risk: systematic review and network meta-analysis. BMJ 2022;376:e064547.
26. Mesiano S, Chan EC, Fitter JT, et al. Progesterone withdrawal and estrogen activation in human parturition are coordinated by progesterone receptor A expression in the myometrium. J Clin Endocrinol Metab 2002;87(6):2924–30.
27. Norman JE, Marlow N, Messow CM, et al. Vaginal progesterone prophylaxis for preterm birth – author's reply. Lancet 2016;388(10050):1160.
28. Blackwell SC, Gyamfi-Bannerman C, Biggio JR Jr, et al. 17-OHPC to prevent recurrent preterm birth in singleton gestations (PROLONG study): a multicenter, international, randomized double-blind trial. Am J Perinatol 2020;37(2):127–36.
29. Romero R, Conde-Agudelo A, Da Fonseca E, et al. Vaginal progesterone for preventing preterm birth and adverse perinatal outcomes in singleton gestations with a short cervix: a meta-analysis of individual patient data. Am J Obstet Gynecol 2018;218(2):161–80.
30. Conde-Agudelo A, Romero R, Nicolaides KH. Cervical pessary to prevent preterm birth in asymptomatic high-risk women: a systematic review and meta-analysis. Am J Obstet Gynecol 2020;223(1):42–65 e2.
31. Conde-Agudelo A, Romero R, Da Fonseca E, et al. Vaginal progesterone is as effective as cervical cerclage to prevent preterm birth in women with a singleton gestation, previous spontaneous preterm birth, and a short cervix: updated indirect comparison meta-analysis. Am J Obstet Gynecol 2018;219(1):10–25.
32. Antonucci R, Zaffanello M, Puxeddu E, et al. Use of non-steroidal anti-inflammatory drugs in pregnancy: impact on the fetus and newborn. Curr Drug Metab 2012;13(4):474–90.

33. Habli M, Clifford CC, Brady TM, et al. Antenatal exposure to nonsteroidal anti-inflammatory drugs and risk of neonatal hypertension. J Clin Hypertens 2018; 20(9):1334–41.

34. Turner JM, Robertson NT, Hartel G, et al. Impact of low-dose aspirin on adverse perinatal outcome: meta-analysis and meta-regression. Ultrasound Obstet Gynecol 2020;55(2):157–69.

35. Landman A, Don EE, Vissers G, et al. The risk of preterm birth in women with uterine fibroids: a systematic review and meta-analysis. PLoS One 2022;17(6): e0269478.

36. Allshouse AA, Jessel RH, Heyborne KD. The impact of low-dose aspirin on preterm birth: secondary analysis of a randomized controlled trial. J Perinatol 2016; 36(6):427–31.

37. Serra R, Penailillo R, Monteiro LJ, et al. Supplementation of omega 3 during pregnancy and the risk of preterm birth: a systematic review and meta-analysis. Nutrients 2021;13(5):1704.

38. Liu Y, Ding C, Xu R, et al. Effects of vitamin D supplementation during pregnancy on offspring health at birth: a meta-analysis of randomized controlled trails. Clin Nutr 2022;41(7):1532–40.

39. Bialy L, Fenton T, Shulhan-Kilroy J, et al. Vitamin D supplementation to improve pregnancy and perinatal outcomes: an overview of 42 systematic reviews. BMJ Open 2020;10(1):e032626.

40. Lamont RF, Jorgensen JS. Safety and efficacy of tocolytics for the treatment of spontaneous preterm labour. Curr Pharmaceut Des 2019;25(5):577–92.

41. Mercer BM, Merlino AA, Society for Maternal-Fetal Medicine. Magnesium sulfate for preterm labor and preterm birth. Obstet Gynecol 2009;114(3):650–68.

42. Mittendorf R, Covert R, Boman J, et al. Is tocolytic magnesium sulphate associated with increased total paediatric mortality? Lancet 1997;350(9090):1517–8.

43. Neilson JP, West HM, Dowswell T. Betamimetics for inhibiting preterm labour. Cochrane Database Syst Rev 2014;(2):CD004352.

44. Gaspar R, Hajagos-Toth J. Calcium channel blockers as tocolytics: principles of their actions, adverse effects and therapeutic combinations. Pharmaceuticals 2013;6(6):689–99.

45. Flenady V, Wojcieszek AM, Papatsonis DN, et al. Calcium channel blockers for inhibiting preterm labour and birth. Cochrane Database Syst Rev 2014;2014(6): CD002255.

46. Mitchell JA, Akarasereenont P, Thiemermann C, et al. Selectivity of nonsteroidal antiinflammatory drugs as inhibitors of constitutive and inducible cyclooxygenase. Proc Natl Acad Sci USA 1993;90(24):11693–7.

47. Reinebrant HE, Pileggi-Castro C, Romero CL, et al. Cyclo-oxygenase (COX) inhibitors for treating preterm labour. Cochrane Database Syst Rev 2015;2015(6): CD001992.

48. Norton ME, Merrill J, Cooper BA, et al. Neonatal complications after the administration of indomethacin for preterm labor. N Engl J Med 1993;329(22):1602–7.

49. Kim SH, Riaposova L, Ahmed H, et al. Oxytocin receptor antagonists, atosiban and nolasiban, inhibit prostaglandin f(2alpha)-induced contractions and inflammatory responses in human myometrium. Sci Rep 2019;9(1):5792.

50. Flenady V, Reinebrant HE, Liley HG, et al. Oxytocin receptor antagonists for inhibiting preterm labour. Cochrane Database Syst Rev 2014;6:CD004452.

51. Moutquin JM, Sherman D, Cohen H, et al. Double-blind, randomized, controlled trial of atosiban and ritodrine in the treatment of preterm labor: a multicenter effectiveness and safety study. Am J Obstet Gynecol 2000;182(5):1191–9.

52. Yoshida M, Sagawa N, Itoh H, et al. Prostaglandin F(2alpha), cytokines and cyclic mechanical stretch augment matrix metalloproteinase-1 secretion from cultured human uterine cervical fibroblast cells. Mol Hum Reprod 2002;8(7):681–7.

53. Pohl O, Chollet A, Kim SH, et al. OBE022, an oral and selective prostaglandin f(2)(alpha) receptor antagonist as an effective and safe modality for the treatment of preterm labor. J Pharmacol Exp Therapeut 2018;366(2):349–64.

54. Pohl O, Marchand L, Gotteland JP, et al. Coadministration of the prostaglandin F2alpha receptor antagonist preterm labour drug candidate OBE022 with magnesium sulfate, atosiban, nifedipine and betamethasone. Br J Clin Pharmacol 2019;85(7):1516–27.

55. Bourguet CB, Claing A, Laporte SA, et al. Synthesis of azabicycloalkanone amino acid and azapeptide mimics and their application as modulators of the prostaglandin F2α receptor for delaying preterm birth. Can J Chem 2014;92(11): 1031–40.

56. Bottcher B, Laterza RM, Wildt L, et al. A first-in-human study of PDC31 (prostaglandin F2alpha receptor inhibitor) in primary dysmenorrhea. Hum Reprod 2014;29(11):2465–73.

57. McDougall ARA, Hastie R, Goldstein M, et al. New medicines for spontaneous preterm birth prevention and preterm labour management: landscape analysis of the medicine development pipeline. BMC Pregnancy Childbirth 2023; 23(1):525.

58. Robertson SA, Hutchinson MR, Rice KC, et al. Targeting Toll-like receptor-4 to tackle preterm birth and fetal inflammatory injury. Clin Transl Immunol 2020; 9(4):e1121.

59. Hutchinson MR, Zhang Y, Brown K, et al. Non-stereoselective reversal of neuropathic pain by naloxone and naltrexone: involvement of toll-like receptor 4 (TLR4). Eur J Neurosci 2008;28(1):20–9.

60. Chin PY, Dorian CL, Hutchinson MR, et al. Novel Toll-like receptor-4 antagonist (+)-naloxone protects mice from inflammation-induced preterm birth. Sci Rep 2016;6:36112.

61. Fox DJ, Reckless J, Lingard H, et al. Highly potent, orally available anti-inflammatory broad-spectrum chemokine inhibitors. J Med Chem 2009;52(11): 3591–5.

62. Shynlova O, Dorogin A, Li Y, et al. Inhibition of infection-mediated preterm birth by administration of broad spectrum chemokine inhibitor in mice. J Cell Mol Med 2014;18(9):1816–29.

63. Coleman M, Orvis A, Wu TY, et al. A broad spectrum chemokine inhibitor prevents preterm labor but not microbial invasion of the amniotic cavity or neonatal morbidity in a non-human primate model. Front Immunol 2020;11:770.

64. Hernandez-Santana YE, Giannoudaki E, Leon G, et al. Current perspectives on the interleukin-1 family as targets for inflammatory disease. Eur J Immunol 2019;49(9):1306–20.

65. Wenthur CJ, Gentry PR, Mathews TP, et al. Drugs for allosteric sites on receptors. Annu Rev Pharmacol Toxicol 2014;54:165–84.

66. Nadeau-Vallee M, Quiniou C, Palacios J, et al. Novel noncompetitive IL-1 receptor-biased ligand prevents infection- and inflammation-induced preterm birth. J Immunol 2015;195(7):3402–15.

67. Brien ME, Gaudreault V, Hughes K, et al. A Systematic review of the safety of blocking the IL-1 system in human pregnancy. J Clin Med 2021;11(1):225.

68. Presicce P, Park CW, Senthamaraikannan P, et al. IL-1 signaling mediates intrauterine inflammation and chorio-decidua neutrophil recruitment and activation. JCI Insight 2018;3(6):e98306.

69. Nadeau-Vallee M, Chin PY, Belarbi L, et al. Antenatal suppression of IL-1 protects against inflammation-induced fetal injury and improves neonatal and developmental outcomes in mice. J Immunol 2017;198(5):2047–62.

70. Kallapur SG, Nitsos I, Moss TJ, et al. IL-1 mediates pulmonary and systemic inflammatory responses to chorioamnionitis induced by lipopolysaccharide. Am J Respir Crit Care Med 2009;179(10):955–61.

71. Habelrih T, Tremblay DE, Di Battista E, et al. Pharmacodynamic characterization of rytvela, a novel allosteric anti-inflammatory therapeutic, to prevent preterm birth and improve fetal and neonatal outcomes. Am J Obstet Gynecol 2023; 228(4):467 e1–e467 e16.

72. Takahashi Y, Takahashi T, Usuda H, et al. Pharmacological blockade of the interleukin-1 receptor suppressed Escherichia coli lipopolysaccharide-induced neuroinflammation in preterm fetal sheep. Am J Obstet Gynecol MFM 2023; 5(11):101124.

73. Geranurimi A, Cheng CWH, Quiniou C, et al. Probing anti-inflammatory properties independent of nf-kappab through conformational constraint of peptide-based interleukin-1 receptor biased ligands. Front Chem 2019;7:23.

74. Bettelli E, Carrier Y, Gao W, et al. Reciprocal developmental pathways for the generation of pathogenic effector TH17 and regulatory T cells. Nature 2006; 441(7090):235–8.

75. Kimura A, Kishimoto T. IL-6: regulator of Treg/Th17 balance. Eur J Immunol 2010; 40(7):1830–5.

76. Hee L. Likelihood ratios for the prediction of preterm delivery with biomarkers. Acta Obstet Gynecol Scand 2011;90(11):1189–99.

77. Romero R, Yoon BH, Kenney JS, et al. Amniotic fluid interleukin-6 determinations are of diagnostic and prognostic value in preterm labor. Am J Reprod Immunol 1993;30(2–3):167–83.

78. Romero R, Avila C, Santhanam U, et al. Amniotic fluid interleukin 6 in preterm labor. Association with infection. J Clin Invest 1990;85(5):1392–400.

79. Silver RM, Schwinzer B, McGregor JA. Interleukin-6 levels in amniotic fluid in normal and abnormal pregnancies: preeclampsia, small-for-gestational-age fetus, and premature labor. Am J Obstet Gynecol 1993;169(5):1101–5.

80. Fang X, Wong S, Mitchell BF. Effects of LPS and IL-6 on oxytocin receptor in non-pregnant and pregnant rat uterus. Am J Reprod Immunol 2000;44(2):65–72.

81. Sebba A. Tocilizumab: the first interleukin-6-receptor inhibitor. Am J Health Syst Pharm 2008;65(15):1413–8.

82. Tanaka T, Narazaki M, Kishimoto T. IL-6 in inflammation, immunity, and disease. Cold Spring Harbor Perspect Biol 2014;6(10):a016295.

83. Mihara M, Hashizume M, Yoshida H, et al. IL-6/IL-6 receptor system and its role in physiological and pathological conditions. Clin Sci 2012;122(4):143–59.

84. Kishimoto T, Kang S. IL-6 Revisited: from rheumatoid arthritis to CART cell therapy and COVID-19. Annu Rev Immunol 2022;40:323–48.

Ethics of Predicting and Preventing Preterm Birth

Wylie Burke, MD, PhD[a,*], Susan Brown Trinidad, MA, PhD[a], Erika Blacksher, PhD[b]

KEYWORDS

- Preterm birth • Ethics • Justice • Social determinants

KEY POINTS

- The disproportionate burden of preterm birth (PTB) among socially disadvantaged women is a concern for justice.
- Theories of disease that incorporate social disadvantage provide a basis for transdisciplinary research aimed at preventing PTB.
- Interventions to prevent PTB must address the social context in which PTB occurs.
- The experience and knowledge of women from groups experiencing high rates of PTB can inform PTB research and the development of effective interventions.
- Research that clarifies the impact of social context on PTB rates can inform policies and programs aimed at reducing PTB.

INTRODUCTION

Spontaneous preterm birth (PTB) is an important and complex problem, leading to higher rates of infant mortality and adverse health outcomes, including disabilities and chronic illness. Caring for a preterm infant can be disruptive, emotionally draining, and expensive for families; prematurity has substantial short-term and long-term costs for society as a whole. As this special issue demonstrates, much productive research is under way, aimed at clarifying risk factors and defining the physiology of normal and preterm labor. This research has demonstrated that PTB involves multiple physiologic functions and likely occurs through multiple biological pathways.[1–4] While many questions remain, innovative approaches offer the potential to develop needed interventions, including predictive tests to identify early labor and new pharmaceutical agents to prevent or delay PTB.[1,3,5–7]

[a] Department of Bioethics and Humanities, University of Washington, Box 357120, Seattle WA 98195, USA; [b] Center for Practical Bioethics, 1111 Main Street, Suite 500, Kansas City, MO 64105-2116, USA
* Corresponding author. Department of Bioethics and Humanities, University of Washington, Box 357120, Seattle WA 98195.
E-mail address: wburke@uw.edu

Clin Perinatol 51 (2024) 511–519
https://doi.org/10.1016/j.clp.2024.02.007   perinatology.theclinics.com

Yet PTB is not only a societal and scientific challenge but also a moral challenge. Globally, rates of PTB range from 4% to 16%, with the highest rates occurring in countries with widespread poverty and limited health care infrastructures.[8] Developed countries fare better, but a troubling social gradient is evident. For example, in Europe, PTB rates range from 5% to 10%, but rates are up to 2 times higher among disadvantaged groups.[9–12] The overall rate of PTB in the United States (10.49%) is among the highest seen in any developed country,[8,13] and PTB rates are substantially higher among Black and Indigenous women and women of all races who live and work in poverty.[14,15] The disproportionate burden of PTB among socially disadvantaged women is a concern for justice.

BACKGROUND: THE ETHICS OF PRETERM BIRTH INEQUALITIES

The association of PTB with social disadvantage reflects a persistent and predictable pattern that applies to many health outcomes: the more disadvantaged people are, the more likely they are to experience poor health and premature death. The case of PTB is particularly salient morally because it affects individuals across the life course and because early disadvantage all too often begets disadvantage in the next generation.

Arguments vary widely as to why health generally and some health inequalities in particular are a matter of justice—that is, when an *inequality* constitutes an *inequity*. There is, however, a shared concern across otherwise diverse arguments and theories of health justice for those whose life chances are subject to serious and systematic deprivations (see, eg, references[16–22]). Women who experience the highest incidence of PTB fit that description. In the United States and globally, PTB disproportionately afflicts women who are racialized and minoritized; subject to chronic poverty, social instability, violence, and environmental toxins; and lack reliable access to the kinds of social and health care resources that support the health and well-being of women.[8,14,23–27] That these women are more likely to have begun their lives in poverty and to persist in poverty adds to the view that health inequalities in PTB and related inequalities, such as differences in access to prenatal care and differing rates of maternal and infant death,[27–29] are unjust.

These conditions and exposures are neither natural nor inevitable. Rather, they reflect the norms and collective choices of societies, as reflected in a host of policies and practices that influence how people are treated and what access they have to safe housing and neighborhoods, education, employment, health care, transportation, and nutrition. The clear social gradients in PTB—the persistent and predictable patterning described earlier—support the plausibility of a causal role for social, material, economic, and environmental conditions in the physiology of PTB.[30] The contribution of these factors to PTB disparities underscores the moral significance of research and policy-making efforts to address them.

DISCUSSION: RESEARCH TO ADDRESS PRETERM BIRTH

The scope of research on PTB is broad, ranging from epidemiologic studies of PTB and related pregnancy outcomes to physiologic studies of gestation and to the evaluation of novel clinical interventions to reduce PTB and promote the health of premature and low-birthweight infants. As with other scientific efforts aimed at solving difficult multidimensional problems, conceptualizations of justice are implicit in this effort.[31] On the view that a more explicit recognition of the ethical dimensions of PTB may help to focus scientific study and ultimately enhance it, we suggest here 3 considerations that are particularly relevant.

Framing the Problem

If PTB is framed as a problem that increases when women's lives and choices are constrained by poverty and racism—as opposed to framing it, for example, as a problem of dysfunctional gene regulation, cell signaling, or inflammatory processes—the social disadvantage that affects women's health prior to and during pregnancy becomes visible. This framing motivates the development of more complex theories of disease, which in turn can shape novel research questions and expand the range of data collection and measurement.

Theories of disease that incorporate social context, for example, such as the ecosocial model, embodiment, and weathering,[32,33] can elucidate why some groups have higher rates of PTB and foreground the social conditions and lived realities that contribute to this outcome. Importantly, these theories lead to testable hypotheses. For example, the theory of weathering, or allostatic load, proposes that cumulative stress resulting from prolonged exposure to psychosocial or physical challenges such as food insecurity, violence, racism, unsafe housing and the like has biological effects that harm health and longevity.[32,34]

Two lines of biomedical research support this theory. The first concerns chromosomal telomeres, the nucleoprotein complexes occurring at the ends of chromosomes, which shorten with aging. Accelerated shortening occurs among populations exposed to chronic social stress.[35] The second has identified several neuroendocrine, metabolic, cardiovascular, and inflammatory biomarkers that can differentiate levels of health risk related to chronic stress. Findings from these studies support the idea that allostatic load is a key driver of health disparities.[27,32,34]

The need for transdisciplinary research on PTB is well recognized,[36,37] and disease theories such as weathering provide a powerful framework for expanding the scope of such collaborations. For example, studies have assessed the association of allostatic load with PTB; these have produced conflicting results, potentially reflecting differences in how or when allostatic load was measured in study design.[38] Further transdisciplinary research may resolve the question. In another example, telomeres have been proposed to play a key role in gestational timing: placental telomeres expand at the beginning of pregnancy and then progressively shorten, potentially creating a gestational clock.[39] A testable hypothesis posits that PTB is mediated by accelerated placental telomere shortening in disadvantaged populations.[39,40] Effective investigation of this hypotheses would require collaboration among basic and social scientists and clinicians and would likely be enhanced by community-based participatory research methods that engage affected communities in the research process. Similar hypotheses, related to the effect of weathering on other determinants of gestational timing, might also emerge from transdisciplinary discussion. More fundamentally, theories of disease that incorporate social contexts are more likely to yield insights and results that can be used to develop social solutions that act on the conditions driving PTB inequities.

Acknowledging the Need for Interventions that Act on Social Conditions

If social conditions (broadly construed) are implicated in PTB inequities, then advancing health equity requires policies and interventions that address those conditions.[41–43] By extension, a complete research agenda will include identification and evaluation of opportunities to address the social determinants of PTB. Biomedical interventions, such as better tests to identify premature labor and better pharmaceutical agents to arrest or delay labor, clearly can offer benefits in obstetric care and remain an important object of research, but they are downstream, reacting to the problem once it is manifested. Contextualizing biology and behavior within broader social and political systems, in contrast, points to upstream drivers of disease and health and offers greater potential for discoveries that lead to prevention.

The weathering hypothesis, for example, contains an important implication: meaningful efforts to reduce chronic stress could have beneficial health effects. Two approaches related to pregnancy care suggest benefits consistent with this idea. Several studies have suggested that group prenatal care can, among other positive outcomes, reduce absolute rates of PTB by as much as 3%, resulting in improved health and reduced health care costs.[44-46] However, study results are inconsistent.[46,47] Similarly, some studies suggest that the involvement of a doula (a nonmedical person providing pregnancy support) can have a range of positive effects including reduction in PTB.[48] Limited qualitative data suggest that group care or doula involvement might provide benefit either by increasing women's sense of empowerment or protection or by reducing stress and anxiety.[49-51]

Taken together, these studies suggest that the way in which prenatal care is provided—beyond usual measures of quality or how early prenatal care is initiated—can influence the likelihood of PTB, creating the potential for primary prevention. Many questions and research opportunities arise: Why do these interventions have variable outcomes? What is the mechanism of benefit? Could molecular studies linked to intervention trials help to clarify their effects? Could these interventions be improved if accompanied by explicit structural interventions, such as access to nutritious food, safe shelter, a basic income, or paid family leave? And perhaps most importantly, what do prospective patients think about these kinds of interventions?

Taking Seriously the Lived Realities, Constraints, and Knowledge of Affected Populations

A thick context of lived experience (gathered by varied methods, including public deliberation, key informant interviews, ethnographies, biographies, storytelling, and arts-based techniques) can provide insights into the critical exposures and experiences that influence risk. This information can be used to generate measures for use in transdisciplinary studies, such as epigenetic or gene-environment studies or studies relating lived experience to mechanisms of gestational timing. It also offers guidance regarding implementation, including which kinds of interventions are likely to resonate with affected populations and what factors shape adoption, adherence, and sustainability.

It is important to note that although socioeconomically marginalized and minoritized women experience are more likely to suffer PTB, the majority of women exposed to these conditions do *not* experience PTB. A strength-based community engagement approach recommends seeking their views on what measures help to reduce stress or otherwise provide support to pregnant women. Do they view group care as a useful intervention to study and develop, for example, or do they place a higher priority on other interventions, potentially more fundamental and holistic, such as efforts to improve women's health prior to pregnancy or to support the health of their families and communities? This approach goes beyond seeking advice or gathering data. It respects the *authoritative knowledge* (grounded in lived experience) of those who are subject to health injustice.[52]

From this perspective, "hard science" measures (eg, studies of the physiology of PTB, incorporating gene expression, immune, inflammation, and other molecular processes) remain an essential component of PTB research. But a rich understanding derived from the experience of women and the communities in which they live is also important. This more expansive investigation may help to identify appropriate study measures, participants, and comparisons, leading to the most accurate assessment of health and disease.[33] It is also likely to provide the best information about the feasibility and acceptability of proposed interventions. Incorporating women's knowledge throughout the translational research cycle[53] may yield science and solutions that are best able to reduce PTB inequities, a win for justice. But taking women's lived experience seriously meets the requirements of justice in yet another way, by demonstrating respect for them and their views.[54]

SUMMARY

PTB is a cogent example of a key challenge for researchers and policy makers: how to address an important health problem that has multifactorial causes, including biological effects of the social environment that are not well understood and that contribute to significant health inequities. Attention to justice at key junctures in the discovery research cycle can improve the science, increase the likelihood of progress, and support the development of more effective interventions.[53] An approach to framing PTB that places the physiologic problem in social context offers opportunities to link biomedical, population health, health services, and social science research. Expanding the scope of biomedical inquiry in this way can generate novel hypotheses that might lead to otherwise overlooked preventive strategies.

Policies aimed at dismantling structural racism and eliminating poverty would likely have the greatest effect in reducing the health inequity in PTB now seen in the United States; in this sense, PTB is an exemplar of the myriad health conditions driven by marginalized social status. And it is worth noting that fundamental social changes of this kind would undoubtedly have many health benefits beyond reducing PTB.[55] But social interventions that are less far reaching, and the policies to support them, may still offer substantial benefit.

Biomedical researchers may understandably resist the idea that policy considerations are within their ambit. Regardless of the degree to which researchers take up this charge, however, PTB research that incorporates an understanding of social context will inevitably have policy implications. If results are communicated with an eye to how scientific findings might be taken up outside the research realm—or better yet, communicated in conversation and collaboration with policy-makers—research is likely to have greater beneficial impact. PTB research can make a powerful contribution to more fundamental solutions in 3 ways: by making the social context and disadvantage visible; by adding to knowledge about how social disadvantage drives physiologic processes leading to PTB; and by creating opportunities to conceptualize and test upstream preventive approaches. Some opportunities, grounded in an understanding of social context, may be modest in scope but still substantive: group pregnancy care or doula support might be examples. For others—such as ensuring living wages, expanding Medicaid eligibility, enhancing community safety, reducing intimate partner violence, and providing paid family leave—research may serve primarily to inform policy makers and community-based organizations of salient opportunities to improve pregnancy outcomes. In these ways, PTB researchers have a significant opportunity to promote justice.

DISCLOSURE

The authors have nothing to disclose. The views expressed in this article are those of the authors and do not reflect the official positions of the authors' institutions.

Best Practices
What is the current practice for PTB?
• There is no known best practice for the prevention of PTB.

> **What changes in current practice are likely to improve outcomes?**
>
> Transdisciplinary research offers important opportunities for progress, particularly if:
> - The research is based on theories of disease that incorporate social disadvantage.
> - The research is informed by the experience and knowledge of women from groups experiencing high rates of PTB.
>
> The most effective interventions are likely to be those that act on social conditions.
>
> **Bibliographic Sources:**
>
> Link BG, Phelan J. Social conditions as fundamental causes of disease. J Health Soc Behav 1995;Spec No:80–94.
>
> Commission on Social Determinants of Health. Closing the gap in a generation: health equity through action on the social determinants of health. Final Report of the Commission on Social Determinants of Health. Geneva: World Health Organization 2008.
>
> Woolf SH, Braveman P. Where health disparities begin: the role of social and economic determinants–and why current policies may make matters worse. Health Aff (Millwood) 2011;30(10):1852 to 1859.

REFERENCES

1. Stevenson DK, Winn VD, Shaw GM, et al. Solving the puzzle of preterm birth. Clin Perinatol, this issue.
2. Gomez-Lopez N, Galaz J, Miller D, et al. The immunobiology of preterm labor and birth: intra-amniotic inflammation or breakdown of maternal-fetal homeostasis. Reproduction 2022;164(2):R11–45.
3. Mead EC, Wang CA, Phung J, et al. The role of genetics in preterm birth. Reprod Sci 2023. https://doi.org/10.1007/s43032-023-01287-9.
4. Sultana Z, Qiao Y, Maiti K, et al. Involvement of oxidative stress in placental dysfunction, the pathophysiology of fetal death and pregnancy disorders. Reproduction 2023;166(2):R25–38.
5. Wray S, Arrowsmith S, Sharp A. Pharmacological interventions in labor and delivery. Annu Rev Pharmacol Toxicol 2023;63:471–89.
6. Coler BS, Shynlova O, Boros-Rausch A, et al. Landscape of preterm birth therapeutics and a path forward. J Clin Med 2021;10(13):2912.
7. Jehan F, Sazawal S, Baqui AH, et al. Alliance for maternal and newborn health improvement, the global alliance to prevent prematurity and stillbirth. Multiomics characterization of preterm birth in low- and middle-income countries. JAMA Netw Open 2020;3(12):e2029655.
8. Ohuma EO, Moller AB, Bradley E, et al. National, regional, and global estimates of preterm birth in 2020, with trends from 2010: a systematic analysis. Lancet 2023;402(10409):1261–71.
9. Delnord M, Blondel B, Zeitlin J. What contributes to disparities in the preterm birth rate in European countries? Curr Opin Obstet Gynecol 2015;27(2):133–42.
10. Thomson K, Moffat M, Arisa O, et al. Socioeconomic inequalities and adverse pregnancy outcomes in the UK and Republic of Ireland: a systematic review and meta-analysis. BMJ Open 2021;11(3):e042753.
11. Moster D, Lie RT, Markestad T. Long-term medical and social consequences of preterm birth. N Engl J Med 2008;359(3):262–73.
12. Blumenshine P, Egerter S, Barclay CJ, et al. Socioeconomic disparities in adverse birth outcomes: a systematic review. Am J Prev Med 2010;39(3):263–72.

13. National Vital Statistics Report. Births: final data for 2021. January 31, 2023: 72(1. Available at: https://www.cdc.gov/nchs/data/nvsr/nvsr72/nvsr72-01.pdf. [Accessed 26 November 2023].

14. Braveman PA, Heck K, Egerter S, et al. The role of socioeconomic factors in Black-White disparities in preterm birth. Am J Public Health 2015;105(4):694–702.

15. Centers for Disease Control and Prevention. Preterm birth. Available at: https://www.cdc.gov/reproductivehealth/maternalinfanthealth/pretermbirth.htm. [Accessed 26 November 2023].

16. Marchand S, Wikler D, Landesman B. Class, health, and justice. Milbank Q 1998; 76(3):449–67.

17. Blacksher E. On being poor and feeling poor: low socioeconomic status and the moral self. Theor Med Bioeth 2002;23(6):455–70.

18. Braveman PA, Gruskin S. Defining equity in health. J Epidemiol Community Health 2003;57:254–8.

19. Powers M, Faden R. Social justice: the moral foundations of public health and health policy. New York, NY: Oxford University Press; 2006.

20. Daniels N. Just health: meeting health needs fairly. Cambridge, UK: Cambridge University Press; 2008.

21. Wolff J, de-Shalit A. Disadvantage. New York, NY: Oxford, University Press; 2007.

22. Venkatapuram S. Health justice. Cambridge, UK: Polity Press; 2011.

23. Braveman P, Dominguez TP, Burke W, et al. Explaining the Black-White disparity in preterm birth: a consensus statement from a multi-disciplinary scientific work group convened by the March of Dimes. Front Reprod Health 2021;3:684207.

24. Johnson JD, Green CA, Vladutiu CJ, et al. Racial disparities in prematurity persist among women of high socioeconomic status. Am J Obstet Gynecol MFM 2020; 2(3):100104.

25. Casey JA, Karasek D, Ogburn EL, et al. Retirements of coal and oil power plants in California: association with reduced preterm birth among populations nearby. Am J Epidemiol 2018;187(8):1586–94.

26. Ferguson KK, Rosen EM, Rosario Z, et al. Environmental phthalate exposure and preterm birth in the PROTECT birth cohort. Environ Int 2019;132:105099.

27. Fishman SH, Hummer RA, Sierra G, et al. Race/ethnicity, maternal educational attainment, and infant mortality in the United States. Biodemography Soc Biol 2020;66(1):1–26.

28. Riggan KA, Gilbert A, Allyse MA. Acknowledging and addressing allostatic load in pregnancy care. J Racial Ethn Health Disparities 2021;8(1):69–79.

29. Kindig DA. Using uncommon data to promote common ground for reducing infant mortality. Milbank Q 2020;98(1):18–21.

30. Braveman PA, Kumanyika S, Fielding J, et al. Health disparities and health equity: the issue is justice. Am J Public Health 2011;101(Suppl 1):S149–55.

31. Liboiron M, Liu R, Earles E, et al. Models of justice evoked in published scientific studies of plastic pollution. Facets 2023;8:1–34.

32. Geronimus AT. Deep integration: letting the epigenome out of the bottle without losing sight of the structural origins of population health. Am J Public Health 2013;103(Suppl 1):S56–63.

33. Krieger N, Rowley DL, Herman AA, et al. Racism, sexism, and social class: implications for studies of health, disease, and well-being. Am J Prev Med 1993;9(6): 82–122.

34. Guidi J, Lucente M, Sonino N, et al. Allostatic load and its impact on health: a systematic review. Psychother Psychosom 2021;90(1):11–27.

35. Massey DS, Wagner B, Donnelly L, et al. Neighborhood disadvantage and telomere length: results from the Fragile Families Study. RSF 2018;4(4):28–42.

36. Stevenson DK, Shaw GM, Wise PH, et al. March of dimes prematurity research center at stanford university school of medicine. transdisciplinary translational science and the case of preterm birth. J Perinatol 2013;33(4):251–8.

37. Tough SC. Preterm birth and healthy outcomes team: the science and strategy of team-based investigation. BMC Pregnancy Childbirth 2013;13(Suppl 1):S1.

38. Premji SS, Pana GS, Cuncannon A, et al. Maternal-infant global health team (MiGHT) collaborators in research. Prenatal allostatic load and preterm birth: a systematic review. Front Psychol 2022;13:1004073.

39. Phillippe M. Telomeres, oxidative stress, and timing for spontaneous term and preterm labor. Am J Obstet Gynecol 2022;227(2):148–62.

40. Jones CW, Gambala C, Esteves KC, et al. Differences in placental telomere length suggest a link between racial disparities in birth outcomes and cellular aging. Am J Obstet Gynecol 2017;216(3):294.e1–8.

41. Link BG, Phelan J. Social conditions as fundamental causes of disease. J Health Soc Behav 1995;Spec No:80–94.

42. Commission on Social Determinants of Health. Closing the gap in a generation: health equity through action on the social determinants of health, . Final report of the commission on social determinants of health. Geneva: World Health Organization; 2008.

43. Woolf SH, Braveman P. Where health disparities begin: the role of social and economic determinants – and why current policies may make matters worse. Health Aff (Millwood) 2011;30(10):1852–9.

44. Crockett AH, Heberlein EC, Smith JC, et al. Effects of a multi-site expansion of group prenatal care on birth outcomes. Matern Child Health J 2019;23(10): 1424–33.

45. Gareau S, Lòpez-De Fede A, Loudermilk BL, et al. Group prenatal care results in Medicaid savings with better outcomes: a propensity score analysis of Centering-Pregnancy participation in South Carolina. Matern Child Health J 2016;20(7): 1384–93.

46. Moyett JM, Ramey-Collier K, Zambrano Guevara LM, et al. CenteringPregnancy: a review of implementation and outcomes. Obstet Gynecol Surv 2023;78(7): 490–9.

47. Kettrey HH, Steinka-Fry KT. Effects of March of Dimes supportive pregnancy care on social support and postpartum depression. Health Educ Behav 2021;48(5): 670–9.

48. Ramey-Collier K, Jackson M, Malloy A, et al. Doula care: a review of outcomes and impact on birth experience. Obstet Gynecol Surv 2023;78(2):124–7.

49. Hunter LJ, Da Motta G, McCourt C, et al. Better together: a qualitative exploration of women's perceptions and experiences of group antenatal care. Women Birth 2019;32(4):336–45.

50. Heberlein EC, Picklesimer AH, Billings DL, et al. Qualitative comparison of women's perspectives on the functions and benefits of group and individual prenatal care. J Midwifery Wom Health 2016;61(2):224–34.

51. Arteaga S, Hubbard E, Arcara J, et al. "They're gonna be there to advocate for me so I'm not by myself": a qualitative analysis of Black women's motivations for seeking and experiences with community doula care. Women Birth 2023;36(3): 257–63.

52. Harding S. Rethinking standpoint epistemology: what is "strong objectivity". In: Alcoff L, Potter E, editors. Feminist epistemologies. New York: Routledge; 1993. p. 49–81.
53. Kelley M, Edwards K, Starks H, et al. Values in translation: how asking the right questions can move translational science toward greater health impact. Clin Transl Sci 2012;5(6):445–51.
54. Blacksher E. Redistribution and recognition – pursuing social justice in public health. Camb Q Healthc Ethics 2012;21(3):320–31.
55. Syme SL. Social determinants of health: the community as an empowered partner. Prev Chronic Dis 2004;1(1):A02.

Printed and bound by CPI Group (UK) Ltd, Croydon, CR0 4YY

03/10/2024

01040474-0009